D1580307

Musculoskeletal Trauma

Implications for Sports Injury Management

Gary Delforge, EdD, ATC
Professor Emeritus
Arizona School of Health Sciences

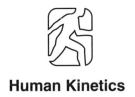

Human Kinetics

Library of Congress Cataloging-in-Publication Data

Delforge, Gary, 1938-
   Musculoskeletal trauma : implications for sports injury management / Gary Delforge.
     p. cm.
   Includes bibliographical references and index.
   ISBN 0-7360-3879-5
    1. Sports injuries. 2. Sports medicine. I. Title.

   RD97 .D457 2002
   617.1'027--dc21   2002017247

ISBN: 0-7360-3879-5

Acquisitions Editor: Loarn D. Robertson, PhD; **Developmental Editor:** Myles Schrag; **Assistant Editor:** Jennifer L. Davis; **Copyeditor:** D.K. Bihler; **Proofreader:** Jim Burns; **Indexer:** Craig Brown; **Permission Manager:** Dalene Reeder; **Graphic Designer:** Fred Starbird; **Graphic Artist:** Yvonne Griffith; **Photo Manager:** Leslie A. Woodrum; **Cover Designer:** Jack W. Davis; **Photographer (interior):** Leslie A. Woodrum, except where noted; **Art Manager:** Carl D. Johnson; **Medical Illustrator:** Jason McAlexander/Interactive Composition Corporation; **Illustrator (Mac):** Kristin Darling; **Printer:** Sheridan Books

Printed in the United States of America   10 9 8 7 6 5 4 3 2 1

Human Kinetics
Web site: www.humankinetics.com

United States: Human Kinetics
P.O. Box 5076
Champaign, IL 61825-5076
800-747-4457
e-mail: humank@hkusa.com

Canada: Human Kinetics
475 Devonshire Road Unit 100
Windsor, ON N8Y 2L5
800-465-7301 (in Canada only)
e-mail: orders@hkcanada.com

Europe: Human Kinetics
Units C2/C3 Wira Business Park
West Park Ring Road
Leeds LS16 6EB, United Kingdom
+44 (0) 113 278 1708
e-mail: hk@hkeurope.com

Australia: Human Kinetics
57A Price Avenue
Lower Mitcham, South Australia 5062
08 8277 1555
e-mail: liahka@senet.com.au

New Zealand: Human Kinetics
P.O. Box 105-231, Auckland Central
09-523-3462
e-mail: hkp@ihug.co.nz

To Julie, Sandy, and Kelly, who taught me what it means to be a dad.

Contents

Preface   ix

Acknowledgments   xi

Part I
Foundations of Sports Injury Management   1

Chapter 1   Introduction to Sports Injury Management   3

The Problem-Oriented Approach   4
Basic Concepts in Sports Injury Management   6
Normal Tissue Structure and Function   11
Essential Elements in Tissue Healing   15
Summary   18
References   19

Chapter 2   Hemorrhage and Hemostasis   21

Primary Hemostasis   22
Secondary Hemostasis   23
Hemorrhagic Manifestations   25
Summary   25
References   26

Part II
Soft Tissue Repair and Therapeutic Intervention   27

Chapter 3   Soft Connective Tissue Repair   29

Inflammation   31
Fibroplasia   38
Scar Maturation   43
Tissue Repair Complications   46
Summary   50
References   51

Chapter 4   Therapeutic Implications: Inflammation and Pain   **53**

Management of Hemorrhage and Edema   54
Alleviation of Pain and Muscle Spasm   60
Summary   82
References   83

Chapter 5   Therapeutic Implications: Scar Formation and Maturation   **87**

Enhancement of Connective Tissue Repair   88
Prevention of Contractures and Adhesions   92
Enhancement of Scar Tissue Structure and Function   97
Summary   110
References   112

Part III
Fracture Healing and Therapeutic Management   115

Chapter 6   Fracture Healing   **117**

Morphology and Histology of Bone   118
Bone Regeneration and Repair   121
Abnormal Bone Healing   128
Summary   130
References   131

Chapter 7   Therapeutic Implications: Fracture Healing   **133**

Basic Concepts in Fracture Management   134
Principles of Fracture Treatment   135
Preservation and Restoration of Function   143
Resumption of Sports Participation   148
Summary   151
References   153

Part IV
Proprioceptive and Sensorimotor Deficits and Therapeutic Intervention   155

Chapter 8   Proprioception and Sensorimotor Function   **157**

The Peripheral Proprioceptive System   159
The Vestibular System   178

The Visual System   182
Summary   184
References   185

Chapter 9 Therapeutic Implications: Proprioceptive and Sensorimotor Deficits   187

Pathology of Proprioceptive Deficits   188
Therapeutic Implications   199
Summary   211
References   213

Part V
Problem Solving in Sports Injury Management   217

Chapter 10 Sports Injury Assessment and Problem Identification   219

The Problem-Oriented Medical Record   220
Summary   226
References   227

Chapter 11 Sports Injury Treatment and Rehabilitation Planning   229

Rehabilitation Goals and Objectives   230
Principles and Concepts in Rehabilitation Planning   232
Summary   238
References   238

Appendix   239
Index   245
About the Author   251

Preface

Historically, sports health care students and clinicians have relied on a vast array of publications in the basic sciences, medicine, and various health care disciplines for development of their knowledge and clinical skills in sports injury management. As the parameters of sports health care became more clearly defined over the years, an increased number of textbooks and reference books have addressed various aspects of sports injury management, including musculoskeletal pathology and medical treatment, use of pharmacologic and physical agents, and rehabilitation techniques. Individually, these publications have made unique contributions to the sports health care clinician's knowledge and skills. This book, however, represents a synthesis of relevant concepts from various disciplines in an attempt to capture an integrated body of knowledge that includes sports injury pathology, musculoskeletal tissue repair, and therapeutic management.

Motivation to write this book evolved gradually, but increased significantly, during my 30 years as a director and classroom instructor in accredited master's degree programs in athletic training and sports health care. Along with the growth of sports health care, the increasing level of professionalism and sophistication among my students presented greater challenges to provide sound rationale for clinical decisions and practices in sports injury management. Experience indicated that the challenge of bringing inquisitive sports health care students to the level of understanding they sought often required time-consuming reference to a wide variety of textbooks and resource materials, many times necessitating reference to the literature in several disciplines. Consequently, this book is written for the busy sports health care student and practitioner who is seeking a convenient source of rationale for contemporary practices in sports injury management.

The purposes of this book are to present a conceptual framework for clinical decision making and problem solving in sports health care and to provide a practical review of the biological events of tissue healing as a basis for therapeutic intervention in injury management. Application of the problem-oriented approach to the management of sports injuries is a predominant theme throughout the book. Inclusion of problem-solving scenarios and questions at the end of selected chapters provides the reader with opportunities to apply clinical problem-solving skills. Ideally, this concept will encourage a coordinated approach to injury management with a focus on identification and resolution of the sports participant's health-related problems, rather than a "modality-oriented" approach. As a basis for decision making and development of therapeutic strategies in sports injury management, the normal biological responses to musculoskeletal trauma and the primary mechanisms of connective tissue repair are reviewed at a clinically applicable level. Accordingly, relevant concepts in anatomy and physiology, tissue biomechanics, and neuroanatomy and neurophysiology are reviewed wherever necessary to provide rationale for therapeutic intervention. This approach is based on the premise that the characteristic tissue responses to musculoskeletal trauma and the vascular and cellular mechanisms of tissue healing provide underlying rationale for therapeutic strategies. A related premise is that the ultimate goal of sports injury management is facilitation of the participant's return to activity as soon as medically indicated, but with minimal risk of reinjury. Given this goal, the sports health care clinician is frequently challenged to select therapeutic agents that are most capable of influencing tissue healing in a positive manner. Consequently, development of effective therapeutic strategies depends on an understanding of sequential tissue-healing mechanisms, including the typical time factors involved.

This book is designed for adoption as a textbook for instructional purposes as well as a reference for practicing clinicians. Educators in accredited entry-level and post-entry-level athletic training curriculums, for example, will find the subject matter to be conducive to their students' development of the Athletic Training Educational Competencies published by the National Athletic Trainers' Association, either as required reading for a course in foundations of sports injury management or as complementary reading for courses in therapeutic and rehabilitation techniques. The educator who adopts this book for instructional purposes will find the chapter and subject matter organization to be conducive to identification and formulation of individualized learning objectives. Inclusion of learning objectives at the beginning of each chapter provides the reader with a guide to identification of major concepts. To facilitate reader comprehension, key terms and concepts are highlighted with incorporation of definitions and explanations as they are presented throughout the context of discussion, thereby minimizing the necessity of referring to additional sources for clarification. Thus, reader comprehension is a positive feature of the book.

Because the problem-oriented approach to sports injury management necessitates a common body of knowledge and coordination of services among health care providers, this book also provides a reference for all members of the sports health care team, particularly practicing certified athletic trainers, physical therapists, team physicians, and physician assistants. Certified strength and conditioning specialists may also find the book valuable in providing rationale for their contributions to rehabilitation of the injured sports participant.

Because of their prevalence in the sports population, management of musculoskeletal injuries involving the connective tissues of the body is the primary focus of this book. Individual parts of the book are devoted to discussion of soft connective tissue injuries, fractures, and proprioceptive and sensorimotor deficits. The book is divided into five parts. Introductory chapters in part I, Foundations of Sports Injury Management, provide an introduction to the problem-oriented approach to injury management and an overview of connective tissue trauma, hemostasis, and tissue-healing mechanisms. Discussion in this part introduces five primary categories of therapeutic intervention that parallel the sequence of events in connective tissue repair. Henceforth, each intervention category becomes a focus for discussion of therapeutic management in part II of the book. Management of proprioceptive and sensorimotor deficits resulting from musculoskeletal trauma is also introduced in part I as a sixth major category of therapeutic intervention. The organizational format for discussion of soft connective tissue injuries, fractures, and proprioceptive and sensorimotor deficits in parts II, III, and IV, respectively, is a unique feature of the book. Initial chapters in each of these parts are devoted to the presentation of relevant anatomy, tissue-healing mechanisms, and related concepts that provide rationale for therapeutic intervention. Subsequently, companion chapters in each part present corresponding implications for therapeutic management. Chapters in part II, Soft Tissue Repair and Therapeutic Intervention, are devoted to the discussion of soft connective tissue healing with corresponding implications for therapeutic management. Part III, Fracture Healing and Therapeutic Management, includes chapters related to fracture healing, medical treatment, and restoration of function. The central topics of part IV, Proprioceptive and Sensorimotor Deficits and Therapeutic Intervention, include the neuroanatomy and neurophysiology of proprioception, pathology of proprioceptive deficits, and proprioceptive and sensorimotor training. Finally, practical application of the problem-oriented approach to musculoskeletal injury management is addressed in part V, Problem Solving in Sports Injury Management, including clinical assessment and problem identification, formulation of rehabilitation goals, and development of treatment plans.

The conceptual strategies in sports injury management presented in this book are intended to foster a coordinated, problem-oriented approach to the treatment of sports injuries. Application of sound principles in clinical decision making and problem solving, combined with a practical understanding of musculoskeletal trauma and tissue healing, will enable each member of the sports health care team to make optimal contributions to the health care of active sports participants.

Acknowledgments

Without doubt, the thirst for knowledge and intellectual curiosity of my former students provided the major incentive for me to compile information for this book. I am grateful not only for the challenge they presented but also for the feedback they provided during classroom presentation of the material. Only with the support of Jackie Kingma, John Parsons, and Erin VanderBunt, my former colleagues in the Department of Sports Health Care, Arizona School of Health Sciences, could completion of this book have become a reality. For this, I am especially thankful.

I would also like to thank Dr. Peg Chilvers, Dr. Patricia Fairchild, Sue Hillman, Jackie Kingma, John Parsons, Dr. Eric Sauers, and Jamie Schwear for their chapter reviews and invaluable input during development of the manuscript. In addition, I want to express my appreciation for the commitment and dedication of Christine Coronado, Betsy Melcher, and Jennie Serenelli in providing word-processing assistance throughout preparation of the manuscript. My thanks are also extended to the dedicated staff at Human Kinetics, who not only provided the opportunity for me to share the information in this book but also worked diligently to finalize the project. Although former students provided the initial incentive for me to write this book, motivation and encouragement to complete the project came, in no small way, from my daughters Julie, Sandy, and Kelly. I will always be grateful for this.

I trust that all of you who have contributed to development of this book will recognize and accept your rightful ownership!

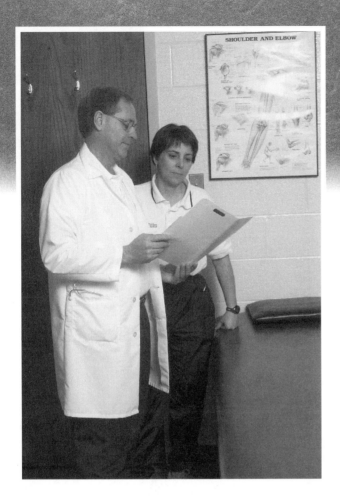

Foundations of Sports Injury Management

Sports health care clinicians are frequently challenged to provide health care services that facilitate a highly motivated injured sports participant's return to activity as soon as possible after injury, but with minimal risk of reinjury. Basic concepts designed to optimize the health care provider's contributions to this goal are introduced in this part of the book. Chapter 1, Introduction to Sports Injury Management, includes an introduction to clinical decision making and problem solving in the management of sports injuries. In addition, an overview of sports trauma and musculoskeletal tissue healing with implications for therapeutic intervention is presented. As a basis for comparison with tissue alterations due to trauma and the healing process, a review of normal connective tissue structure and function is included in this chapter. Further introduction to sports trauma and tissue healing is provided in chapter 2, Hemorrhage and Hemostasis. This chapter includes a review of the characteristic primary and secondary hemostatic responses to hemorrhage in musculoskeletal injuries.

Introduction to Sports Injury Management

CHAPTER 1

The Problem-Oriented Approach
Clinical Decision Making
Problem Identification in Musculoskeletal Injury

Basic Concepts in Sports Injury Management
Overview of Sports Trauma
Categories of Therapeutic Intervention
Mechanisms of Tissue Healing
Tissue-Healing Modifiers

Normal Tissue Structure and Function
Connective Tissue Structure and Function
   Connective Tissue Cells
   Connective Tissue Fibers
   Ground Substance
Connective Tissue Types

Essential Elements in Tissue Healing
Chemical Mediators
Blood Cells
Connective Tissue Cells
Nutrients

Summary

Learning Objectives

After completion of this chapter, the reader should be able to

1. describe the four sequential steps in decision making as applied to problem solving in sports injury management,
2. identify the three primary stages of connective tissue repair,
3. identify six major categories of therapeutic intervention in musculoskeletal injury management,
4. describe the primary differences between tissue regeneration and tissue repair,
5. describe the roles of physical and pharmacologic agents as tissue-healing modifiers,
6. identify the primary structural and functional components of normal connective tissues, and
7. describe the roles of essential chemicals, tissue cells, and nutrients in tissue healing.

Over the past several years, sports health care has become increasingly recognized as a specialty among physicians and other health care providers. Although the principles of sound medical practice and health care that apply to individuals in the general population also apply to the sports participant, effective care of a highly motivated, physically active patient often presents unique challenges to the health care clinician. Typically, the sports participant is motivated to return to activity as soon as possible after injury. Consequently, the sports health care clinician is challenged to provide health care that facilitates attainment of this goal, but which also enhances the patient's resumption of activity with minimal risk of reinjury. These interrelated challenges represent the ultimate goal of sports injury management. Given this goal, sports health care providers are in continual search of the most effective treatment methods and the most efficient means of health care delivery. The purposes of this book are to present a conceptual framework for clinical decision making and problem solving in sports health care and to provide a practical review of the biological events of connective tissue repair as a basis for decision making in sports injury management. Both of these objectives are directed toward enhancement of the health care clinician's contributions to the primary goal of sports injury management.

As an introduction to clinical problem solving, this chapter presents an overview of the decision-making process as related to the problem-oriented approach to injury management. Clinical problem solving is a continuing theme throughout the remaining chapters of the book. This theme is exemplified by inclusion of problem-solving scenarios and questions at the end of selected chapters. These scenarios provide the sports health care clinician with opportunities to apply problem-solving skills to the management of soft connective tissue injuries during the three primary stages of soft connective tissue repair, including inflammation (chapter 4) and scar formation and scar maturation (chapter 5). Clinical problem-solving scenarios pertaining to fracture management and the management of proprioceptive and sensorimotor deficits are included at the end of chapter 7 and chapter 9, respectively. Further emphasis is placed on the problem-oriented approach to sports injury management in chapter 10, Sports Injury Assessment and Problem Identification, and chapter 11, Sports Injury Treatment and Rehabilitation Planning.

Because of the prevalence of sport-related musculoskeletal injuries that involve the connective tissues of the body (e.g., ligaments and joint capsules, tendons, bones), connective tissue healing with corresponding implications for therapeutic intervention is a major focus of this book. As a foundation for discussion in subsequent chapters, basic concepts in sports trauma and injury management are introduced in this chapter, including a discussion of the primary mechanisms of tissue healing and the role of therapeutic agents in injury management. In addition, a review of normal connective tissue structure and function is included as a basis for comparison with alterations associated with tissue trauma. An overview of essential elements in tissue healing (e.g., chemicals, nutrients) is also presented.

The Problem-Oriented Approach

Effective sports injury management necessitates a coordinated, focused approach involving the collective expertise of a number of health care providers. Health care personnel most commonly involved in an injured sports participant's treatment plan include team physicians, orthopedic surgeons, certified athletic trainers, physical therapists, and certified strength and conditioning specialists. Additionally, depending on identification of particular health problems and issues, involvement of various other medical specialists, nutritionists, or sports psychologists may be indicated. Ideally, the respective knowledge and clinical skills of these health care providers are integrated into a comprehensive, coordinated treatment plan that focuses on the patient's health-related problem(s).

Clinical Decision Making

Regardless of the constituents of the sports health care team, a problem-oriented approach to injury management enhances coordination of health care services. Implementation of the problem-oriented approach involves application of fundamental principles inherent in the decision-making process. In a general context, progressive steps in sound decision making include (1) accumulation of information, (2) problem identification and analysis, (3) consideration of alternative actions, and (4) determination of a course of action to resolve the problem. These steps, which represent logical, sequential thought processes leading to problem resolution, are consistent with the problem-solving approach to sports injury treatment and rehabilitation.

As applied to sports injury management, accumulation of information relevant to the patient's health status facilitates an attending physician's determination of the nature and cause of a pathological condition. Hence, a medical diagnosis is established and the fundamental problem to be addressed is identified. After a physician's diagnosis and referral for follow-up care, the sports health care clinician typically synthesizes and analyzes information collected during an initial clinical assessment of the patient's condition. Thus, the clinician's assessment involves accumulation of data in an attempt to identify specific health problems to be resolved during the patient's recovery period. For example, assessment of a musculoskeletal injury may indicate a restriction in normal joint motion, muscle weakness, or a related condition. Implementation of the third basic step in the decision-making process requires the clinician to consider various courses of action to resolve the identified health problem. Typically, clinical decision making at this point involves consideration of alternative therapeutic strategies and, ultimately, determination of specific treatment protocols and methods as a course of action. Determination of a course of action in injury rehabilitation involves two fundamental, sequential steps: (1) establishment of therapeutic objectives (i.e., long-term and short-term goals) and (2) selection of therapeutic agents that most effectively contribute to the identified objectives. The standardized documentation system referred to as the problem-oriented medical record, or SOAP notes, provides a guide to sound clinical decision making as well as an organized format for recording health care information. Chapters 10 and 11 are devoted to application of the SOAP note format to management of sports injuries.

Problem Identification in Musculoskeletal Injury

Sports injuries commonly involve the muscles, tendons, ligaments and joint capsules, and bones of the musculoskeletal system. Although the physiological responses to traumatic disruption of musculoskeletal tissues, including hemostasis and tissue healing, are sometimes taken for granted, a basic understanding of these processes is essential to effective sports injury management. Appropriate clinical decisions regarding development of therapeutic objectives, determination of treatment protocols, and assessment of rehabilitation progress are all predicated on an understanding of the continuum of physiological events that constitute the tissue-healing process. Traditionally, sports health care clinicians are taught to base the development of therapeutic objectives on a clinical assessment and identification of a patient's health-related "problems" (e.g., restricted joint motion). Clinical assessment, however, typically reveals only *signs* (e.g., edema) or *symptoms* (e.g., pain), which become the focuses of therapeutic intervention. Although symptomatic treatment is appropriate and defensible in many cases, clinical signs and symptoms typically represent only the manifestations of underlying pathology. By definition, a pathological condition involves an alteration of the normal structure and function of the cells, tissues, and organs of the body. These alterations, in turn, affect functional systems (e.g., the musculoskeletal system). Commonly, alterations in tissue structure and function are the cause of clinical signs and symptoms. For example, depending on the stage of tissue healing, capsular adhesions and contractures may be the cause of restricted joint motion. Thus, it is suggested that the fundamental problems to be addressed through therapeutic intervention lie at the tissue level where changes occur in response to injury. The sports health care clinician's ability to identify health problems and causative factors is highly dependent on his or her awareness of the typical responses to tissue trauma, knowledge of normal and abnormal tissue repair, and an ability to visualize characteristics of healing tissues at any particular stage of repair. With this insight, a corresponding increase in the clinician's "index of suspicion" contributes significantly to problem identification and analysis. The adage "You see only what you know" seems applicable to identification of the cause(s) of injury complications.

Armed with a practical understanding of the physiological events of tissue healing, sports health care clinicians can more readily establish appropriate and realistic therapeutic objectives. Subsequently, specific therapeutic agents (i.e., physical agents or pharmacologic agents) can be selected on the basis of their ability to influence the vascular and cellular events of tissue healing in a positive manner. The result is a rational treatment plan that avoids a haphazard "modalities-oriented" approach to sports injury management. Continual awareness of sequential healing mechanisms, including the time factors involved, facilitates timely assessment of rehabilitation progress and, if indicated, establishment of new short-term goals. Periodic clinical assessment and modification of therapeutic intervention that parallels the continuum of tissue healing are hallmarks of effective treatment plans.

Basic Concepts in Sports Injury Management

As a foundation for further discussion of musculoskeletal injury management in subsequent chapters, this section provides an overview of tissue responses to sports trauma and identification of five major categories of therapeutic intervention that parallel the sequential stages of connective tissue repair. Management of proprioceptive and sensorimotor deficits that result from musculoskeletal injury is introduced as a sixth major category of intervention. Connective tissue repair and tissue regeneration are reviewed as the two primary healing responses in musculoskeletal trauma. In addition, an introduction to the use of physical and pharmacologic agents as tissue-healing modifiers is included.

Overview of Sports Trauma

With the exception of myofibers (i.e., the contractile element of a muscle), ligaments and joint capsules, musculotendinous structures, and bone represent various types of connective tissues that respond to trauma with similar vascular and cellular reactions. Although the intensity of response typically varies with the type and extent of injury (e.g., stress-related microtrauma or acute macrotrauma), the normal mechanisms of connective tissue repair follow an orderly, predictable pattern. A general overview of connective tissue response to injury is presented in figure 1.1. Commonly, the various vascular and cellular events summarized in figure 1.1 are categorized for discussion purposes as involving three major stages of connective tissue healing: *inflammation, fibroplasia* (scar formation), and *scar maturation* (Bryant 1977). Although these responses reflect the characteristic stages of soft connective tissue repair, fracture healing involves comparable stages, including hematoma formation and inflammation, cellular proliferation and callus formation, and remodeling.

As indicated in figure 1.1, the initial physiological responses to tissue trauma include *hemorrhage* from ruptured blood vessels followed by a series of vascular and cellular

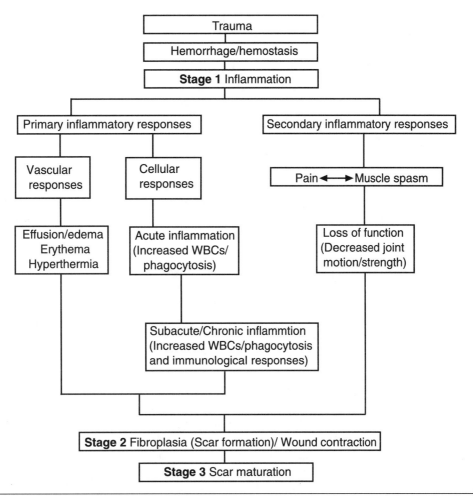

Figure 1.1 Physiological responses to connective tissue trauma. Note the three primary stages of connective tissue repair (inflammation, fibroplasia, and scar maturation).

responses to promote *hemostasis*, the arrest of bleeding. Subsequently, during the acute inflammatory stage of tissue repair, a number of reactions occur that constitute the *primary inflammatory responses* to injury. The primary vascular responses during acute inflammation account for *effusion* (i.e., escape of fluid) and *edema* (swelling), *erythema* (redness), and *hyperthermia* (increased temperature) in the affected tissues. The primary cellular responses that occur during acute inflammation, including proliferation of phagocytic white blood cells, provide the initial nonspecific body defense against invading pathogenic microorganisms. Normally, as these acute inflammatory responses subside, inflammation enters a subacute phase. If not resolved, however, inflammation may progress to a chronic stage during which immunological responses to specific pathogenic agents are elicited. Two additional characteristics of inflammation, *pain* and *muscle spasm*, represent consequential neural responses to tissue damage. Hence, these reactions are referred to as *secondary inflammatory responses*. Pain and muscle spasm, in addition to initial edema formation, can lead to clinical complications associated with *loss of function* (e.g., restricted joint motion, strength deficits). As connective tissue repair continues into the second stage, fibroplasia, fibrous *scar formation* occurs. This stage of tissue repair inherently includes *wound contraction*, or closure, the mechanism through which the size of a tissue defect is reduced. Finally, during the third stage of tissue healing, the connective tissue scar gradually remodels and assumes its ultimate structure and function, a process referred to as *scar maturation*.

Although the overview of physiological responses to tissue injury presented in figure 1.1 provides a useful framework for discussion, further exploration of the primary stages of connective tissue repair is necessary to provide a practical basis for development of effective treatment plans. The primary focus of discussion in subsequent chapters is on those vascular and cellular responses to connective tissue injury that have the greatest implications for therapeutic management of sports injuries. In an attempt to establish a basis for sound decision making in the therapeutic management and rehabilitation of connective tissue injuries, subsequent chapters include a discussion of the primary physiological responses associated with the control of bleeding (chapter 2), soft connective tissue repair (chapter 3), and fracture healing (chapter 6). Companion chapters address implications for therapeutic intervention during acute inflammation (chapter 4), scar formation and maturation (chapter 5), and fracture healing (chapter 7).

Categories of Therapeutic Intervention

A review of the physiological responses to trauma summarized in figure 1.1 indicates several opportunities for therapeutic intervention throughout the three primary stages of connective tissue repair. The characteristic vascular and cellular responses that occur during inflammation, fibroplasia (scar formation), and scar maturation present implications for intervention in five major categories (figure 1.2). Stated as broadly defined therapeutic objectives, these categories of intervention include the use of pharmacologic or physical agents to (1) control the detrimental effects of hemorrhage and edema, (2) alleviate pain and muscle spasm, (3) enhance the physiological mechanisms of connective tissue repair (i.e., fibroplasia), (4) prevent connective tissue contractures and adhesions, and (5) enhance the definitive structural and biomechanical properties of scar tissue (e.g., plasticity, tensile strength). Although stated as therapeutic objectives, these categories of intervention reflect the fundamental "problems" to be addressed throughout the patient's recovery period. Thus, each category represents a focus for discussion of therapeutic intervention in subsequent chapters.

It is important to note that the categories of therapeutic intervention summarized in figure 1.2 parallel the sequence of physiological events in connective tissue repair. Hence, they provide a practical guide to development of progressive sports injury rehabilitation programs, as well as a basis for selection of appropriate therapeutic agents. For example, the two primary therapeutic objectives during the inflammatory stage of connective tissue repair are to control hemorrhagic effusion and edema (i.e., primary inflammatory responses) and to alleviate the pain-spasm-pain cycle (i.e., secondary inflammatory responses). Therapeutic strategies to achieve these objectives are discussed in chapter 4. With the beginning of fibroplasia, the second stage of connective tissue repair, therapeutic intervention to enhance the mechanisms of tissue repair becomes a primary objective. During this stage, management of contractures and adhesions associated with abnormal

- Control of hemorrhage and edema
- Alleviation of pain and muscle spasm
- Enhancement of tissue repair mechanisms
- Prevention of contractures and adhesions
- Enhancement of scar tissue structure and function

Figure 1.2   Major categories of therapeutic intervention in connective tissue repair.

wound contraction or excessive scar formation may also become necessary. Finally, during scar maturation, optimal restoration of the structural and functional properties of the connective tissue matrix becomes a primary therapeutic objective. Therapeutic intervention during scar formation and scar maturation, the second and third stages of connective tissue repair, is addressed in chapter 5.

In addition to the primary indications for therapeutic intervention during connective tissue repair, proprioceptive and sensorimotor deficits resulting from musculoskeletal injuries commonly present an indication for intervention during the recovery period. As discussed further in chapter 8, proprioceptive deficits represent impairments in perception of joint position and movement that may result from disruption of musculoskeletal tissues (e.g., ligaments, joint capsules) that house the sensory nerve endings for proprioception. In this event, restoration of proprioceptive and sensorimotor function also becomes a primary therapeutic objective, especially as related to safe and successful resumption of sports participation. In contrast to the use of therapeutic agents to influence the physiological mechanisms of connective tissue repair, intervention to enhance proprioception is focused on restoration of the sensory input that provides the basis for neuromuscular control and functional patterns of motor performance. Therapeutic intervention to restore these functions is referred to as *proprioceptive training*. Because proprioceptive training is directed to reestablishment of neuromuscular control and motor function, it is commonly associated with sport-specific *functional rehabilitation*, the final phase of sports injury management. However, if permitted by an acceptable degree of tissue healing, introduction of proprioceptive training activities during earlier phases of rehabilitation may be indicated in an attempt to preserve or enhance the proprioceptive input necessary for motor control (e.g., postural control, balance). Thus, carefully monitored proprioceptive activities commonly parallel therapeutic protocols designed to facilitate connective tissue repair. Based on the premise that proprioceptive deficits represent a pathological component of musculoskeletal injuries, implications for management of proprioceptive and sensorimotor dysfunction are discussed in chapter 9 as a sixth major category of therapeutic intervention in sports injury rehabilitation.

Mechanisms of Tissue Healing

Healing has been defined as the natural response to injury through which dead or lost tissue is replaced by living tissue. The healing process restores the anatomical and structural continuity of body tissues that have been disrupted by injury (Martinez-Hernandez and Amenta 1990). Despite similarities in healing among various body tissues, the specific physiological mechanisms and the resulting tissue matrix vary according to the type of tissue involved. In general, injured tissues heal through one of two primary mechanisms: *regeneration* or *repair* (Martinez-Hernandez 1994). Either regeneration or repair may become the predominant healing mechanism, depending on the particular type of injured tissues. In some body parts, soft tissue healing occurs through a combination of regeneration and repair. Regeneration refers to the restoration of tissue that is identical in structure and function to the tissue that has been destroyed, thus qualifying as ideal tissue healing (Leadbetter 1994). Restoration of normal tissues results from a division of cells with regeneration capability that have survived tissue trauma and remained functional. In contrast, tissues that are subjected to an unfavorable healing environment or are composed of cells with limited regeneration capability undergo repair, the healing pattern in connective tissues that is characterized by replacement of damaged tissues with fibrous scar tissue (Martinez-Hernandez and Amenta 1990). Although normal connective tissue repair typically restores the anatomical continuity of damaged tissues, functional restoration may be incomplete, resulting in less than ideal healing (Leadbetter 1994). As discussed further in chapter 3, soft connective tissue repair may be augmented significantly by wound contraction, the process through which the size of a tissue defect is reduced.

Whether regeneration or repair becomes the primary healing mechanism in musculoskeletal injuries depends, in part, on the predominant cell type in the particular type of tissue affected. The cells of the body are classified according to their ability to divide, and thus regenerate after injury. This classification system includes *labile cells, stable cells,* and *permanent cells* (Cotran, Kumar, and Robbins 1989). Labile cells, such as those found in the bone marrow and the epidermis, undergo continual division and replication. Thus, body tissues composed of labile cells have excellent regeneration potential. Injured bone tissue, for example, heals through the process of regeneration (see chapter 6). Stable cells, by comparison, demonstrate a low level of replication but may divide rapidly in response to an abnormal stimulus, including tissue injury. For example, fibroblasts, the type of cells from which connective tissues are derived, proliferate in response to tissue disruption. However, the characteristic healing pattern in connective tissues is scar formation rather than replacement of normal tissue.

In contrast to labile cells and stable cells, permanent cells (e.g., neurons of the central nervous system) lack the ability to divide, and thus do not regenerate after injury. Although skeletal muscle cells (i.e., myofibers) are classified as permanent cells, they have the potential for regeneration by virtue of reserve cells called *satellite cells,* which are contained within the basement membrane of skeletal muscle fibers. When stimulated by muscle trauma, these normally quiescent cells undergo division, proliferation, and migration to the site of injury where replacement of necrotic muscle fibers occurs (MacDougall 1992). Because muscle fibers and muscle fiber bundles are surrounded by connective tissue sheaths that are repaired by fibrous scar formation, muscle injuries heal through a combination of regeneration and repair, although repair is typically the predominant healing mechanism in moderate to severe injuries. This tissue-healing pattern is discussed further in chapter 3.

Tissue-Healing Modifiers

Because of their potential to influence the vascular and cellular events of tissue healing, therapeutic agents used to achieve the primary objectives of intervention are referred to collectively as *modifiers.* Tissue-healing modifiers are classified into two broad categories: (1) pharmacologic agents (i.e., oral, injectable, or topical medications) and (2) physical agents, including therapeutic modalities (e.g., thermotherapy, cryotherapy, electrotherapy) and therapeutic exercise (Leadbetter, Buckwalter, and Gordon 1990). This broad classification of modifiers encompasses the array of therapeutic agents available to the sports health care clinician for intervention throughout the sequential stages of tissue healing. Judicious selection of specific therapeutic agents is based on at least four preliminary considerations: (1) the characteristic vascular and cellular responses during a particular stage of healing, (2) the specific physiological or neurological response to be modified, (3) the capability of the therapeutic agent to effect the desired response (i.e., indications), and (4) the potential detrimental effect of the therapeutic agent on normal, diseased, or surgically repaired tissues (i.e., contraindications).

Selection of appropriate therapeutic agents sometimes requires a clear distinction between the physiological effect of a particular modality and its therapeutic effect. Although a therapeutic agent may have a demonstrated ability to influence a particular vascular or cellular response to tissue trauma, it does not necessarily follow that the response is therapeutic. In some cases, the therapeutic effect depends on the stage of tissue healing during which a particular modality is used. For example, heat applications that increase tissue temperature, thus producing vasodilation and increased local blood flow, may be therapeutic during the fibroplastic stage of healing. Premature stimulation of these vascular responses, however, may exacerbate hemorrhage and edema formation. Thus, heat applications are typically contraindicated during the acute inflammatory stage. In other instances, a modality may enhance a therapeutic physiological response but, at same time, elicit a detrimental reaction. For example, as discussed further in chapter 5, the nonthermal, mechanical effects of ultrasound have been shown to have a positive influence on various cellular activities of connective tissue repair (e.g., collagen synthesis). On the other hand, the mechanical effects of ultrasound may disrupt blood-clotting mechanisms, thus increasing hemorrhagic effusion if applied too soon after injury (Gieck and Saliba 1990). As these two examples suggest, selection of appropriate therapeutic agents is not only a matter of identifying specific indications and contraindications but also a matter of judicious timing.

Normal Tissue Structure and Function

All tissues of the human body are composed of basic structural and functional units called *cells* (e.g., blood cells, nerve cells, muscle cells, connective tissue cells). When grouped by their embryonic origin or function, cells combine to form *tissues,* the next highest level of structural organization. Body tissues are classified into four primary types according to their structure and function. These tissue types include (1) epithelial tissue, (2) nervous tissue, (3) muscle tissue, and (4) connective tissue (Tortora and Grabowski 1993). In the hierarchical structural organization of the body, one or more tissue types form the organs that constitute the major functional *systems* of the body (e.g., skeletal system, muscular system, nervous system, cardiovascular system).

Although sports health care clinicians may be confronted with injuries involving any one, or a combination, of the various tissue types and functional systems of the body, injuries to tissues constituting the skeletal system and the muscular system are among the most common. Injuries to these systems, collectively referred to as *musculoskeletal injuries,* typically involve muscles, tendons, ligaments and joint capsules, and bone. Thus, closed soft tissue injuries of the musculoskeletal system may involve muscle tissue, connective tissue, or a combination of both. Because bone is considered a specialized type of connective tissue, fractures also represent connective tissue injuries. Damage to epithelial cells that form the endothelium of vascular walls is characteristically associated with injuries to the musculoskeletal system. On occasion, peripheral nerve injuries involving damage to nervous tissue may accompany musculoskeletal injuries of the upper or lower extremities. Despite potential injury to associated tissue types, however, most sports injuries inherently involve connective tissue damage.

Connective Tissue Structure and Function

Because soft connective tissues heal by fibrous scar formation, or *fibrosis,* the repair process typically alters the normal connective tissue architecture. The structural and functional alterations that result from connective tissue repair are best understood when compared with the characteristic structure and function of normal, uninjured tissues. Although bone is classified as connective tissue, the architecture of bone obviously differs from that of soft connective tissues. The structural composition of bone, as a specialized type of connective tissue, is addressed in chapter 6. Discussion in this section is focused on the composition of soft connective tissues that form such structures as ligaments, joint capsules, and tendons. The repair of soft connective tissue injuries, as well as the resulting structural and functional alterations, is addressed in chapter 3.

The primary function of connective tissue is to connect and bind body cells, other tissue types, and organs, thereby providing mechanical support, strength, and form to the various structures of the body. In many cases, connective tissues function to compartmentalize body structures, as exemplified by the connective tissue sheaths that surround muscle fibers (i.e., endomysium) and muscle fiber bundles (i.e., perimysium). Mature connective tissue is formed by three basic structural components including cells, *fibers,* and *ground substance* (Junqueira, Carneiro, and Kelly 1995). The major components of connective tissue are summarized in figure 1.3. Because they are located outside the cells, connective tissue fibers and ground substance form what is referred to as the *extracellular matrix.* Thus, connective tissue cells are embedded in the extracellular matrix and separated by its various components. The structural relationship of these basic components in loose connective tissue is illustrated in figure 1.4. In addition to the primary components of the extracellular matrix, connective tissues contain a small amount of *tissue fluid* that continually filtrates through the capillary walls into the interstitial spaces. Under normal conditions, tissue fluid is returned to the bloodstream through the lymphatic system (i.e., lymph vessels). As discussed in chapter 3, however, excess interstitial fluid results in edema, or tissue swelling.

Connective Tissue Cells

The primary cell types in soft connective tissues are *mast cells, macrophages, plasma cells,* and *fibroblasts* (see figure 1.4). Derived from embryonic cells called *mesenchymal cells,* mature connective tissue cells play vital roles in the maintenance of normal tissue structure and function and in the repair of connective tissue injuries. Mast cells, for example, are a major source of vasoactive mediators (i.e., chemicals) in acute inflammation. During later stages of inflammation, macrophages become important phagocytic cells. Both macrophages and plasma cells have significant immunological functions in the body's defense against specific pathogenic microorganisms. In addition, macrophages play an important role in the proliferation and cellular functions of fibroblasts during connective tissue repair. Fibroblasts, one of the most abundant cells found in connective tissues, are the cells responsible for synthesis of collagen and other components of the extracellular tissue matrix during the repair process.

Connective Tissue Fibers

The fibrous components of the extracellular connective tissue matrix include *collagen, elastic,* and *reticular* fibers. These fiber types are found in varying proportions in different types of connective tissue, thus providing such structures as ligaments, joint capsules, and tendons with specific functional properties. Collagen fibers, which provide strength and stiff-

Cells
    Mast cells
    Macrophages
    Plasma cells
    Fibroblasts
Fibers
    Collagen
    Elastic
    Reticular
Ground substance
    Water
    Glycoproteins

Figure 1.3   Major components of connective tissue.

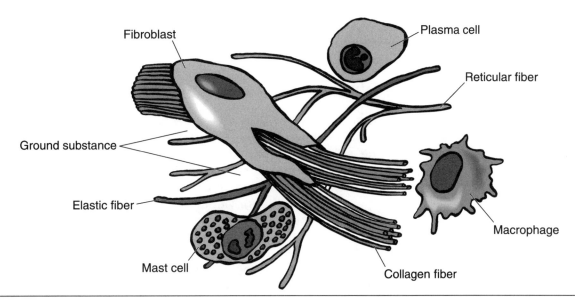

Figure 1.4   Relationship of cells, fibers, and ground substance in loose connective tissue.

Adapted from G.J. Tortora and S.R. Grabowski, 1993, *Principles of anatomy and physiology,* 7th ed. (New York: Harper Collins College Publishers), 112. Copyright © 1993, John Wiley & Sons, Inc. This material is used by permission of John Wiley & Sons, Inc.

ness, are the largest and typically the most abundant fiber type in the musculoskeletal structures of the body. Connective tissue collagen fibers are formed by collagen, a type of protein that represents approximately 30% of the dry weight of the human body (Junqueira, Carneiro, and Kelly 1995). Although smaller than collagen fibers, elastic fibers also contribute to the tensile strength of connective tissues. Because of their ability to stretch and recoil, however, the primary biomechanical property of elastic fibers is elasticity. Thus, elastic fibers are found predominantly in pliable tissues such as the skin and blood vessels. Reticular fibers, the third connective tissue fiber type, are very thin fibers that provide a supporting framework for various body organs and glands (e.g., lymph nodes, liver, spleen). These fibers, however, are not typically prevalent in the dense connective tissues of the musculoskeletal system that require tensile strength to resist tissue loading.

Ground Substance

Ground substance, the second major component of the extracellular connective tissue matrix, is an amorphous (i.e., without form) gelatinous material that occupies the spaces between the cells and the fibrous components of soft connective tissues. Functionally, ground substance not only provides a supporting framework for cells but also acts as a lubricant to reduce friction between connective tissue fibers, thereby permitting tissue mobility (Junqueira, Carneiro, and Kelly 1995). Ground substance contains a mixture of water and large protein and carbohydrate molecules known as *glycoproteins.* Protein and carbohydrate compounds referred to as *structural glycoproteins* (e.g., fibronectin) are associated with binding of cells to various components of the extracellular matrix and cross-linkage of collagen fibrils and fibers. Thus, they contribute structure and strength to the connective tissue matrix during the early stages of connective tissue repair (Martinez-Hernandez 1994). Glycoproteins with a high carbohydrate content are called *proteoglycans.* Proteoglycans, which consist of a protein core and carbohydrate chains called *glycosaminoglycans* (GAGs), have a high affinity for water. Thus, this hydrophilic proteoglycan aggregate plays an important role in tissue lubrication. Combined with water, GAGs form a lubricating semifluid gel that maintains distance between collagen fibers, thereby preventing excessive collagen fiber cross-linkage, loss of collagen fiber gliding functions, and consequential restriction of connective tissue mobility (Harrelson 1991). Loss of GAGs and water as the result of immobilization and restricted activity after connective tissue injury is discussed in chapter 5.

Connective Tissue Types

Connective tissue has been classified broadly as *embryonic connective tissue* and *mature connective tissue* (Tortora and Grabowski 1993). Embryonic connective tissue, the name given to connective tissue in the embryo and fetus, is composed in part of a tissue type referred to as *mesenchyme*, which contains mesenchymal cells. Mesenchymal cells are the cells from which other types of connective tissue cells are derived (e.g., fibroblasts, osteoblasts). Mature connective tissue is the term used to describe the connective tissues of the body beginning at birth. The primary types of mature connective tissues have been classified as *connective tissue proper, bone, cartilage,* and *blood* (Junqueira, Carneiro, and Kelly 1995; Tortora and Grabowski 1993).

Connective tissue proper is further categorized as *loose connective tissue* and *dense connective tissue,* depending to a large extent on its architectural structure and function. Unlike loose connective tissue, which is composed of comparatively thin, loosely woven fibers, the fibers in dense connective tissue are thicker and stronger but less flexible. Although all three major fiber types (i.e., collagen, elastic, and reticular) may be found in both loose and dense connective tissue, collagen is the predominant fiber type in dense connective tissues, thus providing strength to ligaments, joint capsules, tendons, and other supportive structures of the musculoskeletal system.

When collagen fibers in dense connective tissue are arranged in a random, nonlinear pattern without definite orientation, the tissue type is referred to as *dense irregular connective tissue* (figure 1.5). This irregular fiber pattern provides resistance to tissue loading from all directions. Joint capsules, which are composed partially of dense irregular connective tissue, are an example of supporting structures designed to resist multidirectional loading. In contrast to dense irregular connective tissue, the tissue type in which closely packed collagen bundles are arranged in a linear, parallel pattern is called *dense regular connective tissue* (figure 1.6). As exemplified by tendons, this fiber orientation pattern provides optimal resistance to tissue loading from one direction. Ideally, tissue healing in musculoskeletal injuries would restore the normal structure and biomechanical properties of the types of connective tissue that form each particular body part. However, connective tissue repair, which occurs through fibrous scar formation, typically alters the normal architecture and thus the characteristic behavioral properties of connective tissues.

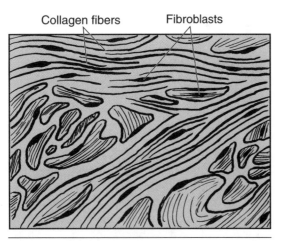

Figure 1.5   Dense irregular connective tissue (dermis of skin).

Adapted from G.J. Tortora and S.R. Grabowski, 1993, *Principles of anatomy and physiology*, 7th ed. (New York: Harper Collins College Publishers), 114. Copyright © 1993, John Wiley & Sons, Inc. This material is used by permission of John Wiley & Sons, Inc.

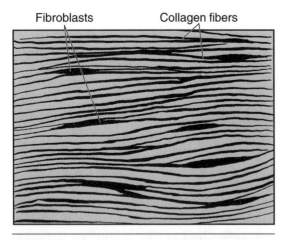

Figure 1.6   Dense regular connective tissue (tendon).

Adapted from G.J. Tortora and S.R. Grabowski, 1993, *Principles of anatomy and physiology*, 7th ed. (New York: Harper Collins College Publishers), 114. Copyright © 1993, John Wiley & Sons, Inc. This material is used by permission of John Wiley & Sons, Inc.

Essential Elements in Tissue Healing

Although somewhat complicated, normal connective tissue repair follows a predictable sequence of chemically mediated vascular and cellular responses. These responses are initiated at the time of injury and continued throughout the healing process. Many chemicals and several types of blood cells, connective tissue cells, and nutrients play integral, complementary roles in connective tissue repair. An overview of some essential elements in tissue healing should facilitate a fundamental understanding of their role in the healing process. The specific role of various chemicals, blood cells, connective tissue cells, and nutrients is discussed in chapter 3 as their primary functions become relevant to the physiological events of connective tissue repair.

Chemical Mediators

When traumatic forces are applied abruptly to body tissues, a number of chemicals are released from damaged blood cells and connective tissue cells at the site of injury. Because these chemicals regulate and control the numerous vascular and cellular events of tissue healing, they are referred to as *mediators* (Fantone 1990). Chemical mediators that influence healing function as *enzymes,* organic catalysts that effect changes in other substances without being changed themselves. Chemical mediators may have singular or multiple actions. Some mediators function as antagonists to counteract the action of other mediators. Chemical mediators may also interact in a synergistic manner to facilitate the physiological mechanisms of tissue healing (American Academy of Orthopaedic Surgeons 1991).

The integral role of chemical mediators in connective tissue repair can be illustrated by a few examples. Chemical mediators that promote hemostasis (i.e., arrest of escaping blood) after injury are serotonin, which mediates initial vasoconstriction, and adenosine diphosphate (ADP), which promotes platelet adhesion and platelet aggregation. These two early responses to tissue injury are essential to the control of bleeding (Kloth and Miller 1990; Koester 1993; Tortora and Grabowski 1993). Vasodilation and increased vascular permeability, which follow vasoconstriction in damaged tissues, are mediated by histamine, bradykinin, prostaglandins, and other vasoactive chemicals. Thus, these chemical mediators contribute significantly to edema formation (Calabrese and Rooney 1986; Ciccone 1990; Fantone 1990). Through their synergistic interaction with other chemical mediators, prostaglandins also increase the sensitivity of nociceptors in damaged tissues, thereby contributing to inflammatory pain (Ciccone 1990). Other chemicals, leukotrienes for example, function as chemotactic agents to attract phagocytic white blood cells (e.g., neutrophils) to the damaged tissues during acute inflammation (Koester 1993). As connective tissue repair progresses beyond the inflammatory stage to fibroplasia, or scar formation, various chemicals mediate the many vascular and cellular responses involved. For example, some chemicals that have been identified as mediators of cellular response during fibroplasia are leukotriene B4, prostaglandins, and bradykinin (Kloth and Miller 1990; Postlethwaite 1990).

Blood Cells

Blood is composed of intercellular fluid, or *plasma,* and *formed elements,* including *platelets, leukocytes* (white blood cells), and *erythrocytes* (red blood cells). The components of whole blood are listed in figure 1.7. Various cellular components of blood, the formed elements, function to influence hemostasis and inflammation. Platelets, for example, are a major source of chemical mediators (e.g., serotonin) that promote vasoconstriction. Platelets are also the primary component of the hemostatic plug that forms in damaged blood vessels

---

Plasma

Formed elements
    Leukocytes (WBCs)
        Granular (granulocytes)
            Neutrophils
            Eosinophils
            Basophils
        Agranular (agranulocytes)
            Monocytes
            Lymphocytes

    Erythrocytes (RBCs)
    Platelets

Figure 1.7 Composition of whole blood.

after injury. As discussed further in chapter 2, formation of a temporary platelet plug is a critical vascular response in the control of bleeding.

Because of their phagocytic and immunological functions, white blood cells are essential to tissue healing in the event of pathogenic microorganism invasion. The morphological classification of white blood cells includes granular leukocytes, or *granulocytes* (neutrophils, basophils, and eosinophils), and agranular leukocytes, or *agranulocytes* (monocytes and lymphocytes). Granular leukocytes, primarily neutrophils, perform an important phagocytic function during acute inflammation, thus providing an essential component of the initial nonspecific defense against pathogenic agents. Agranular leukocytes, monocytes and lymphocytes, function in both nonspecific and specific body defense systems during later stages of inflammation. During the inflammatory process, monocytes emigrate through the vascular wall and develop into large phagocytic macrophages that eventually become the primary phagocytic cells in the nonspecific defense against invading pathogenic microorganisms. Lymphocytes, some of which produce antibodies in response to specific pathogens, are essential components of the immune system that constitutes the specific body defense against pathogenic agents. The role of various blood cells in inflammation is discussed further in chapter 3.

Connective Tissue Cells

As previously indicated, the primary types of soft connective tissue cells are mast cells, macrophages, plasma cells, and fibroblasts. Each of these cell types is activated in response to connective tissue injury. Hence, they become active participants in the repair process. Mast cells are a source of chemical mediators that influence the early vascular responses to injury. Among these chemical mediators are serotonin (a vasoconstrictor), histamine (a vasodilator), and leukotrienes, which attract white blood cells to the damaged area (Thomas 1993). Macrophages are the primary phagocytic agents during subacute and chronic inflammation. In addition to their phagocytic function, macrophages mediate certain immunological responses in the specific defense system of the body. Plasma cells, which produce antibodies in response to specific pathogenic agents, are also essential components of the immune system. As tissue repair progresses, macrophages release chemotactic agents (i.e., chemicals) that attract fibroblasts to the damaged tissues. In addition, macrophages are a source of various growth factors that stimulate the cellular functions of fibroblasts during the early phase of tissue healing. As connective tissue repair proceeds, fibroblasts become the essential cell in collagen synthesis and fibrous tissue formation. Wound contraction, or closure, is a function of *myofibroblasts,* specialized connective tissue cells with contractile properties and migration capabilities. Whereas fibroblasts are essential to the repair of soft tissue injuries, fracture healing relies on their cellular counterparts in osseous tissue. The specific role of osteoblasts, chondroblasts, and other bone cells in fracture healing is discussed in chapter 6.

Nutrients

By definition, a *nutrient* is a substance that promotes tissue growth, or replacement of damaged tissues, through normal metabolic activities. Essential nutrients include minerals, vitamins, proteins, carbohydrates, lipids, and water. In addition to water, which is essential to a multitude of metabolic functions, several other nutrients become essential elements in tissue healing. Certain minerals, for example, assume various roles in connective tissue repair that begin at the time of injury and continue throughout the repair process (Tortora and Grabowski 1993). Calcium, which is released from platelets at the time of vascular disruption, mediates development of hemostatic plugs and functions as an essential coagulation factor in blood clotting (see chapter 2). Without sufficient calcium, blood will not clot (Thomas 1993). As fibroplasia begins, zinc becomes essential to the synthesis of collagen by fibroblasts. As an additional example, successful regeneration and remodeling of bone following fractures is highly dependent on calcium. Deposition of calcium in the bony matrix during fracture healing is essential to hard callus formation and solid bony union. During remodeling, continued mineralization is an important function through which bone density, hardness, and stiffness are gradually restored.

In addition to certain minerals, several vitamins play essential roles in tissue healing. Most vitamins act as *coenzymes,* activators of enzymes that function as catalysts to regulate the metabolic processes of the body (Tortora and Grabowski 1993). Vitamins K, C, and D are among those vitamins that influence specific metabolic activities in connective tissue repair. Vitamin K, for example, is necessary for synthesis of prothrombin, an essential coagulation factor in blood clotting. As tissue healing begins, vitamin C becomes essential to the cellular functions of fibroblasts in collagen synthesis and fibrous tissue formation. In addition, synthesis of collagen that provides strength to newly formed capillaries during tissue healing is dependent on vitamin C. Another vitamin, vitamin D, regulates absorption of calcium and phosphorus from the intestinal tract, thereby facilitating mineral deposition in the bony matrix during fracture healing (Thomas 1993; Tortora and Grabowski 1993). In general, deficiencies in vitamins that mediate tissue healing can be expected to impair the specific physiological activity for which a particular vitamin is responsible. For example, a deficiency in vitamin K may result in delayed clotting time and prolonged bleeding after vascular disruption. Decreased collagen production associated with vitamin C deficiency may delay soft connective tissue repair and bone healing. In the event of vitamin D deficiency, mineralization and development of a hard bony callus during fracture healing may be negatively affected.

Proteins, carbohydrates, and lipids represent three categories of organic compounds that are essential to the normal metabolic functions of the body. Collectively, these nutrients assume a multitude of roles throughout the various stages of connective tissue repair. For example, immunoglobulins represent a family of proteins that act as antibodies to neutralize or destroy pathogenic agents (i.e., antigens) in the body's specific defense system, thereby providing an important immunological function in the event of persistent inflammation. Proteins derived from dietary sources provide the essential amino acids for synthesis of other proteins, including collagen, which provides the major structural component of the fibrous tissue matrix that forms during connective tissue repair. Hence, proteins are essential to the repair of damaged tissues during fibroplasia, the second primary stage of healing (Tortora and Grabowski 1993). In addition to proteins, carbohydrates play various roles in the physiological events of tissue healing. For example, carbohydrates combine with proteins to form glycoproteins, a group of noncollagenous macromolecules that contribute to the structural integrity and strength of the extracellular connective tissue matrix (Martinez-Hernandez 1994).

Summary

A problem-oriented approach to sports injury management, including application of the fundamental steps in clinical decision making, represents a logical strategic model for injury treatment and rehabilitation. After a physician's referral for follow-up treatment, clinical assessment and identification of an injured sports participant's health-related problem(s) are early fundamental steps in clinical decision making. While a clinical assessment commonly reveals relevant signs and symptoms of underlying pathology that become a focus of therapeutic intervention, alterations in tissue structure and function due to trauma and tissue healing are typically the source of clinical signs and symptoms. As such, they represent the fundamental problems to be addressed during therapeutic intervention.

Sport-related musculoskeletal injuries commonly involve the connective tissues of the body, including ligaments and joint capsules, musculotendinous tissues, and bones. Rational decisions in the therapeutic management of these injuries stem from an understanding of the normal physiological responses to tissue trauma. Initially, these reactions include vascular and cellular responses to promote hemostasis, or control of bleeding. Subsequently, the continuum of normal connective tissue repair includes the three primary stages of inflammation, fibroplasia (fibrous scar formation), and scar maturation. Five primary indications for therapeutic intervention that parallel the three stages of connective tissue repair include (1) control of hemorrhage and edema, (2) alleviation of pain and muscle spasm, (3) enhancement of connective tissue repair mechanisms, (4) prevention of contractures and adhesions, and (5) enhancement of the structural and biomechanical properties of scar tissue. Therapeutic agents used to facilitate achievement of these objectives include both physical agents and pharmacologic agents, referred to collectively as tissue-healing modifiers. Management of proprioceptive and sensorimotor deficits associated with musculoskeletal injuries represents a sixth primary area of therapeutic intervention.

Injured body tissues heal through one or both primary mechanisms: regeneration and repair. Whereas regeneration restores the normal structure and function of damaged tissues, repair involves fibrous scar formation that alters the normal structure and biomechanical properties of the affected tissues. Connective tissue repair is augmented by wound contraction, the mechanism that reduces the size of a tissue defect, thus decreasing the amount of tissue that needs to be repaired. Whether regeneration or repair becomes the predominant healing mechanism depends, in part, on the cellular composition of the damaged tissues. Cells referred to as labile cells have good regeneration capability, whereas stable cells demonstrate a low level of replication but may divide rapidly in response to a traumatic stimulus. Cells classified as permanent cells are incapable of regeneration (e.g., nervous tissue) with the exception of muscle cells, which have the capacity to regenerate by virtue of specialized satellite cells. Physical and pharmacologic agents used to influence the vascular, cellular, or neural responses in tissue healing are referred to collectively as modifiers.

The alterations in connective tissue structure and function that result from fibrous scar formation are best understood when compared with the structural components of normal, uninjured connective tissues (i.e., cells, fibers, and ground substance). Further insight regarding the structural and functional consequences of fibrous scar formation can be gained by a comparison with the normal characteristics of various connective tissue types, particularly the dense connective tissues that form tendons, ligaments and joint capsules, and other supportive structures of the musculoskeletal system. Basic elements necessary to restore or replace damaged tissues in these structures include various chemicals, specific blood and connective tissue cells, and nutrients.

References

American Academy of Orthopaedic Surgeons. 1991. *Athletic training and sports medicine,* 2nd ed. Park Ridge, Ill.: American Academy of Orthopaedic Surgeons.

Bryant, W.M. 1977. *Wound healing.* Reading, Mass.: CIBA Pharmaceutical Co.

Calabrese, L.H., and T.W. Rooney. 1986. The use of nonsteroidal anti-inflammatory drugs in sports. *The Physician and Sportsmedicine* 14:89-97.

Ciccone, C.D. 1990. *Pharmacology in rehabilitation.* Philadelphia: Davis.

Cotran, R.S., V. Kumar, and S.L. Robbins. 1989. *Robbins pathological basis of disease,* 4th ed. Philadelphia: W.B. Saunders.

Fantone, J.C. 1990. Basic concepts in inflammation. In *Sports-induced inflammation,* edited by W.B. Leadbetter, J.A. Buckwalter, and S.L. Gordon. Park Ridge, Ill.: American Academy of Orthopaedic Surgeons.

Gieck, J.H., and E.N. Saliba. 1990. Therapeutic ultrasound: Influence on inflammation and healing. In *Sports-induced inflammation,* edited by W.B. Leadbetter, J.A. Buckwalter, and S.L. Gordon. Park Ridge, Ill.: American Academy of Orthopaedic Surgeons.

Harrelson, G.L. 1991. Physiologic factors of rehabilitation. In *Physical rehabilitation of the injured athlete,* edited by J.R. Andrews and G.L. Harrelson. Philadelphia: W.B. Saunders.

Junqueira, L.C., J. Carneiro, and R.O. Kelly. 1995. *Basic histology,* 8th ed. Norwalk, Conn.: Appleton and Lange.

Kloth, L.C., and K.H. Miller. 1990. The inflammatory response to wounding. In *Wound healing: Alternatives in management,* edited by L.C. Kloth, J.M. McCulloch, and J.A. Feeder. Philadelphia: Davis.

Koester, M.C. 1993. An overview of the physiology and pharmacology of aspirin and nonsteroidal anti-inflammatory drugs. *Journal of Athletic Training* 28:252-59.

Leadbetter, W.B. 1994. Soft tissue athletic injuries. In *Sports injuries: Mechanisms, prevention, treatment,* edited by F.H. Fu and D.A. Stone. Baltimore: Williams and Wilkins.

Leadbetter, W.B., J.A. Buckwalter, and S.L. Gordon, eds. 1990. *Sports-induced inflammation.* Park Ridge, Ill.: American Academy of Orthopaedic Surgeons.

MacDougall, J.D. 1992. Hypertrophy or hyperplasia. In *Strength and power in sport,* edited by P.V. Komi. Cambridge, Mass.: Blackwell Science.

Martinez-Hernandez, A. 1994. Repair, regeneration, and fibrosis. In *Pathology,* 2nd ed., edited by E. Rubin and J.L. Farber. Philadelphia: J.B. Lippincott.

Martinez-Hernandez, A., and P.S. Amenta. 1990. Basic concepts in wound healing. In *Sports-induced inflammation,* edited by W.B. Leadbetter, J.A. Buckwalter, and S.L. Gordon. Park Ridge, Ill.: American Academy of Orthopaedic Surgeons.

Postlethwaite, A.E. 1990. Failed healing responses in connective tissue and a comparison of medical conditions. In *Sports-induced inflammation,* edited by W.B. Leadbetter, J.A. Buckwalter, and S.L. Gordon. Park Ridge, Ill.: American Academy of Orthopaedic Surgeons.

Thomas, C.L., ed. 1993. *Taber's cyclopedic medical dictionary,* 17th ed. Philadelphia: Davis.

Tortora, G.J., and S.R. Grabowski. 1993. *Principles of anatomy and physiology,* 7th ed. New York: Harper Collins College Publishers.

Hemorrhage and Hemostasis

Primary Hemostasis	Hemorrhagic Manifestations
Secondary Hemostasis	Summary

Learning Objectives

After completion of this chapter, the reader should be able to

1. describe the vascular and cellular responses that characterize primary and secondary hemostasis,
2. describe the "cascade" concept of coagulation as a function of hemostasis,
3. describe the relationship between hemostasis and the early inflammatory responses to soft tissue trauma, and
4. describe the primary clinical manifestations of soft tissue hemorrhage.

When body tissues are injured, blood vessels are disrupted and hemorrhagic effusion (i.e., escape of fluids) occurs in the damaged tissues. Control of hemorrhage is referred to as *hemostasis,* which is defined as "the arrest of bleeding, either by physiological properties of vasoconstriction and coagulation or surgery" (Dorland 1988). The specific physiological processes of hemostasis can be categorized as *primary hemostatic mechanisms,* including vasoconstriction and temporary hemostatic plug formation, and *secondary hemostatic mechanisms,* which include coagulation (i.e., blood clotting) and clot retraction (Cotran, Kumar, and Robbins 1989; Tortora and Grabowski 1993). Although these hemostatic responses are overlapped in time by interrelated vascular and cellular changes associated with acute inflammation, hemostasis and inflammation represent two distinguishable early responses to tissue injury (Bryant 1977). Discussion in this chapter is focused on the continuum of physiological events associated with primary and secondary hemostasis. The normal inflammatory responses to trauma that represent the first stage of tissue healing are discussed in chapter 3.

Primary Hemostasis

The initial hemostatic mechanisms, which occur within seconds after blood vessel trauma, include (1) vasoconstriction and (2) development of a temporary hemostatic plug in the damaged vessels (figure 2.1). Stimulated by blood vessel disruption, platelets accumulate along the walls of the damaged vessels and become activated as the result of morphological and functional changes. Through a process called *platelet release reaction,* various hemostatic mediators are released from the activated platelets. Among these substances are serotonin, thromboxane, adenosine diphosphate (ADP), and calcium (Fantone and Ward 1994). These platelet-derived mediators, in conjunction with other substances released from damaged connective tissue cells, assume various roles in activation of primary and secondary hemostatic mechanisms.

When trauma occurs, the smooth muscle fibers of the vascular wall contract, leading to constriction of small blood vessels (i.e., the arterioles) at the site of injury. Vasoconstriction is mediated by the action of serotonin, a potent vasoconstrictor released from activated platelets and from mast cells found in adjacent connective tissues. Thromboxane

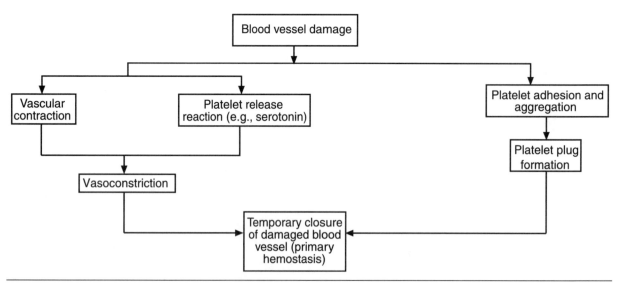

Figure 2.1   Primary hemostatic mechanisms (vasoconstriction and platelet plug formation).

A$_2$, another vasoconstrictor, is also released from activated platelets. Initial vasoconstriction of local blood vessels is transient, usually lasting from a few seconds to a few minutes, after which vasodilation and increased blood flow occur in the injured area (Cotran, Kumar, and Robbins 1989). In some cases, vasoconstriction may completely occlude an arteriole or small artery depending on the extent and type of blood vessel damage (Ganong 1995). Occlusion of larger arteries, however, does not occur to the extent that the need for subsequent hemostatic responses is precluded.

Paralleling vasoconstriction, a temporary hemostatic plug develops in the damaged blood vessels within one to three minutes after injury (see figure 2.1). This plug, formed by masses of activated platelets along the walls of the disrupted vessels, constitutes a second mechanism of primary hemostasis. Initially, the platelets adhere to subendothelial connective tissue (i.e., collagen), which has been exposed during trauma to the inner lining of the blood vessel. This process is referred to as *platelet adhesion*. Platelets also adhere to each other, a process called *platelet aggregation*. Adhesion and aggregation of large numbers of platelets account for the main mass of the plug that forms in the disrupted blood vessel. Formation of the hemostatic plug is mediated, in part, by ADP and thromboxane A$_2$, two substances that promote platelet aggregation (Fantone and Ward 1994). The initial platelet plug that develops in damaged blood vessels forms the basis for subsequent clot formation. Because the platelet plug is unstable and easily disrupted, it must be reinforced by the formation of an insoluble fibrin network that develops during coagulation.

Secondary Hemostasis

Coagulation, or blood clotting, is the secondary hemostatic mechanism through which the initial platelet plug in damaged vessels is reinforced. Overlapping in time with vasoconstriction and platelet plug formation, coagulation is initiated by the release of hemostatic mediators from damaged tissues and disrupted blood vessels. Ultimately, coagulation results in formation of a stable insoluble fibrin clot in the damaged vessels. Coagulation occurs through a series of catalytic reactions during which normally inactive *coagulation factors* are activated. Traditionally, each coagulation factor has been designated by a Roman numeral in order of its discovery. These coagulation factors, along with their corresponding Roman numerals, are listed in figure 2.2. Most substances that function as coagulation factors are produced in the liver and released into the circulating blood, although some are released from activated platelets (e.g., calcium). One coagulation factor, thromboplastin (factor III), is released from damaged tissue cells at the time of injury (Tortora and Grabowski 1993).

I	Fibrinogen	VIII	Antihemophilic factor
II	Prothrombin	IX	Christmas factor
III	Thromboplastin (tissue factor)	X	Stuart-Prower factor
IV	Calcium ions	XI	Plasma thromboplastin antecedent (PTA)
V	Proaccelerin	XII	Hageman factor
VII	Proconvertin	XIII	Fibrin stabilizing factor (FSF)

Figure 2.2   Coagulation factors.
Data from Thomas 1993.

Stage 1

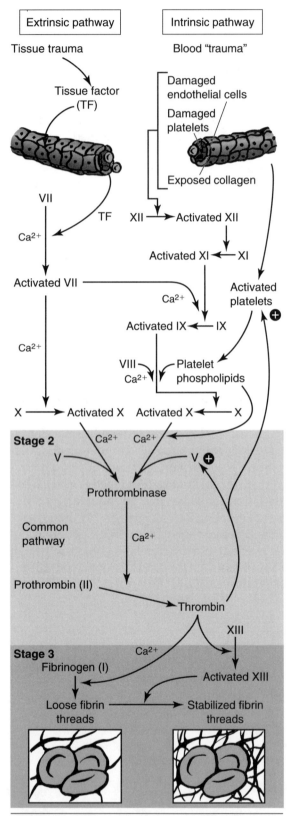

Figure 2.3   Primary stages of coagulation (blood-clotting cascade).

The "cascade" concept of coagulation holds that an activated coagulation factor functions as an enzyme, an organic catalyst, to activate the next factor, which in turn functions to activate the next. This series of enzymatic reactions continues until blood clotting is complete. Commonly, coagulation is described as having three main stages: (1) formation of prothrombinase, (2) conversion of prothrombin into thrombin, and (3) conversion of soluble fibrinogen into insoluble fibrin (Tortora and Grabowski 1993). These stages are summarized in figure 2.3.

The first stage of coagulation is initiated by release of coagulation factors through two pathways, an *extrinsic pathway* and an *intrinsic pathway.* In the extrinsic pathway, the protein thromboplastin (factor III), also called tissue factor, infiltrates the blood from damaged tissues outside, or extrinsic to, the blood vessel. Initiated by thromboplastin, sequential activation of factors VII and X, in the presence of calcium ions (factor IV), occurs within seconds. In the more complex intrinsic pathway, the Hageman factor (factor XII) is activated by exposure to subendothelial collagen within, or intrinsic to, the blood vessel. Initiated by the activated Hageman factor, sequential activation of factors XI, IX, VIII, and X occurs. The presence of calcium ions is also an essential element in these catalytic actions. Completion of the first stage of coagulation is marked by formation of the active enzyme prothrombinase, the prothrombin activator, which results from the interaction of factor X and factor V in both the extrinsic and the intrinsic pathway (Tortora and Grabowski 1993).

Clotting mechanisms in the second and third stage of coagulation occur through a common pathway. In the second stage of coagulation, in the presence of calcium ions, prothrombinase catalyzes the conversion of prothrombin (factor II) into thrombin. Finally, during the third stage, thrombin converts fibrinogen (factor I) into fibrin and a loose threadlike network of soluble fibrin filaments is developed. As this network is reinforced and strengthened by the fibrin-stabilizing factor (factor XIII), a stable insoluble clot, or *coagulum,* is formed. Finally, *clot retraction* occurs within a few minutes after clot formation. Fibrin threads attached to the damaged blood vessel contract and pull the edges of the blood vessel together, thus further strengthening the clot and preparing the blood vessel for repair. Eventually, the clot is dissolved as the fibrin threads are degraded by proteolytic enzymes, a process referred to as *fibrinolysis* (Ganong 1995).

In addition to its hemostatic function, the fibrin network formed during blood clotting establishes a structural framework for localization of the formed elements in the blood (e.g., red blood cells, white blood cells) and connective tissue cells (e.g., fibroblasts). White blood cells are essential to resolution of inflammation during the first stage of tissue healing, whereas fibroblasts are responsible for collagen synthesis and fibrous tissue formation in the second stage of healing. Thus, the fibrin network formed during coagulation establishes an essential link between hemostasis and subsequent tissue repair processes. The phagocytic function of white blood cells and the role of fibroblasts in fibrous tissue formation are discussed in chapter 3.

Hemorrhagic Manifestations

Despite the effectiveness of normal hemostatic mechanisms in arresting blood loss from damaged vessels, varying degrees of hemorrhage and effusion into the affected tissues can be expected, especially with moderate to severe tissue injury. Soft tissue hemorrhage in extraarticular structures (e.g., muscles) is commonly manifested as a *hematoma*, a localized collection of blood in the damaged area. Two types of hematoma formation in muscle tissues have been described (Kellett 1986; Leadbetter 1994). A localized accumulation of blood that remains confined by an intact connective tissue sheath (i.e., the epimysium) is referred to as an *intramuscular hematoma*. In contrast, an *intermuscular hematoma* involves localized hemorrhage, but without confinement. In this type of hematoma, blood remains free to extravasate throughout a muscle unit. Commonly, over a period of a few days, the blood gravitates distally to appear as *ecchymosis*, a bluish-black or greenish-yellow discoloration of the skin. Injuries to synovial joints may result in hemorrhagic effusion that is confined within an intact joint capsule. Such intracapsular effusion is referred to as *hemarthrosis*. More severe articular injuries, however, may involve capsular disruption with escape of blood into extracapsular tissues. Clinical techniques to assist hemostasis and control hemorrhagic effusion and edema are discussed in chapter 4.

Summary

Hemostasis, or arrest of bleeding, following an acute soft tissue injury involves a sequence of physiological responses that include primary hemostatic mechanisms and secondary hemostatic mechanisms. The primary hemostatic mechanisms include vasoconstriction and formation of a temporary hemostatic plug. Initially, within seconds following injury, chemically mediated vasoconstriction occurs. Concurrently, platelet adhesion occurs. In this process, masses of platelets accumulate along the vascular wall and adhere to subendothelial collagen that is exposed during vascular disruption. Platelet aggregation, the adherence of platelets to other platelets, also occurs within seconds. These processes result in formation of a temporary hemostatic plug within one to three minutes following injury.

Secondary hemostatic mechanisms include coagulation and clot retraction. During this phase of hemostasis, the unstable temporary platelet plug that forms in damaged blood vessels is subsequently reinforced by formation of a fibrin clot. Coagulation, or clotting, occurs through a series of enzymatic reactions during which normally inactive coagulation factors are activated. In accordance with the "cascade" concept, sequential activation of coagulation factors occurs until a stable coagulum, or clot, is formed. Finally, clot retraction provides further stability and strength. In addition to its hemostatic function, the fibrin threadlike network that forms during coagulation provides a structural framework for localization of white blood cells, fibroblasts, and other cells that are essential to connective tissue repair. Despite normal hemostatic mechanisms, varying degrees of hemorrhagic effusion can be expected in most soft tissue injuries. Hemorrhage in muscle injuries may be manifested as an intramuscular or an intermuscular hematoma. Hemorthrosis occurs when bleeding is confined within a joint capsule.

References

Bryant, W.M. 1977. *Wound healing.* Reading, Mass.: CIBA Pharmaceutical Co.

Cotran, R.S., V. Kumar, and S.L. Robbins. 1989. *Robbins pathological basis of disease,* 4th ed. Philadelphia: W.B. Saunders.

Dorland's illustrated medical dictionary, 27th ed. 1988. Philadelphia: W.B. Saunders.

Fantone, J.C., and P.A. Ward. 1994. Inflammation. In *Pathology,* 2nd ed., edited by E. Rubin and J.L. Farber. Philadelphia: J.B. Lippincott.

Ganong, W.F. 1995. *Review of medical physiology,* 17th ed. Norwalk, Conn.: Appleton and Lange.

Kellett, J. 1986. Acute soft tissue injuries—A review of the literature. *Medicine and Science in Sports and Exercise* 18:489-99.

Leadbetter, W.B. 1994. Soft tissue athletic injuries. In *Sports injuries: Mechanisms, prevention, treatment,* edited by F.H. Fu and D.H. Stone. Baltimore: Williams and Wilkins.

Thomas, C.L., ed. 1993. *Taber's cyclopedic medical dictionary,* 17th ed. Philadelphia: Davis.

Tortora, G.J., and S.R. Grabowski. 1993. *Principles of anatomy and physiology,* 7th ed. New York: Harper Collins College Publishers.

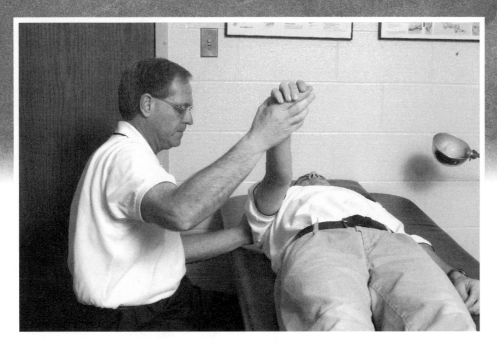

Soft Tissue Repair and Therapeutic Intervention

Inflammation, fibroplasia (scar formation), and scar maturation are commonly considered three primary phases in the continuum of soft connective tissue repair. The purposes of this part are to review the normal mechanisms of connective tissue repair and to present implications for therapeutic intervention throughout the repair process. Chapter 3, Soft Connective Tissue Repair, includes a review of the primary vascular and cellular events that characterize each of the three sequential stages of normal connective tissue healing. Additionally, manifestations of tissue repair complications are identified and reviewed. Two companion chapters in this part are devoted to therapeutic intervention during the tissue repair process. Chapter 4, Therapeutic Implications: Inflammation and Pain, is focused on the management of primary inflammatory responses (hemorrhage and edema) and secondary reactions (pain and muscle spasm) to acute musculoskeletal injury. Therapeutic management during the second and third stages of connective tissue repair is discussed in chapter 5, Therapeutic Implications: Scar Formation and Maturation. Collectively, the three chapters in this part provide a comprehensive review of soft connective tissue repair with corresponding implications for therapeutic management.

Soft Connective Tissue Repair

Inflammation
Acute Inflammation
Vascular Changes
Cellular Responses
Subacute and Chronic Inflammation
Subacute Inflammation
Chronic Inflammation
Fibroplasia
Proliferation of Fibroblasts
Collagen Synthesis and Fibrogenesis
Formation of Granulation Tissue
Type III Collagen Formation
Neovascularization
Wound Contraction
Fibrous Scar Formation
Type I Collagen Formation
Increased Collagen Deposition
Resorption of Blood Vessels

Scar Maturation
Collagen Turnover
Collagen Cross-Linkage
Realignment of Collagen Fibers
Tissue Repair Complications
Granulomatous Inflammation
Retardation of Muscle Fiber Regeneration
Contractures and Adhesions
Contractures
Adhesions
Hypertrophic Scars and Keloids
Summary

Learning Objectives

After completion of this chapter, the reader should be able to

❶ identify the three primary stages of soft connective tissue repair,

❷ describe the primary vascular and cellular events associated with acute, subacute, and chronic inflammation,

❸ describe the continuum of vascular and cellular responses that characterize scar formation,

❹ describe the characteristic cellular responses and connective tissue adaptations associated with scar maturation, and

❺ identify and describe the primary complications and clinical manifestations of abnormal connective tissue repair.

Sports injuries to the musculoskeletal system commonly involve ligaments and joint capsules, musculotendinous tissues, and bone. With the exception of myofibers (i.e., the contractile element of a muscle), these structures represent various types of connective tissues that heal through an orderly sequence of physiological events. Although bone is classified as a type of connective tissue, fracture healing occurs through distinguishable, yet analogous mechanisms as compared to the repair of soft tissue injuries. Fracture healing and the clinical implications for therapeutic intervention are addressed in chapters 6 and 7. Discussion in this chapter is devoted to a review of the mechanisms associated with normal soft connective tissue repair. In addition, several conditions that represent alterations in the normal repair process are discussed. Implications for therapeutic intervention throughout the various stages of soft tissue repair, including management of tissue-healing complications, are presented in chapters 4 and 5.

Damaged connective tissues heal through a process of fibrous scar formation, or repair, rather than by regeneration, which restores normal tissue structure and function. Because the vascular and cellular events of tissue healing, as well as the sequence in which they occur, are essentially the same in all soft connective tissues, the repair process is relatively nonspecific to the particular type of tissue involved. As described by Bryant (1977), soft connective tissue repair involves three primary stages: (1) inflammation, (2) fibroplasia, and (3) scar maturation (figure 3.1). Although the processes are the same, Daly (1990) used somewhat different descriptive terminology and classified the stages of tissue healing as inflammation, granulation tissue formation, and matrix formation and remodeling. Martinez-Hernandez and Amenta (1990) described a similar classification involving

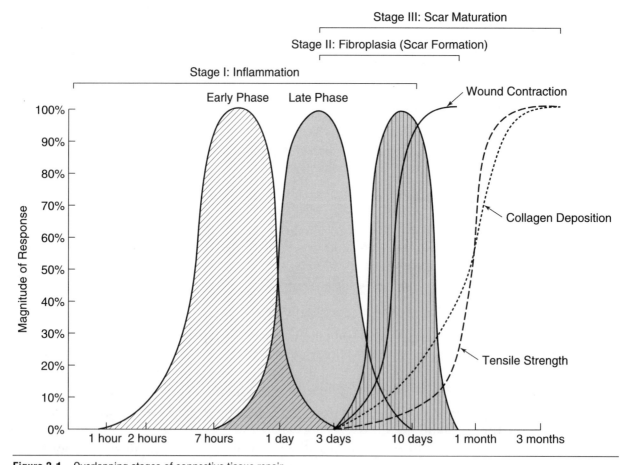

Figure 3.1   Overlapping stages of connective tissue repair.

Adapted, by permission, from T.J. Daly, 1990, The repair phase of wound healing—re-epithelialization and contraction. In *Wound healing: Alternatives in management*, edited by L.C. Kloth, J.M. McCulloch, and J.A. Feeder (Philadelphia: F.A. Davis), 15.

inflammation, proliferation, and maturation. Wound contraction, the process through which the size of a tissue defect is reduced, overlaps in time with fibrous tissue formation, or fibroplasia. Thus, wound contraction is an important contributor to connective tissue repair during the second stage of tissue healing. Although the traditional classification of connective tissue repair into three primary stages facilitates discussion, it is important to note that tissue healing occurs on a continuum of interrelated events. Each stage overlaps in time with the preceding stage. Whereas the mechanisms of tissue healing and the time frames in which they occur are fairly predictable under normal physiological conditions, tissue healing may be affected by several factors. Tissue-healing time, as well as the quality of repair, may vary according to such factors as the type of injured tissue, the extent of tissue damage, regional vascularity in the injured area, and the age and general nutrition of the injured person (Leadbetter 1994). As discussed shortly, persistent inflammation may also affect the rate and quality of connective tissue repair.

Inflammation

Inflammation, which represents the first stage of connective tissue repair, is the normal, nonspecific response of vascularized tissues to an irritant, including the types of musculoskeletal injuries commonly associated with sports participation. Whether injury results from macrotrauma with acute tissue disruption or microtrauma due to repetitive tissue loading, the inflammatory response is essentially the same. Traditionally, inflammation has been categorized as acute or chronic, primarily on the basis of characteristic vascular and cellular responses and the nature and duration of clinical signs and symptoms. In a new injury, the *acute inflammatory response* typically lasts for three to four days (see figure 3.1). As signs and symptoms gradually subside, inflammation enters a *subacute phase* of approximately two weeks. If not resolved, the local inflammatory response may become generalized, or systemic. Systemic inflammation is exemplified by *lymphangitis* (inflammation of the lymph vessels), *lymphadenitis* (inflammation of the lymph nodes), and generalized symptoms such as fever and malaise. Unresolved acute inflammatory responses, recurrent microtrauma, or persistent irritation from foreign material in the tissues may lead to *chronic inflammation* that may last for months or longer (Kloth and Miller 1990).

Acute Inflammation

When injury to connective tissues invokes an inflammatory response, a multitude of chemically mediated vascular changes and cellular reactions occurs. Acute inflammation is the initial response to injury that functions to localize and destroy pathogenic agents and foreign material. As such, the phagocytic activities that characterize acute inflammation represent the body's first line of defense against invading pathogens (i.e., microorganisms capable of producing disease). As this primary function indicates, acute inflammation is a normal, essential component of connective tissue repair. To the extent that the complimentary vascular and cellular events of acute inflammation are successful in eliminating pathogenic agents, foreign material, and necrotic tissue debris, a favorable environment for uncomplicated tissue repair is created.

Acute inflammation is of relatively short duration. Typically, acute inflammatory responses reach a peak within a few hours after tissue injury but may last for three to four days (see figure 3.1). During this period, acute inflammation is characterized by (1) vascular responses that result in excess fluid accumulation in the affected tissues (i.e., edema) and (2) cellular responses that include proliferation of white blood cells and phagocytosis. Although these primary inflammatory responses are discussed separately, it is important to note the many physiological interrelationships between the vascular and cellular reactions in acute inflammation.

Vascular Changes

The sequential vascular responses associated with acute inflammation include (1) vasodilation and increased blood flow, (2) increased vascular permeability, and (3) increased blood viscosity with slowing of blood flow (Cotran, Kumar, and Robbins 1989). Collectively, these hemodynamic changes result in increased interstitial fluid, or edema, in the injury area. In addition to the hemodynamic changes that occur in the blood vessels, obstruction of local lymph vessels with decreased lymphatic drainage of interstitial fluid also contributes to edema. Despite their seemingly negative effects, these vascular changes are an essential prelude to the phagocytic functions of white blood cells, as discussed shortly.

Following initial transient vasoconstriction of damaged blood vessels within a few minutes after injury, vasodilation and increased blood flow occur in the injured area. Coincident with these vascular responses, increased vascular permeability also occurs (figure 3.2b-c). At the time of injury, histamine, which is known to cause vasodilation and increased vascular permeability, is released from mast cells, basophils, and platelets. Histamine-mediated contraction of endothelial cells in the walls of small blood vessels accounts for the initial increase in vascular permeability. As cellular contraction occurs, the endothelial cells separate, creating intercellular gaps in the vascular wall. Enhanced by an increase in intravascular hydrostatic pressure, fluid filtrates through these gaps into the interstitial spaces, a process called *transudation* (figure 3.2b). Accumulation of excess fluid in the interstitial spaces is referred to as *edema*, the clinical manifestation of increased vascular permeability. The initial increase in vascular permeability mediated by histamine is relatively short-lived, lasting less than one hour. Increased vascular permeability attributable to other vasoactive mediators, however, may last for several hours beyond the duration of histamine action. Other chemicals that have been associated with increased vascular permeability include prostaglandins, bradykinin, leukotrienes, and complement proteins (Stevens and Lowe 1995).

Initially, the fluid that escapes through the permeable vascular wall consists primarily of water, contains very few blood cells, and is relatively low in protein content. This fluid is called *transudate* (figure 3.2b). As vascular permeability increases, blood cells (e.g., leukocytes) and plasma proteins are allowed to escape, causing the extravascular fluid to become more viscous in nature. This vascular response, referred to as *exudation*, results in excess interstitial fluid called *exudate*, the hallmark of acute inflammatory edema (figure 3.2c). With exudation of fluids into the interstitial spaces, red blood cells become concentrated in the small blood vessels, the viscosity of the blood increases, and a slowing of blood flow (i.e., stasis) occurs (Cotran, Kumar, and Robbins 1989). As stagnation of blood flow develops, contact of circulating white blood cells with the inner lining of the vascular wall is facilitated. Thus, the white blood cells are positioned for emigration through the intercellular gaps in the vascular wall. Although increased vascular permeability leads to edema, the intercellular gaps that occur also allow emigration of phagocytic white blood cells (e.g., neutrophils) into the injured tissues. As a result, an important link is established between the vascular responses in acute inflammation and the phagocytic activities of white blood cells that follow.

Under normal physiological conditions, the intravascular fluid that continually moves through the vascular wall into the interstitial spaces is balanced by drainage into the lymphatics (i.e., the lymph vessels) and edema does not occur. With tissue injury, however, exudation of fluids into the damaged tissues may exceed drainage by the lymph vessels, thereby localizing the inflammatory response. Should invasion of pathogenic microorganisms (e.g., bacteria) occur, localization permits phagocytosis by white blood cells in the exudate, thus preventing transportation of pathogenic agents to other body parts. In this manner, lymphatic obstruction, along with the phagocytic function of white blood cells, serves as an early nonspecific defense against invading pathogens. Although lym-

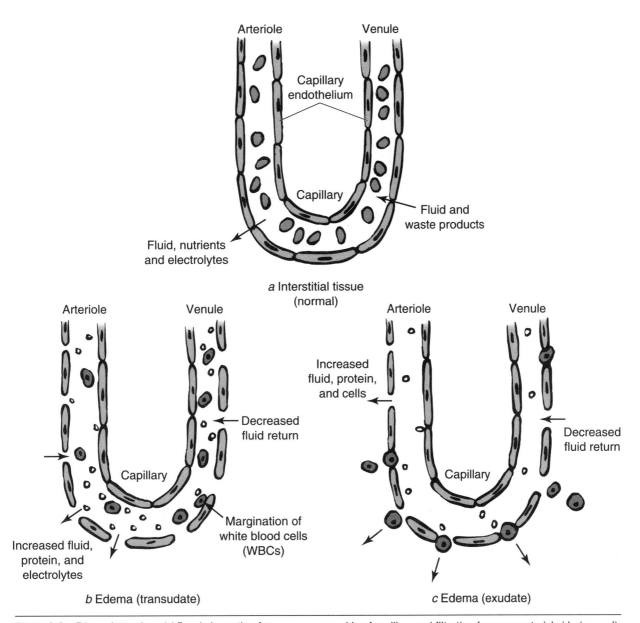

Figure 3.2   Edema formation. *(a)* Equal absorption forces on venous side of capillary and filtration forces on arterial side (normal). *(b)* Margination of white blood cells, increased capillary permeability, transudate (fluid) leakage into extravascular spaces. *(c)* Exudate (fluid, proteins, and blood cells) leakage into extravascular spaces.

Adapted, by permission, from L.C. Kloth and K.H. Miller, 1990, The inflammatory response to wound healing. In *Wound healing: Alternatives in management*, edited by L.C. Kloth, J.M. McCulloch, and J.A. Felder (Philadelphia: F.A. Davis), 6.

phatic blockage contributes to edema, premature resolution may result in a spread of inflammation, such as that seen in lymphangitis and lymphadenitis (Cotran, Kumar, and Robbins 1989).

The vascular responses that occur in acute inflammation are primarily responsible for producing three of the *five cardinal signs of inflammation* (see chapter 1, figure 1.1). Local vasodilation and increased blood flow account for increased tissue temperature (hyperthermia) and redness (erythema), whereas increased vascular permeability with exudation of fluids into the interstitial spaces results in swelling (edema). In addition to these manifestations, cellular necrosis may occur as a complication of early vascular responses to tissue injury. As edema forms in the affected tissues, interstitial pressure increases, leading to impairment of local circulation (i.e., ischemia) and a diminished oxygen supply (i.e., hypoxia). As a result, ischemic cellular necrosis occurs. This phenomenon is referred to as *secondary hypoxic injury* (Knight 1990). To the extent that secondary hypoxic injury occurs, in addition to tissue destruction caused by the initial trauma, the degree of necessary tissue repair increases. Early therapeutic intervention, including the use of cold applications, to decrease the oxygen demands of local tissues and minimize cellular necrosis is discussed in chapter 4. The fourth cardinal sign of inflammation, *pain*, can also be attributed to vascular changes involving circulatory impairment (i.e., ischemic pain) or edema formation with increased pressure on nociceptive nerve endings (i.e., pain receptors) in the injured tissues (Kloth and Miller 1990). Pain is commonly accompanied by protective *muscle spasm*, which in turn exacerbates the pain. *Loss of function*, sometimes considered the fifth cardinal sign of inflammation, may be attributed to the resulting pain-spasm-pain cycle, the congestive effect of edema, or both. Therapeutic intervention to alleviate pain and muscle spasm is discussed in chapter 4.

Cellular Responses

The response of white blood cells during inflammation provides both nonspecific and specific body defenses against invading pathogenic microorganisms. Nonspecific defenses, which constitute the *innate defense system*, provide generalized protection against a wide spectrum of pathogenic agents. Physical barriers (e.g., skin, mucous membranes), as well as mechanical and chemical barriers, provide an initial nonspecific defense. Should pathogen invasion occur, however, phagocytosis and destruction of pathogenic agents by white blood cells represent a second line of nonspecific defense during acute inflammation. In the presence of persistent pathogens, specific immunological responses that constitute the *adaptive defense system* may be invoked (Cotran, Kumar, and Robbins 1989). Immunological responses to specific pathogens, as related to chronic inflammation, are discussed in a following section of this chapter.

The cellular responses of the nonspecific, innate defense system that occur during acute inflammation are characterized by proliferation of white blood cells (i.e., leukocytes) and phagocytosis of pathogenic microorganisms. The initial cellular response is increased production of leukocytes by red bone marrow, a process called *hemopoiesis*. Release of leukocytes from the bone marrow results in *leukocytosis*, an increased accumulation of white blood cells in the blood. Within a few hours, leukocytes accumulate in the injured area in large numbers. Granular leukocytes (i.e., neutrophils, eosinophils, and basophils) and nongranular leukocytes (i.e., monocytes and lymphocytes) are attracted to the affected tissues in proportion to their concentration in the circulating blood. Proportionally, neutrophils are the most numerous type of leukocytes in whole blood. Hence, they represent the most prevalent type of white blood cell at the site of injury during the early phase of acute inflammation. Following proliferation at the injury site, the sequence of leukocyte activity includes (1) margination, (2) adhesion, (3) emigration, (4) chemotaxis, and (5) phagocytosis (Cotran, Kumar, and Robbins 1989). The mechanisms of leukocyte margination, adhesion, emigration, and chemotaxis are depicted in figure 3.3.

As previously indicated, slowing of blood flow in damaged vessels (i.e., stasis) facilitates contact of circulating leukocytes with the endothelial lining of the vascular wall. The process through which leukocytes move from the central portion of the blood vessel and accumulate along the endothelial surface is called *margination* (see figure 3.3). After margination, leukocytes become attached to the vascular wall through a mechanism referred to as *adhesion*, or *pavementing*. Leukocyte attachment to the vascular wall is attributed, in part, to a group of chemicals referred to as *adhesion molecules* (e.g., glycoproteins) that act on the surface of the leukocyte, the endothelium, or both (Cotran, Kumar, and Robbins 1989; Fantone and Ward 1994). As the result of margination and adhesion, the endothelial surface of the vascular wall becomes covered with leukocytes within a few hours after injury.

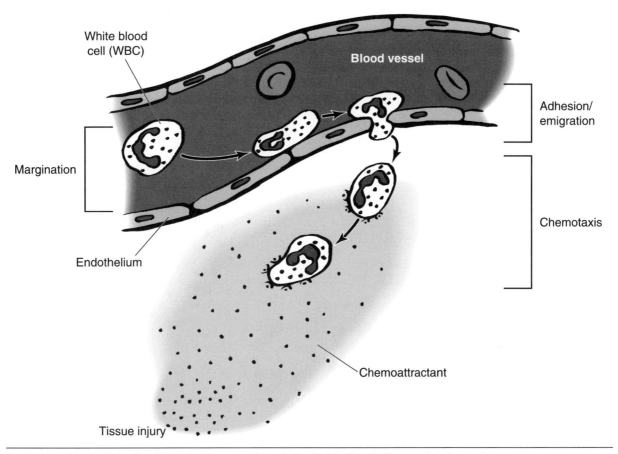

Figure 3.3 Margination, adhesion, emigration, and chemotaxis of white blood cells in acute inflammation.

Adapted, by permission, from R.S. Cotran, V. Kumar, and S.L. Robbins, 1989, *Robbins pathological basis of disease*, 4th ed. (Philadelphia: W.B. Saunders), 45.

Following margination and adherence, increased vascular permeability allows leukocytes to move through intercellular gaps in the vascular wall into interstitial spaces where they migrate to the damaged tissues (see figure 3.3). Movement of leukocytes through the vascular wall is referred to as *emigration,* or *diapedesis* (Hettinga 1990). Because the escaping fluid now contains blood cells, as well as plasma proteins, it is referred to as *exudate.* After emigration, leukocytes are attracted to the damaged tissues by various chemicals referred to collectively as *chemotactic factors* (i.e., chemoattractants) in preparation for phagocytosis (see figure 3.3). This process is called *chemotaxis,* the unidirectional movement of cells toward a chemical attractant (Fantone and Ward 1994). The predominant phagocytic cells during early acute inflammation are classified as *polymorphonuclear leukocytes* (i.e., neutrophils, basophils, eosinophils). Neutrophils are the most active phagocytic cells during the first 24 hours of acute inflammation. Although several chemoattractants for neutrophils have been identified, components of the complement system (i.e., blood proteins), products of arachidonic acid metabolism (e.g., leukotrienes), and cytokines (e.g., interleukins) have been cited as particularly significant (Cotran, Kumar, and Robbins 1989; Fantone and Ward 1994). In comparison to *mononuclear leukocytes* (monocytes and lymphocytes), neutrophils are short-lived. Neutrophils appear to reach their maximum phagocytic effectiveness within 6 to 12 hours, after which they disintegrate and disappear within 24 to 48 hours. Within 48 hours, monocytes replace neutrophils as the primary phagocytic cells during the late acute and subacute stages of inflammation (Cotran, Kumar, and Robbins 1989; Hettinga 1990). The role of mononuclear phagocytes is discussed shortly.

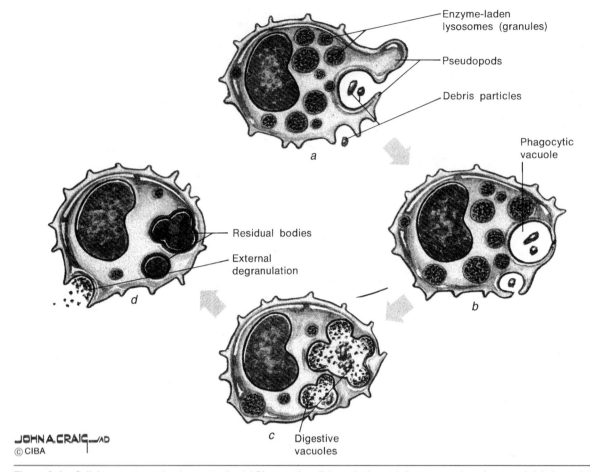

Figure 3.4 Cellular responses in phagocytosis. *(a)* Phagocytic cell (e.g., leukocyte) forms pseudopods around debris particles. *(b)* Membranes of pseudopods fuse, enclosing debris in phagocytic vacuole (phagosome). *(c)* Phagocytic cell undergoes degranulation: Lysosomes fuse with phagocytic vacuole and extrude enzymes into the resulting digestive vacuole. *(d)* At completion of phagocytosis, cell shows few lysosomes and dense residual bodies of digested debris.

As neutrophils proliferate in damaged tissues, they begin the process of *phagocytosis* (figure 3.4). Phagocytosis is the nonspecific cellular response whereby pathogenic microorganisms, foreign material, and tissue debris are disposed of in preparation for fibroplasia, the subsequent phase of connective tissue repair. The primary mechanisms of phagocytosis are described as (1) *recognition* of the invading pathogenic microorganism (e.g., bacteria) and *adherence*, or attachment, of the phagocytic cell to the surface of the pathogenic agent, (2) *engulfment*, or ingestion, of the microorganism by extensions of the phagocytic cell membrane (i.e., pseudopodia), and (3) *degradation*, or digestion, of the pathogenic agent (Cotran, Kumar, and Robbins 1989; Fantone and Ward 1994). Accumulation of polymorphonuclear leukocytes (e.g., neutrophils) in response to bacterial invasion may result in formation of a purulent exudate called *pus*, the thick liquid product of suppurative inflammation that contains degenerated or dead leukocytes (Fantone and Ward 1994).

Subacute and Chronic Inflammation

A primary function of the cellular responses during acute inflammation is to localize and destroy invading pathogenic microorganisms. To the extent that the early phagocytic activity of white blood cells is successful, the signs and symptoms of acute inflammation subside, the inflammatory response enters a subacute phase, and a favorable environment for connective tissue repair continues to develop. If, on the other hand, phagocytic activity fails to destroy persistent pathogenic agents, inflammation may enter a chronic stage during which specific immunological responses are elicited. The primary biological responses inherent in the subacute and chronic stages of inflammation are reviewed in the following sections of this chapter.

Subacute Inflammation

Successful phagocytosis normally marks the end of the acute stage of inflammation. Most of the signs and symptoms associated with the acute inflammatory response typically subside within three to four days following injury. During the subsequent two-week period, the *subacute phase,* clinical signs and symptoms continue to diminish and eventually disappear (see figure 3.1). With the disappearance of neutrophils, within a few days after injury, mononuclear leukocytes (i.e., monocytes) become the primary phagocytic cells during the late acute and subacute phase of inflammation. When monocytes emigrate through the intercellular gaps in the vascular wall into interstitial spaces, they enlarge and mature into long-lived, highly phagocytic cells known as *macrophages* (Hettinga 1990). Macrophages became the predominant phagocytic cells beginning approximately three days after injury and continuing for about two weeks. Some macrophages, called *wandering macrophages*, move freely throughout the tissues and accumulate at the site of pathogen invasion. These cells, in combination with *fixed macrophages* that are found in loose connective tissues and other organs, are components of the nonspecific defense system known as the *mononuclear phagocyte system*, formerly referred to as the *reticuloendothelial system* (Cotran, Kumar, and Robbins 1989; Tortora and Grabowski 1993).

Chronic Inflammation

With successful phagocytosis of invading pathogenic agents by neutrophils and macrophages, the early inflammatory reactions to tissue injury are typically resolved. Persistent pathogenic microorganisms, however, may provoke a chronic inflammatory response. Chronic inflammation, which may last for months or longer, occurs when damaged tissues are contaminated with pathogenic agents or foreign material that cannot be phagocytized during the acute inflammatory stage of tissue healing. In this regard, chronic inflammation represents an extension of the acute inflammatory response, which may be further prolonged by recurrent injury to the affected tissues (Reed 1996). In other cases, chronic inflammation may be characterized by a gradual insidious onset that eventually becomes symptomatic. Examples of persistent inflammatory responses commonly seen in the sports population are tenosynovitis, bursitis, and synovitis. In addition to the continued presence of macrophages, which regulate a variety of chronic inflammatory responses, an increased number of lymphocytes in damaged tissues is a characteristic cellular response in chronic inflammation. Lymphocytes, which are found in lymphatic tissues (e.g., lymph nodes, spleen) as well as the circulating blood, are the primary nonphagocytic cells responsible for the specific body defenses against invading pathogens. In contrast to nonspecific defense mechanisms, which combat a broad scope of pathogenic agents, specific body defenses provide protection, or *immunity*, against specific pathogens. Pathogenic microorganisms that are capable of invoking a specific immune response are called *antigens*. As previously indicated, the defense mechanisms that respond to specific antigens are components of the *adaptive defense system* (Cotran, Kumar, and Robbins 1989).

Specific immune responses are mediated by two types of lymphocytes known as B cells and T cells. Unlike the phagocytic white blood cells of the nonspecific defense system (i.e., neutrophils, macrophages), which respond to a wide variety of pathogenic agents, each type of lymphocyte is predisposed to recognize and respond only to a specific antigen.

When activated by a foreign antigen, lymphocytes respond through complex processes of proliferation and differentiation into various cell types. These responses produce two types of immunity, *humoral immunity* and *cellular immunity*. Humoral immunity results from differentiation of B cells into plasma cells that produce *antibodies*, the immunoglobulins that neutralize or destroy specific pathogenic agents. Cellular immunity, in contrast, results from differentiation of T cells into various cell types that destroy foreign antigens directly, or indirectly through regulation of B cell activity. Because these immunological responses may take several days or longer, the specific immune system functions as a second line of defense against invading pathogenic agents. Thus, it functions when nonspecific defenses (i.e., phagocytosis) fail to provide adequate protection. Although there are various interactions between the cellular responses of the nonspecific and the specific defense system, the specific immune defenses eventually become dominant in the presence of persistent pathogens (Cotran, Kumar, and Robbins 1989).

Fibroplasia

With successful phagocytosis of pathogenic agents, foreign material, and tissue debris at the site of injury, damaged tissues are prepared for the second stage of connective tissue repair referred to as *fibroplasia*. During this stage, fibrous scar tissue formation occurs through a continuum of cellular and vascular events characterized by (1) proliferation of fibroblasts, (2) collagen synthesis and fibrogenesis, (3) formation of granulation tissue, (4) wound contraction, and (5) dense fibrous scar formation. Although fibroplasia is commonly identified as the second stage of connective tissue repair, it is important to note that the cellular responses leading to fibrous scar formation (e.g., proliferation of fibroblasts) begin within a few hours after injury, thus overlapping the vascular and cellular events of inflammation (see figure 3.1). This overlap, if prolonged by severe, persistent inflammatory responses (e.g., chronic inflammation), may create a tissue-healing environment that interferes with fibrous tissue formation, thus adversely affecting the quality of scar formation. The detrimental effects of persistent inflammation are discussed in a subsequent section of this chapter.

Proliferation of Fibroblasts

An increase in the number of fibroblasts in damaged tissues signals initiation of the fibroplastic stage of tissue healing. Fibroblasts, which arise from undifferentiated mesenchymal cells, are the connective tissue cells responsible for formation of *collagen*, the main supportive protein of connective tissues (i.e., ligaments and joint capsules, tendons). In uninjured tissues, continually active fibroblasts synthesize collagen and other elements of the extracellular connective tissue matrix. Through the simultaneous processes of collagen *synthesis* (i.e., buildup) and *lysis* (i.e., degradation), the normal tissue matrix is maintained by a continual, relatively constant rate of collagen turnover. When injury to connective tissue occurs, however, there is an increased demand for collagen deposition in order that a new tissue matrix can be developed at the injury site. Thus, the initial phase of the connective tissue repair is characterized by proliferation of fibroblasts in the damaged tissues. During this phase, macrophages release a number of chemicals, some of which function as chemotactic agents to attract fibroblasts to the damaged area. As discussed in chapter 2, the fibrin network formed during blood clotting provides a structural framework for localization of fibroblasts at the site of injury. Within a few hours after injury, fibroblasts migrate to the damaged area and become entrapped in the fibrin threads of the clot. Hence, fibroblasts are positioned to synthesize collagen for fibrous tissue formation and development of a new tissue matrix. Proliferation of fibroblasts in the damaged tissues is well established within 48 hours, thus overlapping the acute stage of inflammation (Groner and Weeks 1992; Koester 1993).

Collagen Synthesis and Fibrogenesis

Restoration of the extracellular connective tissue matrix in damaged tissues is dependent on collagen synthesis and *fibrogenesis*, or collagen fiber formation. Because the mechanical properties of collagen are critical to the tensile strength of scar tissue, collagen synthesis is an essential component of connective tissue repair. The sequence of collagen synthesis and collagen fiber formation is illustrated in figure 3.5. Collagen synthesis is a primary function of fibroblasts, the connective tissue cells that have migrated to the damaged area. Thus, collagen synthesis begins at the cellular level with formation of three coiled polypeptide alpha chains (i.e., union of amino acids) that form a triple helix *procollagen molecule*, the collagen precursor. The chemical composition of polypeptide chains that form the procollagen molecule determines the particular type of collagen to be formed. Of the several types of collagen that have been identified, Types I, II, and III are the types in which collagen fibrils are formed (Junqueira, Carneiro, and Kelly 1995). Hence, these collagen types are referred to as the *fibrillar collagens* (Cotran, Kumar, and Robbins 1989). The importance of Type I and Type III collagen fibers, as related to soft connective tissue repair, is discussed in the following section of this chapter.

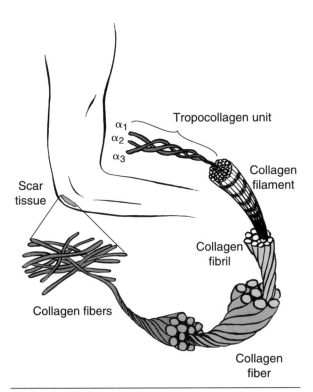

Figure 3.5 Collagen synthesis and fibrogenesis.

Adapted, by permission, from B.V. Reed, 1996, Wound healing and the use of thermal agents. In *Thermal agents in rehabilitation*, 3rd ed., edited by S.L. Michlovitz (Philadelphia: F.A. Davis), 10.

As biosynthesis of fibrillar collagen continues, modified procollagen molecules are secreted from the cell (i.e., fibroblast) into the extracellular matrix where procollagen bundles are linked together to form *tropocollagen*, the basic molecular unit of collagenous tissues (Junqueira, Carneiro, and Kelly 1995). Outside the cell, tropocollagen molecules are joined by comparatively weak *hydrogen bonds*. Although weak compared to collagen cross-linkage that subsequently develops, these hydrogen bonds provide initial strength and stiffness to the collagen molecule. Aggregation of tropocollagen molecules initiates fibrogenesis, the process through which collagen fibers are eventually formed. Initially, tropocollagen molecules combine to form *fibrils*, which are reinforced by comparatively strong *covalent bonds*. These covalent bonds contribute significantly to the strength and structural integrity of developing collagen fibrils. With continued fibrogenesis, fibrils combine to form progressively larger and stronger collagen *fibers* (see figure 3.5). As discussed shortly, comparatively weak Type III collagen is the collagen type that forms during the initial phase of fibroplasia, followed by deposition of stronger Type I collagen. Finally, as fibrogenesis continues, groups of collagen fibers combine to form collagen *bundles*, or *fasciculi*, which become the major structural components of tendons, ligaments, and other connective tissues of the body. The organizational structure of collagen fibrils, fibers, and bundles in a tendon is illustrated in figure 3.6.

The intramolecular bonds and intermolecular cross-links that develop during collagen synthesis and fibrogenesis are major factors in the structural stability and strength of the developing extracellular tissue matrix during connective tissue repair. The tensile strength of collagen has been attributed to intramolecular bonding of the polypeptide chains of the tropocollagen molecule, as well as to intermolecular cross-linkage of collagen fibrils and

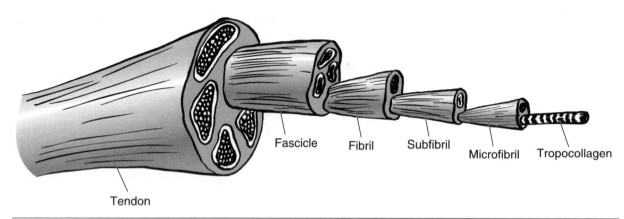

Fascicle   Fibril   Subfibril   Microfibril   Tropocollagen

Tendon

Figure 3.6   Structural organization of a tendon.

Reprinted, by permission, from W.C. Whiting and R.F. Zernicke, 1998, Biological tisssue: classification, structure, and function. In *Biomechanics of musculoskeletal injury* (Champaign, Ill.: Human Kinetics), 31.

fibers in the connective tissue matrix. Bonding of tropocollagen molecules as a primary source of tensile strength is indicated by structural failure of stressed tendons at the tropocollagen level (American Academy of Orthopaedic Surgeons 1991). With excessive loading, covalent bonds and collagen cross-links are disrupted, leading to subsequent tendon rupture (Leadbetter 1994). The importance of collagen cross-linkage as related to scar formation and maturation is discussed further in subsequent sections of this chapter.

Formation of Granulation Tissue

As collagen synthesis and fibrogenesis initiate fibrous tissue formation, a temporary connective tissue matrix begins to develop at the site of injury. The initial type of tissue that develops is referred to as *granulation tissue*. Although immature and structurally weak, granulation tissue represents a normal function of connective tissue healing and is an indication that the repair process is proceeding. Compared to more mature tissue that eventually develops during fibrous scar formation, granulation tissue has several distinguishing structural and functional characteristics. These characteristics are exemplified by two primary coinciding vascular and cellular responses: (1) synthesis of Type III collagen with random organization of collagen fibers and (2) neovascularization, or formation of a new vascular network in the developing tissue matrix. Both of these responses are mediated by macrophages, a prevalent cell type during granulation tissue formation. Macrophages release a number of growth factors, chemicals that stimulate the cellular functions of fibroblasts and vascular endothelial cells.

Type III Collagen Formation

As previously discussed, the chemical composition of the procollagen molecule determines the type of collagen to be formed during collagen synthesis. Of the several collagen types that have been identified in various body tissues, Types I and II are predominant in the musculoskeletal structures of the body (Martinez-Hernandez and Amenta 1990). Type II collagen is found primarily in cartilaginous tissues (e.g., hyaline articular cartilage, intervertebral disks), whereas Type I is the predominant collagen type in tendons, ligaments, and joint capsules. Thus, synthesis of Type I collagen is critical to optimal repair of the types of soft connective tissue injuries commonly associated with sports participation.

Despite the importance of Type I collagen to the tensile strength of soft connective tissues, the initial collagen deposited in new soft tissue injuries is Type III, a comparatively weak, fragile collagen type. Synthesis of Type III collagen begins within 24 hours after injury with significant deposition in the damaged area within four days (Martinez-

Hernandez 1994). Thus, Type III collagen is a primary characteristic of the granulation tissue that forms during the initial stage of connective tissue repair. Normally found in pliable body tissues such as blood vessels and the skin, Type III collagen lacks the strength and stability of Type I collagen. This lack of tensile strength, as compared to Type I collagen, is attributed to smaller fiber size, fewer intermolecular cross-links, and a random organization of fibers. Despite these features, deposition of Type III collagen is a normal mechanism of early connective tissue repair. Along with glycoproteins (see chapter 1), Type III collagen is a primary component of the temporary extracellular matrix that develops in healing tissues within approximately one week after injury (Groner and Weeks 1992). As the scar matrix in healing tissues continues to form, Type III collagen synthesis is eventually replaced by synthesis of Type I collagen. This transition, as well as other factors contributing to dense fibrous scar formation, is discussed in a following section of this chapter.

Neovascularization

As granulation tissue develops, a new vascular network begins to form in the tissue matrix within 48 to 72 hours after injury, thus coinciding with the formation of Type III collagen fibers (Martinez-Hernandez 1994). Formation of new blood vessels, referred to as *angiogenesis*, results from a division of vascular endothelial cells and endothelial budding, or sprouting of new capillaries from uninjured blood vessels in adjacent tissues. Within a few days after injury, the developing capillaries branch out and connect, or *anastomose*, to form the new vascular bed. Meanwhile, Type III collagen fibers continue to form and a highly vascular matrix of fibrous granulation tissue develops. Similarly, a new network of lymph vessels also forms in the developing matrix. With continued capillary proliferation, granulation tissue assumes a characteristic red, granular appearance as the result of the newly formed vascular bed. In addition, granulation tissue may show evidence of persistent edema due to the inherent permeability of the new capillaries that permits escape of fluids into the interstitial spaces (Cotran, Kumar, and Robbins 1989). With time, many of the newly formed capillaries are resorbed as the metabolic demands of the new tissues diminish. Consequently, the ultimate result is a comparatively pale, avascular scar (Martinez-Hernandez and Amenta 1990).

Wound Contraction

The mechanism through which the size of a tissue defect is reduced is referred to as *wound contraction*, a healing response that can significantly decrease the amount of damaged tissue in need of repair. Because of overlapping physiological responses, wound contraction is typically addressed as a component of fibroplasia, the second stage of connective tissue repair. Nevertheless, the mechanisms of wound contraction are distinct and unique. Whereas the actual process of tissue repair involves formation of new connective tissue fibers (i.e., fibrogenesis), wound contraction involves approximation of newly formed or existing fibers in the wound margins. Thus, soft connective tissue injuries typically heal through the two complementary mechanisms of repair and contraction.

Wound contraction is a primary function of specialized connective tissue cells known as *myofibroblasts*. These cells have been found to have contractile properties similar to those of muscle cells (i.e., myofibers). Myofibroblasts appear in the wound area within three to four days after injury and become predominant within six or seven days (Martinez-Hernandez and Amenta 1990). Hence, they are particularly active during the formation of granulation tissue, the first type of tissue that develops in a new injury. Wound contraction begins within a few days after injury and appears to reach a peak at about two weeks (see figure 3.1). Typically, however, wound contraction continues for an extended period into the late phase of fibroplasia (Daly 1990).

The contractile property of myofibroblasts is attributed to a high intracellular concentration of actin and myosin, two proteins that combine to form *actomyosin*. These proteins, which are typically associated with muscle contraction, are also thought to be responsible for contraction of myofibroblasts. It has been suggested that a contractile unit is formed by an interaction between myofibroblasts and newly formed collagen fibers in the extracellular matrix (Daly 1990). This contractile unit develops when myofibroblasts extend pseudopodia and attach to the collagen fibers, thus providing an adhesive basis for wound contraction (Price 1990). Subsequently, the migration capability of myofibroblasts produces centripetal pulling of new collagen fibers in the damaged area toward the center of the defect, thereby effecting tissue approximation, or wound closure, and a reduction in the size of the tissue defect (Bryant 1977; Daly 1990). In some cases, wound contraction can reduce the size of a tissue defect by as much as 70%, thus greatly decreasing the extent of necessary tissue repair (Martinez-Hernandez and Amenta 1990). For example, the restoration of ligament integrity due to wound contraction has been cited as rationale for a conservative, nonoperative approach to the medical management of grade I and grade II ligament injuries (American Academy of Orthopaedic Surgeons 1991). Despite the positive contributions of normal wound contraction to connective tissue repair, inhibited wound contraction may contribute to excessive scar formation, whereas excessive contraction can lead to tissue shortening and contractures. These clinically significant complications are addressed in a following section of this chapter.

Fibrous Scar Formation

Whereas the early stage of fibroplasia is characterized by formation of granulation tissue and wound contraction, subsequent scar formation occurs as the tissue matrix gradually assumes the characteristics of dense fibrous connective tissue (see chapter 1). It is significant to note, however, that scar formation never duplicates the structural or biomechanical properties of normal connective tissue. Connective tissue repair involves abnormal formation of fibrous tissue, the process referred to as *fibrosis*. Despite the ultimate result, the transition from granulation tissue to dense fibrous tissue involves three identifiable vascular and cellular events that contribute to optimal scar formation. These responses are (1) a transition from Type III to Type I collagen synthesis, (2) an increase in overall collagen deposition, and (3) resorption of small blood vessels in the vascular bed.

Type I Collagen Formation

Synthesis of Type I collagen represents a significant cellular response that characterizes the transition from formation of granulation tissue to development of dense fibrous scar tissue. Ideally, with regard to tensile strength, collagen synthesis during the early stages of fibroplasia would result in deposition of Type I collagen. As discussed earlier, however, formation of granulation tissue is characterized by deposition of comparatively weak Type III collagen. Significantly, synthesis of Type III collagen following connective tissue injury is temporary. As fibrous scar tissue develops, Type III collagen is replaced by Type I collagen, the stronger component of mature connective tissue. Because of its strength and abundance, Type I collagen is the major structural element in the normal connective tissue matrix (Martinez-Hernandez and Amenta 1990). Thus, the transition from Type III to Type I collagen synthesis during fibroplasia may be viewed as an attempt to achieve normalcy in fibrous connective tissue formation.

Synthesis of Type I collagen becomes dominant at about one week following injury, after which the proportion of Type I collagen, compared to Type III collagen, continues to increase (Martinez-Hernandez 1994). With increased deposition of Type I collagen, dense collagen bundles form in the damaged tissues and the tensile strength of the scar matrix increases. Although the most rapid increase in Type I collagen occurs during the early stages of fibroplasia, the transition to Type I collagen may last for several months or years

(Price 1990; Martinez-Hernandez and Amenta 1990). Continued synthesis of Type I collagen with simultaneous degradation of weaker Type III collagen has been associated with scar maturation, as discussed shortly. Ultimately, the tensile strength of the scar matrix is determined, in part, by the increased proportion of Type I to Type III collagen fibers. To a large extent, the comparatively greater strength of Type I fibers is attributed to a higher number of intermolecular cross-links that provide resistance to connective tissue tensile loading. Examination of normal connective tissue structures reveals that the extent of intermolecular cross-linkage in Type I collagen varies according to the mechanical functions of specific body tissues. For example, Type I collagen in tissues typically subjected to high tension forces (e.g., tendons) or weight-bearing loads (e.g., anterior cruciate ligament) exhibit the greatest number of cross-links (Eyre 1990).

Increased Collagen Deposition

In addition to the transition from Type III to Type I collagen synthesis, the overall rate of collagen production and fibrogenesis increases rapidly during the early stage of scar formation, beginning at about one week after injury (Groner and Weeks 1992). Hence, the increasing tensile strength of developing scar tissue is related not only to the type of collagen fibers that develop but also to the total amount of collagen deposited in the healing tissues. As scar formation progresses, increased collagen synthesis continues at a steady rate, usually reaching a plateau that lasts from two to four weeks. Collagen synthesis that exceeds collagen degradation may continue for six to eight weeks or longer, however (Kellett 1986). Connective tissue repair associated with healing of muscle injuries typically requires approximately three weeks. Tendons, on the other hand, normally heal at a slower rate with fibroplasia continuing for four to six weeks (Martinez-Hernandez and Amenta 1990). If fibroplasia continues in an uneventful manner, the concentration of fibroblasts in the damaged tissues gradually diminishes as a sufficient amount of collagen is produced to effect tissue repair. Disappearance of active fibroblasts, as well as myofibroblasts, in the injured area typically signals the end of fibrous scar formation, or fibroplasia, and the beginning of scar maturation, the third stage of connective tissue repair (Bryant 1977).

Resorption of Blood Vessels

Resorption of small blood vessels in the vascular network of granulation tissue represents a third characteristic event in the transition to dense fibrous scar tissue. As noted earlier, an extensive network of new capillaries develops in granulation tissue in order to meet the nutritional demands of newly formed tissues. Not all of these capillaries, however, develop into functional blood vessels with a definite blood flow. Consequently, they are preferentially resorbed (Martinez-Hernandez 1994). As an organized pattern of blood flow develops in the scar matrix, capillaries with minimal blood flow undergo degeneration and resorption (Cotran, Kumar, and Robbins 1989). The net result of decreased vascularization is transformation of richly vascularized granulation tissue into pale, avascular scar tissue. This transition continues as a characteristic of scar maturation, the third stage of connective tissue repair.

Scar Maturation

Because development of the scar tissue matrix that forms in response to connective tissue injury occurs on a continuum, a differentiation between scar formation and scar maturation is somewhat arbitrary. Nevertheless, several identifiable structural and functional changes begin to occur in the scar matrix at about three weeks after injury, especially as related to an increase in tensile strength. These changes mark the beginning of the third major stage of connective tissue healing, commonly referred to as *scar maturation* (see figure 3.1). During scar maturation, the ultimate structure, strength, and biomechanical properties of the scar tissue matrix are gradually determined. Scar maturation may continue for months, a year, or longer.

During fibroplasia, the tensile strength of healing tissues is directly proportional to the rate of collagen synthesis. Hence, the most rapid increase in strength occurs during fibroplasia when collagen synthesis is at the highest level. Despite an early, rapid increase in tensile strength, the newly formed scar matrix is weak compared to mature scar tissue. At this stage, the immature scar is susceptible to reinjury during tensile loading. As the scar matrix matures, however, the tensile strength of newly formed tissues continues to increase despite a decrease in fibroblastic activity and collagen synthesis. Thus, tensile strength increases at a rate greater than net collagen production during scar maturation.

Although the strength of the scar matrix increases significantly during maturation, scar tissue typically lacks the tensile strength of normal connective tissue. Ultimately, the tensile strength of scar tissue may be as much as 30% less than that of the original, uninjured tissues (American Academy of Orthopaedic Surgeons 1991). Within these parameters, the tensile strength of scar tissue increases through a combination of interrelated remodeling mechanisms. Although several mechanisms contribute to scar maturation, the primary factors appear to be (1) the rate of collagen turnover, (2) an increased number of stronger collagen cross-links, and (3) linear alignment of collagen fibers. These three processes, along with a continued decrease in the vascularity of the scar tissue matrix, characterize the maturation phase of connective tissue repair.

Collagen Turnover

The term *collagen turnover* refers to the continual, simultaneous processes of collagen production (i.e., synthesis) and collagen degradation (i.e., lysis). When balanced, the normal collagen turnover rate maintains the structural and functional properties of uninjured connective tissues. In the event of injury, however, collagen synthesis increases rapidly during early tissue healing in order to restore the connective tissue matrix. Thus, collagen synthesis exceeds collagen degradation. As scar tissue continues to form, however, the rate of collagen turnover gradually approaches normal levels (American Academy of Orthopaedic Surgeons 1991). Despite a significant decrease in fibroblast activity and collagen synthesis toward the end of fibroplasia, the balance of collagen turnover nevertheless favors synthesis, rather than lysis, for an extended period (Martinez-Hernandez and Amenta 1990). It has been proposed that scar maturation is, in part, related to progressive restoration of the normal rate of collagen turnover (Bryant 1977).

Collagen degradation, in particular, has been associated with connective tissue maturation (Cotran, Kumar, and Robbins 1989). Whereas collagen synthesis is a function of fibroblasts, collagen degradation, or lysis, is attributed to protein-degrading enzymes referred to as *proteases*. Although resistant to most nonspecific proteases, the fibrillar collagens (i.e., Types I, II, III) are susceptible to degradation by *collagenase*, an enzyme secreted by fibroblasts, macrophages, and other connective tissue cells (Cotran, Kumar, and Robbins 1989; Martinez-Hernandez 1994). Although all three types of fibrillar collagens are susceptible to degradation by collagenase, the rate of degradation differs with each type. It has been suggested that the weaker Type III randomly organized collagen fibrils deposited during granulation tissue formation are preferentially degraded, whereas comparatively strong, linear-oriented Type I fibers that are under tension are less susceptible to degradation (Martinez-Hernandez 1994). These observations suggest that if Type I collagen production continues during scar maturation while Type III collagen is selectively degraded, the tensile strength of the scar matrix continues to increase.

Collagen Cross-Linkage

The tensile strength of scar tissue increases at a rate that exceeds net collagen production as the scar approaches maturity. During scar maturation, tensile strength increases as the result of collagen cross-linkage in the scar matrix (Cotran, Kumar, and Robbins 1989;

Martinez-Hernandez 1994). Cross-links that develop within and between collagen molecules significantly enhance the stability of maturing scar tissue (Whiting and Zernicke 1998). During granulation tissue formation and early scar development, intramolecular linkage is formed by comparatively weak chemical bonds (i.e., hydrogen bonds). As scar tissue matures, however, stronger intermolecular bonds (i.e., covalent bonds) develop (Price 1990). These bonds, or cross-links, have been attributed to binding of glycosaminoglycan molecules (i.e., carbohydrates) to collagen fibers in the extracellular matrix of connective tissues (Junqueira, Carneiro, and Kelly 1995). As the result of more stable collagen cross-linkage, mature scar is more dense but less pliable than immature scar. Thus, the increased tensile strength of mature scar tissue, as compared with immature scar tissue, not only results from a greater number of Type I collagen fibers but also occurs as the result of an increase in the number and stability of intermolecular cross-links (Price 1990).

Realignment of Collagen Fibers

In addition to continued Type I collagen fiber deposition and cross-linkage, the increase in tensile strength that occurs during scar maturation is attributed to a gradual linear alignment of collagen fibers in the scar matrix. In normal, uninjured connective tissues, tensile strength is directly related to the structural organization of collagen fibers. Typically, collagen fiber orientation differs among the various types of connective tissues. An examination of normal tendons and ligaments reveals that the characteristic collagen fiber orientation in each type of tissue is conducive to its respective function (figure 3.7). For example, collagen fibers in tendons are arranged in an orderly, parallel fashion that provides optimal resistance to unidirectional

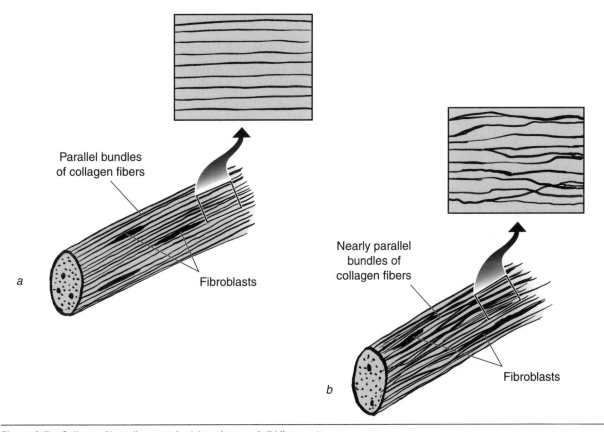

Figure 3.7   Collagen fiber alignment in *(a)* tendons and *(b)* ligaments.

Reprinted, by permission, from C.A. Carlstedt and M. Nordin, 1989, Biomechanics of tendons and ligaments. In *Basic biomechanics of the musculoskeletal system*, 2nd ed., edited by M. Nordin and V.H. Frankel (Philadelphia: Lea and Febiger), 61.

tensile forces. Although most collagen fibers in ligaments are also aligned in a predominant direction, some fibers have a nonparallel orientation that provides resistance to multidirectional tissue loading (Carlstedt and Nordin 1989). Microscopic examination of connective tissues has also revealed variations in collagen fiber alignment within a particular tissue type. For example, the structural orientation of collagen fibers has been found to vary among ligaments, seemingly in accordance with their function as mechanical restraints to particular joint motions (Leadbetter 1994).

The ultimate goal of connective tissue repair includes not only the replacement of disrupted collagen fibers but also the restoration of normal collagen fiber alignment in order to maximize the tensile strength of each respective tissue type. Reorganization of collagen fibers occurs during scar maturation as tensile loading is applied to the scar matrix. Initially, as granulation tissue forms during fibroplasia, collagen fibers are randomly oriented, resulting in a fragile, structurally weak connective tissue matrix. During scar maturation, however, the early matrix becomes increasingly organized as the collagen fibers gradually assume a more linear, parallel structural orientation. Consequently, they become more resistant to tensile loading in the direction of applied forces.

Understandably, it is difficult to pinpoint the initiation or the duration of collagen fiber realignment. In all probability, the duration of fiber realignment varies with the type of connective tissue involved, as well as the extent of tensile forces imposed on the remodeling tissues. Histological examination of surgically repaired medial collateral ligaments in rabbit models has indicated random organization of collagen fibers at six months after surgery with longitudinal orientation from six months to one year and beyond (Frank et al. 1983). Other investigators have reported functional linear alignment of collagen fibers in ligaments and tendons within two to four months after injury (Leadbetter 1994). Despite collagen realignment, optimal recovery of ligamentous structures may take a year or longer with an ultimate tensile strength deficit of 30 to 50% (American Academy of Orthopaedic Surgeons 1991).

A review of the literature regarding connective tissue repair reveals a preponderance of evidence emphasizing the importance of controlled tensile loading in scar maturation, especially as related to collagen fiber alignment and tensile strength. Although typically associated with remodeling of osseous tissue, Wolff's law is also applicable to remodeling of soft connective tissues. As applied to scar maturation, Wolff's law holds that the scar tissue matrix remodels in accordance with mechanical forces imposed on the healing tissues (Price 1990). When continuous tensile loading is applied, through normal activity or therapeutic exercise, collagen fibers assume a linear, or longitudinal, orientation as new collagen is deposited along the lines of tension (American Academy of Orthopaedic Surgeons 1991; Price 1990). As a result, tensile strength increases in the direction of the applied force, thus contributing to restoration of normal connective tissue function (Kellett 1986). Collagen fiber realignment that occurs in response to extrinsic tensile loading is an example of *adaptation*, a process whereby tissues respond positively to changing conditions without injury (Leadbetter 1994). Therapeutic techniques to promote collagen fiber realignment and tensile strength are discussed in chapter 5.

Tissue Repair Complications

Under normal physiological conditions, connective tissue repair results in characteristic fibrous scar formation without undue complications. In some cases, however, deviations in the normal vascular and cellular responses during tissue repair may alter the structural and functional development of scar tissue, thereby presenting clinically significant complications. Complications arising from altered connective tissue healing may be associated with a persistent inflammatory response, excessive scar formation, abnormal wound contraction, or a combination of these factors. In the event of persistent inflammation, the continued presence of pathogenic agents or foreign material in the damaged tissues may interfere with fibrous tissue formation, resulting in a comparatively weak scar matrix. In other circumstances, a persistent inflammatory response may promote prolonged fibroblast proliferation and collagen synthesis that results in excessive scar formation (Wahl and Renstrom 1990). Because of the inelastic qualities of scar tissue, undue limitations in tissue mobility may result. Excessive scar formation may also result from inhibited wound contraction. In these cases, a greater amount of scar formation is necessary to repair the tissue defect that would normally be reduced in size by wound contraction. Conversely, exaggerated wound contraction may contribute to permanent tissue shortening and loss of tissue mobility. Whereas these complications result from deviations in normal connective tissue repair, they may be exacerbated by the use of inappropriate therapeutic techniques (e.g., improper or prolonged immobilization). The effect of immobilization on connective tissue mobility is discussed in chapter 5.

Clinically significant complications that may be associated with altered connective tissue repair include (1) granulomatous inflammation, (2) retardation of muscle fiber regeneration, (3) contractures and adhesions, and (4) hypertrophic scars or keloids. To the extent that these complications are associated with sports injuries, they present significant therapeutic challenges to the sports health care clinician. As a prelude to discussion of therapeutic management in chapters 4 and 5, the primary characteristics of particular connective tissue repair deviations are addressed in the following sections of this chapter.

Granulomatous Inflammation

In some circumstances, persistent pathogenic agents or foreign material in damaged tissues may provoke a chronic inflammatory response called *granulomatous inflammation* (Cotran, Kumar, and Robbins 1989). The primary characteristic of granulomatous inflammation is the development of small, discrete nodules in the affected tissues referred to as *granulomas*. These granular nodules result from the failure of macrophages, the predominant phagocytic cell in late stages of inflammation, to destroy pathogenic agents or foreign materials. Granuloma formation occurs as clusters of macrophages undergo structural transformation and become known as *epithelioid cells*, so named because of their resemblance to epithelial cells. These cells surround and enclose the undigested pathogens or foreign bodies, thereby forming the granuloma. In addition to undigested foreign material, granulomas may incorporate other connective tissue cells (e.g., macrophages, fibroblasts) and white blood cells (e.g., lymphocytes) that are characteristically present in chronic inflammation. Because fibroblasts typically proliferate in damaged tissues before chronic inflammation is resolved, collagen synthesis may produce fibrous tissue that encapsulates the granuloma. With persistent tissue irritation, multiple granulomas may develop, leading to a condition known as *granulomatosis*. The result is a pattern of weak, granulomatous scar tissue (Cotran, Kumar, and Robbins 1989; Fantone and Ward 1994). Although granulomas are most commonly associated with chronic infectious diseases (e.g., tuberculosis, syphilis), granulomatous tissue may be observed around sutures, splinters, or other foreign objects that have penetrated the skin. Granulomas that form in reaction to a foreign body are referred to as *foreign body granulomas*.

Retardation of Muscle Fiber Regeneration

Persistent inflammation or other conditions that promote excessive scar formation may be counterproductive to optimal healing of muscle injuries that heal through the simultaneous processes of myofiber (i.e. muscle fiber) regeneration and connective tissue repair. As discussed in chapter 1, myofibers have the potential for regeneration by virtue of satellite cell division and replacement of normal cells. Muscle injuries may involve the myofibers, their surrounding connective tissue sheaths (i.e., endomysium), or both, depending on the extent of injury. The anatomical relationship of myofibers to surrounding endomysium is illustrated in figure 3.8. In mild strains, only the myofibers are damaged and regeneration typically occurs within 7 to 14 days, provided that the basal membrane remains intact (Stauber 1990). More commonly, however, both the myofibers and their surrounding connective tissue sheaths are damaged. In these cases, regeneration of myofibers and simultaneous scar tissue formation in connective tissue sheaths represent two competing processes (Wahl and Renstrom 1990). Should connective tissue sheaths be damaged, in addition to the myofibers, the resulting scar tissue may create a barrier to myofiber regeneration.

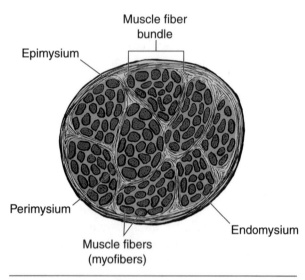

Muscle fiber bundle
Epimysium
Perimysium
Endomysium
Muscle fibers (myofibers)

Figure 3.8 Cross section of a skeletal muscle. Note three types of connective tissue sheaths covering muscle fibers (the endomysium), muscle fiber bundles (the perimysium), and the entire muscle (the epimysium).

Despite the potential for myofiber regeneration, most muscle injuries heal with a predominance of scar formation (Leadbetter 1994; Malone 1988). Although some myofiber regeneration may occur, depending on the extent of tissue disruption, collagen deposition and fibrous scar formation occurs in the connective tissue sheaths that surround individual myofibers (i.e., endomysium) and myofiber bundles (i.e., perimysium), and the entire muscle (i.e., epimysium). These structures are illustrated in figure 3.8. It has been suggested that the connective tissue sheaths, rather than the myofibers, are the limiting factors in muscle stretching (Malone 1988). Thus, excessive scar formation in these fibrous sheaths not only interferes with muscle fiber regeneration but also creates tissue shortening that limits extensibility of the muscle unit (Leadbetter 1994). The clinical implications of this tissue-healing pattern, with specific reference to therapeutic stretching techniques, are discussed in chapter 5.

Contractures and Adhesions

Whereas normal wound contraction contributes significantly to the structural integrity and strength of healing tissues, adverse complications can arise if wound contraction is altered. Clinically significant complications may be associated with deficient or incomplete wound contraction as well as excessive wound contraction. If wound contraction is inhibited, optimal closure may not occur. Tension, or lack of mobility, in surrounding tissues limits the ability of a wound to contract (Bryant 1977). The effect of adjacent soft tissue immobility can be observed clinically in an open wound of the anterior leg, for example. In this case, tension in the surrounding skin and subcutaneous tissues may limit wound contraction. To the extent that tension exists in deep tissue structures (e.g., tendons, ligaments, joint capsules), wound contraction may be similarly affected. Restricted tissue approximation requires the damaged tissues to heal with a greater amount of fibrous scar formation. Because of the characteristic inelasticity of scar tissue, excessive scar formation due to deficient wound contraction may limit segmental tissue mobility.

Contractures

Although the contributing mechanism is different from that of deficient wound contraction, excessive wound contraction may also limit tissue mobility. As discussed in a previous section of this chapter, wound contraction is a function of sustained myofibroblast contraction and centripetal migration toward the center of the damaged area. If these processes progress in an uninhibited manner, optimal wound closure occurs and shortening of the developing scar tissue may result (Martinez-Hernandez 1994). Permanent shortening of scar tissue associated with excessive wound contraction and fibrotic tissue formation is referred to as a *contracture*. Whereas tension in surrounding tissues inhibits wound contraction, lack of tension in tissues adjacent to the injured area facilitates excessive wound contraction and development of contractures. For example, injured tissues that have been casted or splinted in their shortened, relaxed range may have an increased propensity to development of contractures. The effects of inappropriate or prolonged immobilization on soft tissue mobility, including contractures and adhesions, is discussed further in chapter 5.

Adhesions

In the presence of persistent inflammation or prolonged immobilization of injured tissues, abnormal binding and adhesion of adjacent tissues may occur. Fibrous adhesions may develop as the result of traumatized musculotendinous tissues or joint capsules and ligaments, thereby restricting tissue mobility. Examples of these complications can be seen in cases of adhesive capsulitis (e.g., the glenohumeral joint) and adhesive tenosynovitis. As noted by Reed (1996), optimal functioning of articulating and gliding tissues requires a delicate balance between tensile strength and tissue mobility. Prolonged inflammatory responses are detrimental to restoration of this balance because they predispose the injured area to excessive scar tissue that lacks both strength and extensibility. With regard to repair of ruptured tendons, Bryant (1977) noted that successful healing requires two inherently contradictory conditions, dense fibrous union for strength and freedom from adhesions to permit tendon excursion.

Trauma to adjacent tissues is a related factor in formation of adhesions associated with persistent inflammation. Injury to a particular structure (e.g., ligament, joint capsule, tendon) seldom involves an isolated lesion. Structures immediately adjacent to the tissue in which the primary lesion occurs may also be disrupted. Hence, all disrupted tissues in the damaged area are incorporated within the same repair process. With reference to tendon healing, Bryant (1977) noted that a loss of tendinous excursion is a potential consequence of tissue healing involving injured tendons and adjacent tissues (e.g., synovial tendon sheaths). Loss of mobility due to adhesion of adjacent structures can also be observed clinically in synovial joints. For example, capsular fibrosis and adherence to the underlying head of the humerus has been observed in chronic adhesive capsulitis of the glenohumeral joint. Other observers have attributed post-traumatic loss of motion in the knee to articular adhesions (e.g., capsular adhesion to the femoral condyle), as well as adhesions in extraarticular structures (e.g., adhesion of the vastus lateralis to the femoral condyle). In addition to persistent inflammatory responses, prolonged immobilization following injury or surgery to synovial joints further contributes to articular fibrosis and capsular adhesions (Wahl and Renstrom 1990).

Hypertrophic Scars and Keloids

Excessive collagen production during fibroplasia may result in one of two types of abnormal fibrous tissue formations: *keloids* or *hypertrophic scars*. Throughout the tissue-healing process, simultaneous collagen synthesis and lysis occurs which, if appropriately balanced, produces a scar with optimal extensibility and tensile strength. In the early stages of fibrous scar formation, synthesis of collagen exceeds collagen lysis in order to provide strength to the developing scar. Toward the end of fibroplasia, collagen production lessens and a gradual return to normal collagen turnover occurs. If the normal balance of collagen synthesis and lysis is disturbed, however, with synthesis exceeding lysis in the later stages of fibrosis, the overproduction of collagen can result in excessive, abnormal scar formation. Abnormal scar formation may be manifested either as a hypertrophic scar or a keloid. Hypertrophic scars are those in which excessive collagen deposition is confined to the area of the original lesion, whereas a keloid involves deposition of collagen that extends beyond the margins of the damaged area into ordinarily normal, healthy tissue (Price 1990). The composition of these types of scars, which includes an abnormal number of fibroblasts and an abundance of irregular collagen bundles, suggests an arrest of scar maturation (Martinez-Hernandez 1994). Hypertrophic scars and keloids are most readily observed as localized masses on the skin resulting from abnormal healing of open wounds.

Summary

Damaged soft connective tissues of the musculoskeletal system heal through a process of fibrous scar formation, or repair. Although tissue healing occurs on a continuum, connective tissue repair is commonly described as having three primary stages: inflammation, fibroplasia, and scar maturation. The initial stage, inflammation, represents a normal response of vascularized body tissues to trauma. Acute inflammatory responses, which typically last for three to four days after injury, are characterized by vascular changes including vasodilation, increased vascular permeability, and accumulation of excessive interstitial fluid, or edema. Edema formation may be exacerbated by local lymphatic obstruction. As edema develops, impairment of local circulation and a diminished oxygen supply may lead to cellular necrosis, or secondary hypoxic injury, in adjacent tissues. Proliferation of phagocytic polymorphonuclear leukocytes, neutrophils in particular, is the primary cellular response during acute inflammation. These white blood cells provide the initial nonspecific defense against invading pathogenic microorganisms. With successful phagocytosis, the signs and symptoms of acute inflammation gradually subside and the inflammatory response enters a subacute phase during which macrophages, transformed monocytes, become the primary phagocytic cells. Persistent pathogenic agents may evoke chronic inflammatory responses during which lymphocytes mediate immunological defenses against specific types of pathogens.

During the second stage of connective tissue repair, fibroplasia, fibrous scar tissue forms through a series of events that includes proliferation of fibroblasts, collagen synthesis and fibrogenesis, granulation tissue formation, wound contraction, and dense fibrous scar formation. Collagen synthesis and fibrogenesis, or collagen fiber formation, is the primary function of fibroblasts. Granulation tissue, the initial type of tissue that develops in a new wound, is characterized by comparatively weak Type III collagen with an unorganized, random alignment of collagen fibers. As granulation tissue develops, a new vascular network forms in the developing tissue matrix. During the early stage of fibroplasia, wound contraction, or closure, occurs. Although normal wound contraction reduces the size of the tissue defect, thereby minimizing the extent of necessary repair, complications may arise if wound contraction is altered. Inhibition of wound contraction may result in excessive scar formation in the damaged tissues, whereas exaggerated wound contraction may lead to limited tissue mobility and development of a contracture. Whereas the early stage of fibroplasia involves granulation tissue formation and wound contraction, subsequent events include a transition from Type III to Type I collagen synthesis, an increase in overall collagen deposition, resorption of small blood vessels in the vascular bed, and development of dense fibrous scar tissue.

The final stage of connective tissue repair is scar maturation, during which changes occur in the composition and strength of the developing scar. During scar maturation, the definitive structure, vascularity, and strength of the tissue matrix are formed. Scar maturation is characterized by a gradual return to the normal rate of collagen turnover, an increase in the number of stronger collagen cross-links, and a realignment of collagen fibers. The tensile strength of the scar matrix increases as collagen fibers assume a linear structural orientation in response to the application of controlled tensile forces.

Deviations in the normal physiological mechanisms of connective tissue repair may result in clinically significant complications that include granulomatous inflammation, retardation of myofiber regeneration, contractures and adhesions, and hypertrophic scars or keloids.

References

American Academy of Orthopaedic Surgeons. 1991. *Athletic training and sports medicine*, 2nd ed. Park Ridge, Ill.: American Academy of Orthopaedic Surgeons.

Bryant, W.M. 1977. *Wound healing*. Reading, Mass.: CIBA Pharmaceutical Co.

Carlstedt, C.A., and M. Nordin. 1989. Biomechanics of tendons and ligaments. In *Basic biomechanics of the musculoskeletal system*, 2nd ed., edited by M. Nordin and V.H. Frankel. Philadelphia: Lea and Febiger.

Cotran, R.S., V. Kumar, and S.L. Robbins. 1989. *Robbins pathologic basis of disease*, 4th ed. Philadelphia: W.B. Saunders.

Daly, T.J. 1990. The repair phase of wound healing—Re-epithelialization and contraction. In *Wound healing: Alternatives in management*, edited by L.C. Kloth, J.M. McCulloh, and J.A. Feeder. Philadelphia: Davis.

Eyre, D.R. 1990. The collagens of musculoskeletal soft tissues. In *Sports-induced inflammation*, edited by W.B. Leadbetter, J.A. Buckwalter, and S.L. Gordon. Park Ridge, Ill.: American Academy of Orthopaedic Surgeons.

Fantone, J.C., and P.A. Ward.1994. Inflammation. In *Pathology*, 2nd ed., edited by E. Rubin and J.L. Farber. Philadelphia: J.B. Lippincott.

Frank, C., S.L-Y. Woo, D. Amiel, M.A. Gomez, F.L. Harwood, and W. Akeson. 1983. Medial collateral ligament healing: A multidisciplinary assessment in rabbits. *American Journal of Sports Medicine* 11:379-89.

Groner, J., and P.M. Weeks. 1992. Healing of hard and soft tissues of the hand. In *Hand injuries in athletes*, edited by J.W. Strickland and A.C. Rettig. Philadelphia: W.B. Saunders.

Hettinga, D.L. 1990. Inflammatory response of synovial joint structures. In *Orthopaedic and sports physical therapy*, 2nd ed., edited by J.A. Gould III. St. Louis: Mosby.

Junqueira, L.C., J. Carneiro, and R.O. Kelly. 1995. *Basic histology*, 8th ed. Norwalk, Conn.: Appleton and Lange.

Kellett, J. 1986. Acute soft tissue injuries—A review of the literature. *Medicine and Science in Sports and Exercise* 18:489-99.

Kloth, L.C., and K.H. Miller. 1990. The inflammatory response to wounding. In *Wound healing: Alternatives in management*, edited by L.C. Kloth, J.M. McCulloch, and J.A. Feeder. Philadelphia: Davis.

Knight, K.L. 1990. Cold as a modifier of sports-induced inflammation. In *Sports-induced inflammation*, edited by W.B. Leadbetter, J.A. Buckwalter, and S.L. Gordon. Park Ridge, Ill.: American Academy of Orthopaedic Surgeons.

Koester, M C. 1993. An overview of the physiology and pharmacology of aspirin and nonsteroidal anti-inflammatory drugs. *Journal of Athletic Training* 28:252-59.

Leadbetter, W.B. 1994. Soft tissue athletic injury. In *Sports injuries: Mechanisms, prevention, treatment*, edited by F.H. Fu and D.A. Stone. Baltimore: Williams and Wilkins.

Malone, T.R., ed. 1988. *Muscle injury and rehabilitation*. Baltimore: Williams and Wilkins.

Martinez-Hernandez, A. 1994. Repair, regeneration, and fibrosis. In *Pathology*, 2nd ed., edited by E. Rubin and J.L. Farber. Philadelphia: J.B. Lippincott.

Martinez-Hernandez, A., and P.S. Amenta.1990. Basic concepts in wound healing. In *Sports-induced inflammation*, edited by W.B. Leadbetter, J.A. Buckwalter, and S.L. Gordon. Park Ridge, Ill.: American Academy of Orthopaedic Surgeons.

Price, H. 1990. Connective tissue in wound healing. In *Wound healing: Alternatives in management*, edited by L.C. Kloth, J.M. McCulloch, and J.A. Feeder. Philadelphia: Davis.

Reed, B. 1996. Wound healing and the use of thermal agents. In *Thermal agents in rehabilitation*, 3rd ed., edited by S.L. Michlovitz. Philadelphia: Davis.

Stauber, W.T. 1990. Repair models and specific tissue responses in muscle injury. In *Sports-induced inflammation*, edited by W.B. Leadbetter, J.A. Buckwalter, and S.L. Gordon. Park Ridge, Ill.: American Academy of Orthopaedic Surgeons.

Stevens, A., and J. Lowe. 1995. *Pathology*. St. Louis: Mosby.

Tortora, G.J., and S.R. Grabowski. 1993. *Principles of anatomy and physiology*, 7th ed. New York: Harper Collins College Publishers.

Wahl, S., and P. Renstrom. 1990. Fibrosis in soft-tissue injuries. In *Sports-induced inflammation*, edited by W.B. Leadbetter, J.A. Buckwalter, and S.L. Gordon. Park Ridge, Ill.: American Academy of Orthopaedic Surgeons.

Whiting, W.C., and R.F. Zernicke. 1998. *Biomechanics of musculoskeletal injury*. Champaign, Ill.: Human Kinetics.

Therapeutic Implications: Inflammation and Pain

CHAPTER

4

Management of Hemorrhage and Edema
- Physical Agents
  - *Cold Applications*
  - *External Compression*
  - *Elevation*
  - *Restricted Movement*
- Pharmacologic Agents

Alleviation of Pain and Muscle Spasm
- Neuroanatomy and Neurophysiology
  - *Sensory Receptors*
  - *Anterolateral System*

Transmission of Pain Impulses
Pain-Spasm-Pain Cycle
Theoretical Bases of Pain
- *Early Pain Theories*
- *Gate Control Theory*
- *Descending Pain Inhibitory Systems*
Therapeutic Strategies and Techniques
- *Physical Agents*
- *Pharmacologic Agents*
- *Psychological Intervention*
Summary

Learning Objectives

After completion of this chapter, the reader should be able to

1. identify the two primary therapeutic objectives in the management of inflammatory responses to soft tissue trauma,

2. identify appropriate therapeutic agents in the management of acute inflammatory responses to soft tissue trauma and relate the therapeutic rationale for each,

3. identify the primary neurological structures and neurophysiological mechanisms associated with pain and the pain-spasm-pain cycle,

4. describe the neurophysiological basis for prevailing pain and pain-control theories, and

5. identify appropriate therapeutic agents for acute pain management and relate the therapeutic rationale for each.

The chemically mediated vascular and cellular responses that occur during acute inflammation, including phagocytosis of pathogenic agents, are essential to creation of a favorable environment for subsequent connective tissue repair. Hence, inflammation is the first stage in the continuum of physiological events that constitute the healing process. Despite the normalcy of inflammation, the primary inflammatory responses to tissue damage include hemodynamic changes (e.g., hemorrhagic effusion and edema formation) that, if excessive or prolonged, may impede the normal mechanisms of connective tissue repair. Although initially protective, pain and muscle spasm, the secondary inflammatory responses to tissue trauma, typically lead to functional impairments (e.g., neural inhibition of strength, loss of joint motion) that may hinder timely recovery. Thus, the primary therapeutic objectives during the acute inflammatory stage of tissue healing are to (1) control the detrimental effects of excessive hemorrhage and edema (primary inflammatory responses) and (2) alleviate pain and muscle spasm (secondary inflammatory responses). These objectives represent the first two major categories of therapeutic intervention in the continuum of connective tissue repair (see chapter 1, figure 1.2).

Intervention during acute inflammation may represent the most advantageous opportunity for the sports health care clinician to influence the vascular and cellular responses to tissue injury, thereby facilitating subsequent tissue-healing mechanisms. As discussed in chapter 3, connective tissue repair proceeds at a fairly predictable rate under normal circumstances. Centuries ago, Hippocrates, the famous Greek physician, noted that tissue healing is a matter of time. As this observation implies, the potential to increase the rate of tissue repair through the use of physical or pharmacologic agents is limited. Although acknowledging that tissue healing is time dependent, Hippocrates nevertheless noted the importance of opportunistic medical intervention in the repair process. In this regard, he viewed the physician's primary responsibility as one of creating favorable conditions for the natural processes of tissue healing to occur (Leadbetter 1990). These observations summarize the overall goal of therapeutic intervention in the acute phase of inflammation.

During the first three to four days after injury, the sports health care clinician's challenge is to minimize the potential impediments to normal tissue healing (e.g., hemorrhage and edema) without interfering with the natural physiological mechanisms of connective tissue repair. This dual challenge implies the need for good judgment in selection of therapeutic agents based on a knowledge of the normal vascular and cellular responses to acute tissue trauma. For example, vasodilation and increased blood flow are recognized vascular responses to increased tissue temperature. Despite the beneficial effect of increased blood flow on connective tissue repair, application of external heat or use of other modalities that promote these vascular responses is contraindicated until hemorrhage and edema are brought under control. Use of pharmacologic agents by the attending physician during acute inflammation also requires discretion. Aspirin and other nonsteroidal anti-inflammatory drugs (NSAIDs), for example, may be indicated because of their analgesic and anti-inflammatory properties. On the other hand, these drugs also have anticoagulation properties that may interfere with normal hemostatic mechanisms. Some authors have noted that the use of aspirin is contraindicated in the treatment of musculoskeletal injuries if there is a risk of local hemorrhage (Buchanan and Rainsford 1990).

Management of Hemorrhage and Edema

An understanding of the hemostatic mechanisms and early vascular responses to injury discussed in chapters 2 and 3 provides rationale for the use of specific therapeutic agents in the management of hemorrhage and edema. When blood vessel damage is minimal, normal hemostatic mechanisms may be sufficient to control bleeding (see chapter 2). With more severe tissue injury and more extensive vascular disruption, however, the natural hemostatic responses are typically inadequate to control hemorrhage and effusion. To the extent that hemorrhage occurs and congestive edema forms, blood flow and oxygen transportation to local tissues is diminished (i.e., ischemia). The resulting *hypoxia*, or oxygen deficiency, leads to *secondary hypoxic injury* during which cellular necrosis occurs in addition to the cellular destruction caused by the original injury. In addition to secondary hypoxia and cell death, excessive accumulation of fluid in the interstitial spaces (i.e., edema) inhibits venous return and lymphatic drainage, which further contributes to tissue swelling (Starkey 1993). Management of these early inflammatory responses represents a primary focus of therapeutic intervention in acute inflammation. Initial intervention may include the use of physical agents, pharmacologic agents, or both.

Physical Agents

Traditionally, control of the potential adverse effects of early vascular responses to injury has been accomplished through the use of cold applications, external compression, and elevation of the affected body part. Restriction of movement in the affected tissues through the use of splints, supportive wraps, or other immobilization devices is also typically indicated. Collectively, these measures are used for the specific purposes of (1) controlling hemorrhage effusion and edema, (2) minimizing secondary hypoxic injury, and (3) protecting traumatized tissues from undue mechanical loading. As discussed shortly, alleviation of pain is a concomitant objective. Because the hemodynamic changes resulting from acute tissue disruption (vasodilation, increased blood flow, etc.) occur within minutes following injury, the beneficial effects of cold application, external compression, and elevation are optimized if these measures are applied as early as possible. Certified athletic trainers, team physicians, and other sports health care clinicians who are present in the sports setting on a daily basis are in a particularly advantageous position for early intervention, thus maximizing a favorable environment for subsequent connective tissue repair.

Cold Applications

Fortunately, if proper precautions are taken and preclusive conditions are identified (e.g., Raynaud's phenomenon, cold urticaria), there are few contraindications to the use of cold applications in the management of early inflammatory responses to injury. Potential benefits, on the other hand, include control of hemorrhage and edema, limitation of secondary hypoxic injury, and alleviation of pain and muscle spasm. The physiological responses to acute tissue trauma and the vascular and neural responses that present indications for intervention with cold applications are summarized in figure 4.1.

Lowering vascular temperature through localized cold application has the overall effect of vasoconstriction and reduction of local blood flow. Consequently, cold applications have traditionally been considered appropriate and effective in the initial management of hemorrhage and edema. Despite a physiological basis for the use of cold for control of edema, however, the effectiveness of cold application alone (i.e., without concomitant external compression and elevation) has been questioned. Wilkerson (1991) noted the paucity of scientific evidence supporting the efficacy of cold applications on edema control following acute tissue injury. Baker and Bell (1991), for example, observed that local blood flow in the calf muscles was not significantly decreased by 20-minute ice pack treatments or ice massage continued to the point of numbness. Although not examined in their study, these investigators suggested that, compared to compression and elevation, the effectiveness of ice packs in edema control may be limited. In view of these observations, the positive effects of cold application following injury may be due to factors other than those directly associated with alteration of vascular responses.

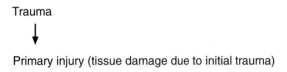

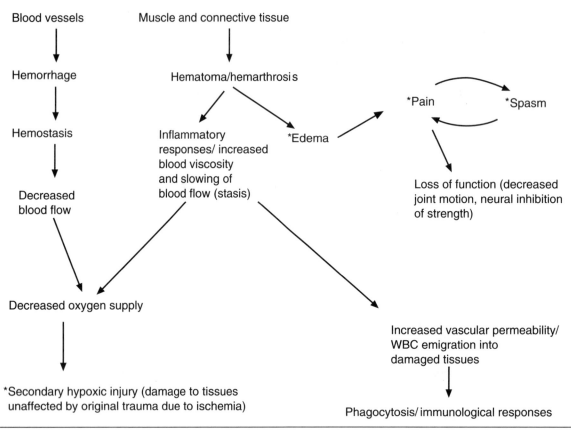

Figure 4.1   Inflammatory responses to acute soft tissue injury with indications for cold applications (indicated by asterisks).

Reprinted, by permission, from K.L. Knight, 1995, Inflammation and wound repair. In *Cryotherapy in sports injury management* (Champaign, Ill.: Human Kinetics), 33.

Compared to the effect on control of edema, cold applications may make a greater contribution to connective tissue repair by limiting the extent of secondary hypoxic injury (Knight 1990). Lowering tissue temperature slows the rate of cellular metabolism, thus reducing the oxygen requirement of local tissues. Consequently, cellular necrosis in tissues that are unaffected by the original injury may be minimized, thereby limiting the extent of necessary tissue repair (Knight 1990; Starkey 1993). Although scientific evidence indicating the time that specific musculoskeletal tissues can survive oxygen deprivation is sparse, it is considered prudent to apply cold within minutes following acute injuries in an attempt to reduce the metabolic needs of surrounding tissue cells.

Given the array of clinical techniques for cold application (e.g., chipped or cubed ice packs, ice massage, commercial cold packs), it is incumbent on the sports health care clinician to identify the specific desired physiological effect and, subsequently, select the most effective method of application. For example, ice massage that is typically applied to a localized area for a period of six to eight minutes may be sufficient for management of mild to moderate pain. On the other hand, deep tissue temperature reduction that is sufficient to lower the rate of cellular metabolism and reduce local tissue oxygen requirements, thereby limiting secondary hypoxic injury, may require a longer period of cold application with techniques that offer greater penetration potential (e.g., chipped ice packs).

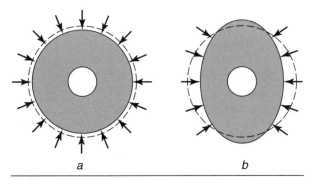

Figure 4.2 Effect of *(a)* circumferential compression and *(b)* collateral compression on soft tissues of an extremity.

Adapted, by permission, from G.B. Wilkerson, 1991, "Treatment of the inversion ankle sprain through synchronous application of focal compression and cold," *Journal of Athletic Training* 26 (3): 222.

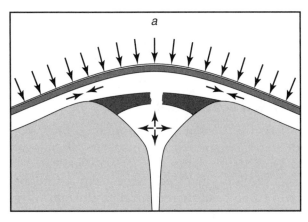
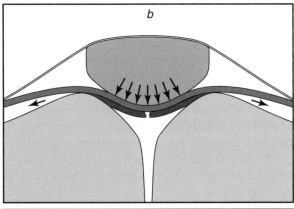

Figure 4.3 Effect of *(a)* uniform compression and *(b)* selective (i.e., focal) compression on edematous tissues.

Adapted, by permission, from G.B. Wilkerson, 1991, "Treatment of the inversion ankle sprain through synchronous application of focal compression and cold," *Journal of Athletic Training* 26 (3): 224.

External Compression

The application of external pressure to an injured body part (e.g., circumferential elastic wraps, felt or sponge pads) is commonly used to control edema. In the presence of increased vascular permeability following injury, increased intravascular hydrostatic pressure facilitates movement of fluids through the vascular wall into interstitial spaces, causing edema. When applied appropriately, external compression counteracts the effect of intravascular pressure and reduces exudation of fluids into the extravascular tissues, thus minimizing edema. External compression, especially when combined with elevation, also encourages venous return and lymphatic drainage (Starkey 1993). Wilkerson (1991) attested to the early application and continued use of external compression as an effective deterrent to excessive edema formation. Contrary to the generally accepted effectiveness of external compression, however, Rucinski et al. (1991) observed an increase in edema in postacute ankle sprains following the use of commercial intermittent compression devices and elastic wraps. These investigators speculated that their unexpected observation may have been due to the uniform external pressure exerted on the ankle by the compression devices, creating a tourniquet-like effect that hindered venous return and lymphatic drainage. This observation attests to the importance of sequential distal to proximal application of external compression with decreasing pressure, thereby avoiding a constrictive tourniquet-like effect while encouraging lymphatic drainage.

Wilkerson (1991) described three types of external compression techniques: (1) circumferential compression with uniform pressure around a body part (e.g., an elastic thigh wrap), (2) collateral compression that produces pressure on each side of a body part (e.g., air-filled "stirrup" ankle braces), and (3) focal compression that concentrates pressure in a localized area (e.g., a U-shaped "horseshoe" pad for the ankle). The effects of circumferential compression and collateral compression on the soft tissues of an extremity are illustrated in figure 4.2. In contrast to circumferential and collateral compression, focal compression provides external pressure to specific, localized body surfaces. Thus, when secured by circumferential wrapping, pressure can be applied more directly to potentially edematous body parts. The use of a U-shaped felt or foam rubber "horseshoe" pad fitted to the contours of the lateral malleolus and secured with a circumferential elastic wrap is a familiar example of focal compression used in the management of acute inversion ankle sprains. In this example, focal compression inhibits excessive interstitial fluid accumulation (i.e., edema) in the lateral ankle. The effect of selective focal compression on edematous tissues compared to the effect of uniform compression is illustrated in figure 4.3.

Elevation

Elevation of an extremity to combat edema is a universally accepted procedure. Elevation employs gravity for positive therapeutic effects. Placement of an extremity in an elevated position counteracts the intravascular pressure in distal body parts, thus inhibiting exudation of fluids into interstitial spaces and minimizing edema. Placement of a limb in a dependent position has the opposite effect with enhancement of edema. The effect of gravity during elevation can effectively promote venous return and lymphatic drainage. Starkey (1993) suggested that the optimal effect of gravity on venous return occurs when an extremity is placed in a position perpendicular to the horizontal (e.g., 90° hip flexion in the supine position). A practical position of 45° is suggested, however (figure 4.4). Rucinski et al. (1991) noted that elevation, with hip flexion to 45°, produced a statistically significant decrease in ankle edema compared to the use of uniform external compression, which resulted in increased edema.

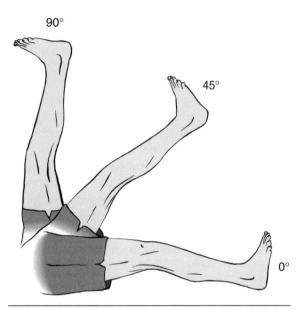

Figure 4.4 Effect of gravity during elevation of the lower extremity. At 90°, the force of gravity is 100%; at 45°, the force of gravity is 71%, and at 0°, the force of gravity is 0%.

Adapted, by permission, from C. Starkey, 1993, *Therapeutic modalities for athletic trainers* (Philadelphia: F.A. Davis), 15.

Restricted Movement

Restriction of movement in an injured body part through use of immobilization devices, ambulatory aids, or other measures is frequently indicated to protect recently damaged tissues from additional trauma. Appropriate immobilization also maximizes sustained approximation of disrupted tissues in the injured area, thus facilitating the repair process. With regard to acute injury management, purposeful restriction of movement in the affected tissues counteracts the potential detrimental effects of vasodilation, increased blood flow, and edema that otherwise would be enhanced by premature active motion. In general, the effects of active motion in acute soft tissue injuries are inconsistent with the desired physiological effects and therapeutic objectives of cold application, external compression, and elevation. Enhancement of venous return and lymphatic drainage, which rely on skeletal muscle contraction, may be an exception, however. In this regard, Wilkerson (1991) presented a convincing case for the early use of a partial weight-bearing crutch gait as an aid to reduction of lymphatic edema in recent ankle sprains. Provided that injured ligamentous structures can be protected from excessive mechanical loading, the controlled muscular contractions associated with partial weight bearing may enhance venous return and lymphatic drainage, thus facilitating edema resolution. Although rationale exists for the use of early active motion in the management of lymphatic edema, this approach should be weighted against the potential adverse affects of increased blood flow and premature alleviation of lymphatic obstruction. Premature resolution of local lymphatic obstruction may enhance the spread of inflammation to other body parts (Cotran, Kumar, and Robbins 1989). Additionally, in injuries involving the lower extremities, early weight bearing may intensify the adverse effects of gravity on lymphatic drainage and edema resolution. Given these considerations, restricted movement, along with cold, compression, and elevation, is the treatment of choice until deleterious hemodynamic responses are brought under control, typically during the first 24 to 48 hours following injury. Thereafter, depending on a clinical assessment of inflammatory responses, venous return and lymphatic drainage may be addressed through such measures as intermittent compression, distal to proximal massage (i.e., effleurage), and controlled active exercise.

Pharmacologic Agents

With some precautions, mediation of the acute inflammatory responses to injury through cold applications, external compression, elevation, and restricted activity can be complemented by the physician's use of pharmacologic agents. Drugs commonly used for this purpose include *anti-inflammatory drugs* and *analgesics*. Nonsteroidal anti-inflammatory drugs (NSAIDs) are a commonly used group of pharmacologic agents in the management of musculoskeletal injuries. Despite common reference to this group of medications as *anti-inflammatory drugs*, NSAIDs have *analgesic* (pain-relieving), *antipyretic* (fever-reducing), and *anticoagulation* properties as well as anti-inflammatory capabilities (Ciccone 1990). Typically, control of excessive inflammatory responses and alleviation of mild to moderate pain are the primary indications for the use of NSAIDs in sports injuries. Examples of NSAIDs used in the treatment of sports injuries are acetylsalicylic acid (Ascriptin, Excedrin), indomethacin (Indocin), tolmetin (Tolectin), phenylbutazone (Butazolidin), ibuprofen (Advil, Motrin, Nuprin), naproxen (Naprosyn), and piroxicam (Feldene). Table 4.1 lists the generic and brand names of NSAIDs according to their classifications.

Although the mechanisms of action associated with NSAIDs are thought to be varied, an anti-inflammatory effect is commonly attributed to their ability to inhibit synthesis of prostaglandins (Abramson 1990; Ciccone 1990; Koester 1993). NSAIDs inhibit production of prostaglandins by inhibiting the catalytic action of cyclooxygenase, an enzyme that mediates conversion of arachidonic acid into prostaglandins (Koester 1993). Kellett (1986) noted the role of prostaglandins in mediation of endothelial cell separation and increased vascular permeability, thus providing rationale for the use of NSAIDs for control of edema in acute inflammation. In addition, it is thought that certain NSAIDs inhibit the release of histamine from mast cells, which occurs at the time of tissue injury (Abramson 1990). Hence, an anti-inflammatory effect of NSAIDs may be due to their ability to combat the vasodilation and increased vascular permeability caused by histamine release.

Aspirin is a commonly prescribed analgesic, anti-inflammatory, and antipyretic drug with specific effects depending on the dosage. As with the newer NSAIDs, the anti-inflammatory and analgesic effects of aspirin are attributed primarily to inhibition of prostaglandin synthesis. Buchanan and Rainsford (1990) and Ciccone (1990) noted that aspirin,

Table 4.1 Classification of Nonsteroidal Anti-Inflammatory Drugs

Generic name	Brand name	Generic name	Brand name
Salicylates		**Mefenamic acid**	
acetylsalicylic acid (aspirin)	Ascriptin, Bayer Bufferin, Excedrin	mefenamic acid	Ponstel
		meclofenamate	Meclomen
salsalate	Disalacid	**Propionic acid derivatives**	
choline magnesium trisalicylate	Trilisate	ibuprofen	Motrin, Advil, Nuprin, Haltran
diflunisal	Dolobid	naproxen	Naprosyn
Indoles		fenoprofen	Nalfon
indomethacin	Indocin	**Pyroxicans**	
sulindac	Clinoril	piroxicam	Feldene
tolmetin	Tolectin	**Phenylacetic acid**	
Pyrazoles		diclofenac	Voltaren
phenylbutazone	Butazolidin		
oxyphenbutazone	Tandearil		

Data from Walder and Hainline 1989.

like other NSAIDs, has an anticoagulation effect that inhibits platelet aggregation, an essential mechanism of hemostasis. Unlike other NSAIDs, which generally affect platelet function for no longer than 24 to 48 hours after the last dose, aspirin decreases platelet aggregation for an extended period and may prolong bleeding time for 10 to 12 days (Stankus 1993). Consequently, early use of aspirin and other drugs with anticoagulation properties may be contraindicated in acute injuries where bleeding may be exacerbated (Walder and Hainline 1989).

To a great extent, the use of NSAIDs has replaced corticosteroids in the management of sports injuries (Leadbetter 1990). Although corticosteroids possess powerful anti-inflammatory properties, they have been shown to inhibit fibroblastic activity and suppress collagen synthesis, thus impairing connective tissue repair (Behrens and Goodwin 1990). Unlike corticosteroids, NSAIDs have demonstrated effectiveness in controlling the adverse effects of inflammation without causing significant negative effects on tissue healing (Abramson 1990). As an alternative to injectable corticosteroids, phonophoresis (i.e., use of ultrasound to drive topical medications into deep tissues) has been used for localized noninvasive introduction of hydrocortisone into inflamed tissues, supposedly avoiding the adverse effects of injectable corticosteroids (Prentice 1990).

Alleviation of Pain and Muscle Spasm

The early vascular changes that result from acute tissue trauma (i.e., vasodilation, increased blood flow, increased vascular permeability) account for swelling, redness, and increased temperature in the affected tissues. As discussed in chapter 3, these three cardinal signs and symptoms are characteristic of the primary inflammatory responses to injury. Associated pain, the fourth cardinal sign of inflammation, and muscle spasm represent the secondary inflammatory responses. Although pain and muscle spasm typically limit the injured sports participant's activity, thus protecting damaged tissues from recurrent injury, persistent pain and muscle spasm may have significant detrimental effects on the recovery process. In addition to the congestive effect of edema, pain and muscle spasm are commonly primary causes of restricted movement and limited joint motion in acute injuries. If prolonged, restrictions in soft tissue mobility may lead to clinically significant complications, including connective tissue contractures and adhesions. In this regard, pain and muscle spasm frequently necessitate specific therapeutic attention in order to minimize the long-term detrimental effects of functional loss. Thus, alleviation of pain and muscle spasm represents the second major focus of therapeutic intervention during the inflammatory stage of connective tissue repair (see chapter 1, figure 1.2).

Pain and muscle spasm are sometimes said to represent a "vicious cycle." In simple terms, pain stimulates protective muscle spasm while spasm, in turn, exacerbates pain. Rationale for effective therapeutic management of pain and muscle spasm is based on an understanding of the neuroanatomy and neurophysiology associated with the conduction of pain impulses, the pathophysiology of the pain-spasm-pain cycle, and prevailing pain theories. Basic concepts associated with each of these considerations are discussed in the following sections of this chapter prior to a discussion of strategies for management of pain and muscle spasm in sports injuries.

Neuroanatomy and Neurophysiology

Comprehension of the neurophysiology of pain is dependent on a basic understanding of sensory receptors and the neural pathways through which pain impulses are transmitted from receptor organs to higher levels of the central nervous system. Peripheral sensory receptors, afferent (sensory) neurons, and ascending neural pathways in the spinal cord, the brain stem, and the brain are the primary neurological structures associated with detection of noxious stimuli and transmission of pain impulses to the cerebral cortex where pain perception occurs. Each of these neural components, including the relevant neuroanatomy of the brain stem and the brain, are reviewed in an attempt to provide a basis for development of pain-management protocols.

Sensory Receptors

Somatosensory nerve fibers have peripheral endings, referred to as *sensory receptors*, that detect environmental stimuli (e.g., mechanical, thermal, chemical alterations) and convert them into electrochemical impulses. These impulses are conducted by afferent (sensory) neurons to the spinal cord with subsequent transmission to the brain via ascending spinal cord pathways. In general, sensory receptors are classified as *exteroceptors, interoceptors,* or *proprioceptors* (Tortora and Grabowski 1993). Sensory receptors that respond to stimuli originating from sources outside the body are called *exteroceptors*. Because exteroceptors in the skin, for example, can be influenced by externally applied therapeutic agents (e.g., heat, cold), they represent clinically significant neurological structures in pain management. Therapeutic intervention directed to stimulation of exteroceptors is discussed in a subsequent section of this chapter. In contrast to exteroceptors, sensory receptors that respond to stimuli originating from within the body are referred to as *interoceptors*. These sensory receptors are primarily associated with changes in the internal environment of the body (e.g., hunger, thirst, visceral pain). In the general classification of sensory receptors, proprioceptors are distinguished from exteroceptors and interoceptors, both anatomically and functionally. Anatomically, they are located in the skin, musculoskeletal structures (muscles, joint capsules, and ligaments), and the vestibular apparatus of the inner ear. Functionally, proprioceptors respond to mechanical stimuli that cause deformation of the tissues in which they are located. Hence, they are associated with detection of body position and movement (see chapter 8).

In addition to their general classification, sensory receptors are commonly categorized functionally according to their sensitivity to particular stimuli. Whereas some sensory receptors are capable of responding to a variety of stimuli, other types of receptors are predominantly sensitive to a single type of stimulus (Hall 1994). For example, sensory receptors that are primarily sensitive to changes in temperature are referred to as *thermoreceptors*. Receptors that respond primarily to mechanical stimuli (e.g., pressure, stretch) are considered *mechanoreceptors* (e.g., proprioceptors). Receptors that are sensitive to chemical stimuli are referred to as *chemoreceptors* (Rowinski 1997). Regardless of the particular stimuli, sensory receptors that respond to a pain stimulus are called *nociceptors*. Although an understanding of all types of sensory receptors is essential to effective management of musculoskeletal injuries, appreciation of the role of nociceptors is important as a basis for effective therapeutic intervention in the pain-spasm-pain cycle.

Nociceptive receptors

Morphologically, nociceptors are classified as *free nerve endings*, as opposed to encapsulated sensory nerve endings which are covered by thin layers of connective tissue (figure 4.5). Nociceptors are characteristically unmyelinated, naked nerve endings with many branches embedded in various tissues throughout the body (e.g., muscles, tendons, joint capsules and ligaments, skin). These receptors represent the terminal ends of A-delta and C fibers, the two types of afferent (sensory) neurons that transmit pain impulses to the spinal cord. Whereas some nociceptors respond selectively to a particular type of stimulus (e.g., thermal, mechanical), other receptors, referred to as *polymodal nociceptors*, are responsive to various kinds of noxious stimuli. The sensory receptors of most afferent C fibers, for example, respond to various types of pain stimuli and, thus, are considered polymodal nociceptors.

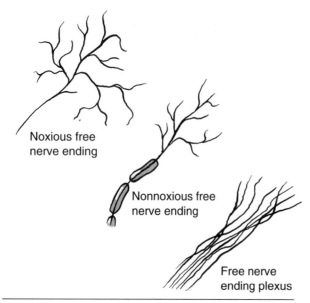

Figure 4.5 Neuroanatomy of free (naked) nerve endings.

Reprinted, by permission, from M.J. Rowinski, 1997, Neurobiology for orthopedic and sports physical therapy. In *Orthopedic and sports physical therapy*, 3rd ed., edited by T.R. Malone, T.G. McPoil, and A.J. Nitz. (St. Louis: Mosby-Yearbook), 51.

Nociceptor stimulation

Clinically, it is important to note that the intensity of a particular stimulus is a primary factor in pain perception. Any stimulus that surpasses a certain threshold of intensity and elicits a pain response is referred as a *noxious stimulus*. At this point, the sensory receptor is considered *nociceptive* (Hall 1994). Clinically applied stimuli (e.g., thermal, mechanical, electrical) may become noxious, and thus counterproductive, if a certain threshold of intensity is surpassed. For example, elevation of tissue temperature to greater than 45°C, the critical heat threshold in humans, may elicit a pain response with a corresponding potential for tissue damage (Rennie and Michlovitz 1996).

Anterolateral System

Stimulation of peripheral somatosensory receptors generates afferent neural impulses that are transmitted to higher centers of the central nervous system through one of two primary ascending pathways: the *dorsal column-medial lemniscal system* and the *anterolateral system*. The dorsal column-medial lemniscal system, which conducts somatosensory impulses for vibration, touch, and proprioception, is discussed in chapter 8 as related to proprioceptive dysfunction and proprioceptive training. The ascending pathway for pain and temperature is the anterolateral system. In both systems, nerve impulses are transmitted to the somatosensory area of the cerebral cortex through three levels of sensory neurons referred to as *first order neurons*, *second order neurons*, and *third order neurons*. These three neurological levels, as related to transmission of pain impulses through the ascending anterolateral system, are illustrated in figure 4.6. A descending neural pathway for pain control, from the brain stem to the spinal cord, is also depicted in figure 4.6. This pathway, as related to descending

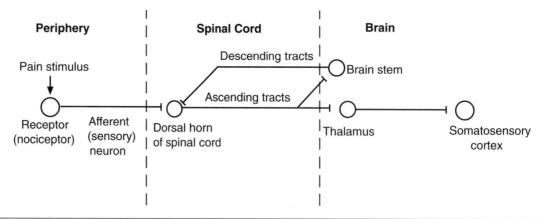

Figure 4.6 Ascending and descending neural pathways for pain. Ascending pathways including peripheral afferent neurons (first order neurons), spinal cord tracts to the thalamus (second order neurons), and thalamic projection to the somatosensory cortex (third order neurons) are illustrated. Descending pathways from the brain stem to the dorsal horn of the spinal cord are also depicted.

Adapted, by permission, from J.L. Hanegan, 1992, Principles of nociception. In *Electrotherapy in rehabilitation*, edited by M.R. Gersch (Philadelphia: F.A. Davis), 27.

pain inhibitory systems, is discussed in a subsequent section of this chapter. The ascending anterolateral system through which pain impulses are transmitted includes three primary components: afferent (sensory) neurons (first order neurons), ascending spinal cord pathways to the thalamus (second order neurons), and thalamic projections to the primary somatosensory cortex (third order neurons). Transmission of pain impulses from one neurological level to the next occurs at a synaptic junction, or synapse.

Afferent (sensory) neurons

Nerve fibers that conduct somatosensory impulses from various peripheral receptors (e.g., nociceptors, mechanoreceptors) to the spinal cord are referred to as *afferent (sensory) neurons*. Afferent neurons are classified as A fibers (i.e., A-alpha, A-beta, A-delta) or C fibers according to their size (i.e., diameter), their rate of nerve impulse conduction, and whether they are myelinated (i.e., covered with a fat-like myelin sheath). Table 4.2 represents a composite of afferent nerve fiber characteristics commonly reported in the literature. With the exception of A-delta fibers, which conduct pain impulses, most A fibers transmit impulses associated with mechanical stimuli. Correspondingly, their sensory receptors are called *mechanoreceptors*. Some A fibers, with receptors classified as thermoreceptors, conduct thermal impulses. Other A fibers convey both mechanical and thermal impulses. Comparatively, A fibers are large-diameter, myelinated neurons with a rapid rate of conduction. Small-diameter unmyelinated C fibers, on the other hand, have the slowest rate of conduction (Hall 1994).

Within the general taxonomy of afferent neurons, A-delta and C fibers are the two types of nerve fibers that conduct pain impulses initiated by noxious stimulation of their sensory receptors. A-delta fibers are the smallest of the three types of A fibers but nevertheless are larger than C fibers. Compared to C fibers, A-delta fibers conduct impulses rapidly. Thus, they are associated with conduction of intense, sharp pain impulses referred to as *fast pain*, or *first pain*. The small, unmyelinated C fibers have the slowest conduction rate and, consequently, are associated with constant, dull, aching sensations called *slow pain*, or *second pain*. The initial, intense pain associated with an acute traumatic incident is thought to be related to A-delta fiber conduction whereas the dull, aching pain that follows is attributed to impulses transmitted by C fibers (Hargreaves 1990). Functionally, the sensory receptors of most C fibers are responsive to a variety of stimuli (i.e., thermal, mechanical, chemical). Thus, they are referred to as *polymodal nociceptors*. Several distinctions among the various types of afferent nerve fibers, especially differences related to specificity of receptor stimulation and rate of conduction, have significant implications for pain management and therapeutic intervention in the pain-spasm-pain cycle. These clinical implications are discussed in subsequent sections of this chapter.

Table 4.2   Classification of Afferent (Sensory) Nerve Fibers

Classification		Fiber size (μm)	Conduction rate (m/sec)	Primary receptor type
Type	Group			
A-alpha	Ia	12-20	70-120	Mechanoreceptor
	Ib	12-20	70-120	Mechanoreceptor
A-beta	II	5-12	30-70	Mechanoreceptor
A-delta	III	2-5	12-30	Nociceptor
C	IV	0.5-1	0.5-2.0	Nociceptor

Data from Donley and Denegar 1990; Hanegan 1992.

Spinal cord connections

As afferent nerve fibers project to the spinal cord, they enter through the dorsal roots on the ipsilateral side. Whereas large-diameter fibers (i.e., A fibers) enter the spinal cord in the dorsal column, small-diameter pain fibers (i.e., A-delta and C fibers) enter the *tract of Lissauer*, a dorsolateral spinal cord tract, before entering the dorsal horn of the gray matter. Most of these fibers terminate and synapse with ascending spinal cord tracts in the dorsal horn (Martin 1996). A basic understanding of the histology and neural functions of the dorsal horn is fundamental to an appreciation of the "gating" mechanisms of pain modulation that are frequently cited as rationale for specific therapeutic protocols. The clinical significance of various dorsal horn connections (i.e., synapses) between first order neurons (afferent nerve fibers) and second order neurons (ascending spinal cord pathways) is discussed shortly.

The dorsal horns, which represent dorsolateral extensions of the gray matter of the spinal cord, are formed by six layers of nerve cells referred to as *Rexed's laminae* (figure 4.7). Named after Bror Rexed, the Swedish neuroanatomist who described them, each of these layers contains neurons with different neural connections and functions (Martin 1996). After entering the overlying tract of Lissauer, some of the small-diameter A-delta and C pain fibers enter the dorsal horn directly, while others divide into short ascending or descending branches before entering. As illustrated in figure 4.7, A-delta and C pain fibers terminate in various layers of the dorsal horn where they synapse, directly or through connecting *interneurons*, with second order neurons that represent the ascending spinal cord pathways for pain and temperature.

Several authors describe the termination of nociceptive A-delta and C fibers in laminae I and V (DePace and Newton 1996; Ganong 1995; Waxman and deGroot 1995). As noted by Kelly (1985), lamina I receives input primarily from small-diameter A-delta and C nerve fibers, but a greater convergence of A-delta and C pain fibers and collaterals from large-diameter A fibers occurs in lamina V. Convergence of various types of afferent nerve

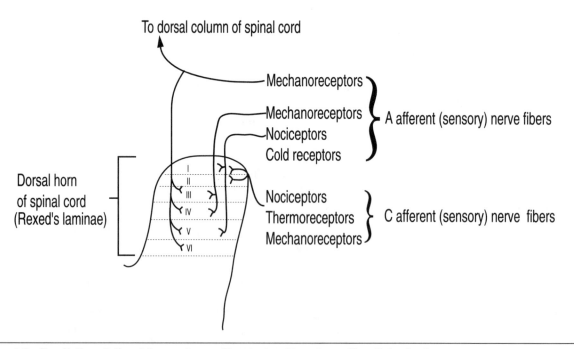

Figure 4.7   Termination of afferent (sensory) nerve fibers in dorsal horn layers (Rexed's laminae).

Adapted from W.F. Ganong, 1995, *Review of medical physiology*, 17th ed. (Norwalk, Connecticut: Appleton & Lange), 122. Reproduced with the permission of The McGraw-Hill Companies.

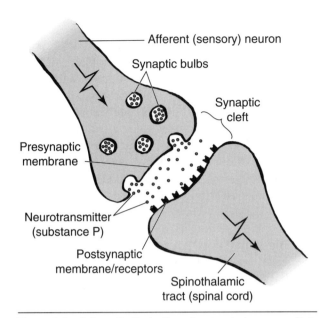

- Afferent (sensory) neuron
- Synaptic bulbs
- Synaptic cleft
- Presynaptic membrane
- Neurotransmitter (substance P)
- Postsynaptic membrane/receptors
- Spinothalamic tract (spinal cord)

Figure 4.8 Schematic illustration of a chemical synapse. Note the release of neurotransmitter (substance P) from afferent (sensory) neuron (first order neuron) in the spinal cord.

Adapted, by permission, from J.A. Paice, 1991, "Unraveling the mystery of pain," *Oncology Nursing Forum* 18 (5): 844.

fibers in lamina V is significant because of their synaptic connections with second order neurons (i.e., ascending spinal cord pathways) that originate in this layer of the dorsal horn. The termination points of various afferent neurons in the dorsal horn, as well as their synaptic connections with ascending spinal cord pathways, represent clinically important sites for pain modulation through the use of pharmacologic or physical agents. It is generally recognized, for example, that the presynaptic terminals of nociceptive afferent neurons (i.e., A-delta and C fibers) release *substance P*, an excitatory neurotransmitter that facilitates transmission of pain impulses across a chemical synapse to postsynaptic neurons of the ascending spinal cord pathways (Ganong 1995; Hanegan 1992). Figure 4.8 represents a dorsal horn chemical synapse with presynaptic release of substance P from an afferent (sensory) neuron. The analgesic effect of certain pharmacologic agents (e.g., opioid analgesics) is attributed to the inhibition of substance P release from afferent neurons in the dorsal horn of the spinal cord (Solomon 1994).

Ascending spinal cord pathways

After entering the dorsal horn of the spinal cord, afferent pain fibers (i.e., A-delta and C fibers) synapse with ascending spinal cord pathways (second order neurons) through which pain impulses are transmitted to higher centers of the central nervous system. These pathways are composed of three ascending spinal cord tracts: the *spinoreticular tract*, the *spinomesencephalic tract*, and the *spinothalamic tract*, each of which terminate in separate regions of the brain stem or the brain (Martin 1996). Respectively, these tracts terminate in the reticular formation of the brain stem (spinoreticular tract), the midbrain tectum and the periaqueductal gray matter (spinomesencephalic tract), and the thalamus (spinothalamic tract). Although these anterolateral tracts function collectively to conduct pain impulses in a highly complex, integrated manner, the spinothalamic tract presents particular implications for pain management through the use of physical agents. Commonly, the spinothalamic tract is considered to have two components: an *anterior spinothalamic tract* and a *lateral spinothalamic tract* (figure 4.9). The lateral spinothalamic tract originates in Rexed's lamina I of the dorsal horn, where it receives input largely from the small-diameter A-delta and C nociceptive fibers, whereas the anterior spinothalamic tract originates from lamina V (Kelly 1985; see figure 4.7). Nerve cells in lamina V are referred to as *wide dynamic range neurons* because they receive input from multiple afferent nerve fibers, including A-delta and C nociceptive fibers (DePace and Newton 1996). The chemical synapses, or synaptic junctions, formed by afferent nerve fibers and wide dynamic range neurons in the dorsal horn of the spinal cord represent important sites for excitatory or inhibitory transmission, or "gating," of nociceptive impulses. As illustrated in figure 4.9, most fibers of the spinothalamic tract decussate (i.e., cross) to the contralateral side of the spinal cord before ascending to the thalamus. Generally considered the classic ascending pain pathway, the lateral spinothalamic tract is thought to conduct sensory impulses associated with acute sharp pain, whereas the anterior spinothalamic tract is associated with transmission of impulses related to dull, aching pain (Kelly 1985).

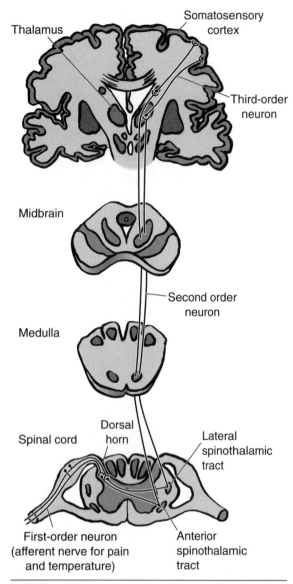

Figure 4.9   Ascending spinothalamic tracts for pain and temperature.

Adapted from G.J. Tortora and S.R. Grabowski, 1993, *Principles of anatomy and physiology*, 7th ed. (New York: Harper Collin's College Publishers), 452. Copyright © 1993, John Wiley & Sons, Inc. This material is used by permission of John Wiley & Sons, Inc.

Thalamus

After ascending through the lateral gray matter of the spinal cord and the brain stem, the spinothalamic tract terminates in the thalamus and synapses with third order neurons that project to the primary somatosensory area of the cerebral cortex (see figure 4.9). The thalamus is composed of several *relay nuclei*, specialized groups of nerve cells that relay information from various areas of the central nervous system to the cerebral cortex (figure 4.10). Relay nuclei that project somatosensory information to the cerebral cortex are referred to as *sensory nuclei*, one of several functional divisions of the thalamus (Waxman and deGroot 1995). Ascending spinal cord tracts in both the dorsal column-medial lemniscal system and the anterolateral system (i.e., the spinothalamic tract) project to the same thalamic nucleus, the *ventral posterior nucleus* (see figure 4.10), although to separate nuclear areas (Waxman and deGroot 1995). Thus, the ventral posterior nucleus is the primary relay station for transmission of proprioceptive as well as nociceptive somatosensory information to the cerebral cortex (Martin 1996). Both types of information are transmitted from the ventral posterior nucleus through the internal capsule of the cerebrum to the primary somatosensory cortex by third order projection, or relay, neurons (Kandel, Schwartz, and Jessell 1995). Relay of proprioceptive information to the primary somatosensory cortex is discussed further in chapter 8.

Because of the functional specificity of thalamic nuclei, the thalamus is thought to play a role in identification of specific types of sensory stimuli, especially pain (Waxman and deGroot 1995). After reaching the thalamus, somatosensory information is selectively transmitted to the cerebral cortex (Hall 1994). Thus, the *modality of sensation* (e.g., pain) is determined by noxious stimulation of sensory receptors (i.e., nociceptors), transmission of neural impulses through the spinothalamic tract to distinct thalamic nuclei (i.e., the ventral posterior nucleus), and projection to discrete areas of the somatosensory cortex where more precise pain perception and localization occurs (Kandel, Schwartz, and Jessell 1995; Waxman and deGroot 1995).

Cerebral cortex

The outermost portion of the cerebrum, the cerebral cortex, represents the highest functional level of the central nervous system. Complete perception of somatosensory stimuli occurs when neural impulses reach the primary somatosensory area of the cerebral cortex located in the postcentral gyrus of the parietal lobe (figure 4.11). The predominant somatosensory input to the primary somatosensory cortex is provided by the ventral posterior nucleus of the thalamus via third order projection neurons. Whereas the role of the primary somatosensory cortex in perception of mechanical stimuli (e.g., touch, pressure) has been documented experimentally, determination of its role in pain perception has

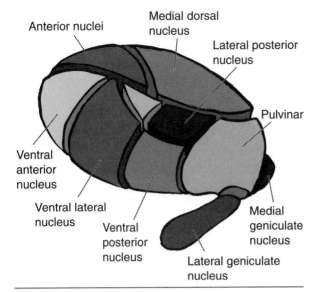

been more elusive. Nevertheless, functional imaging techniques, such as positron-emission tomography (PET), have clarified the role of the primary somatosensory area and other cortical regions in determining the anatomical origin and the intensity of noxious stimuli (Martin 1996). Orderly arrangement of the cerebral cortex is such that three specific functional divisions of the primary somatosensory cortex called *Brodmann's areas* (areas numbered 1, 2, and 3) receive input from different body parts (see figure 4.11). Thus, various body parts are spatially represented, allowing for *localization*, or determination of the anatomical origin of a pain stimulus (Martin 1996). The numbered Brodmann's areas, named after Korbinian Brodmann, the German anatomist who developed the widely published cytoarchitectural map, serve as useful references for discussion of the complex neurophysiology of the cerebral cortex. A more comprehensive discussion of Brodmann's areas, as related to the sensorimotor functions of the cerebral cortex, is presented in chapter 8. Organization of somatic sensory input is

Figure 4.10 Thalamic nuclei. Note the ventral posterior nucleus, which relays somatosensory information (e.g., pain) to the primary somatosensory area of the cerebral cortex.

Reprinted from J.H. Martin, 1996, *Neuroanatomy*, 2nd ed. (Stamford, Connecticut: Appleton & Lange), 77. Reproduced with permission of The McGraw-Hill Companies.

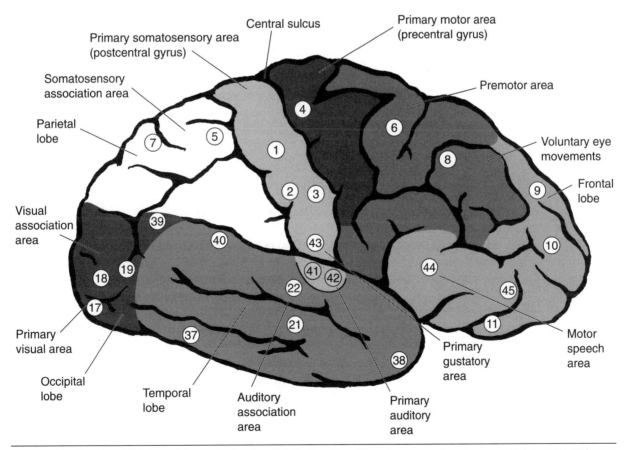

Figure 4.11 Functional divisions of the cerebral cortex. Note the location of the primary somatosensory area in the postcentral gyrus of the parietal lobe (location of Brodmann's areas 1, 2, and 3).

Adapted from G.J. Tortora and S.R. Grabowski, 1993, *Principles of anatomy and physiology*, 7th ed. (New York: Harper Collin's College Publishers), 424. Copyright © 1993, John Wiley & Sons, Inc. This material is used by permission of John Wiley & Sons, Inc.

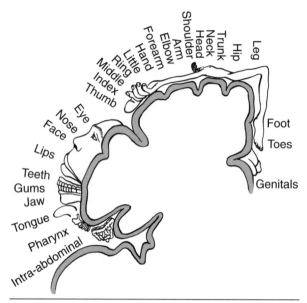

Figure 4.12 Somatotopic organization of the primary somatosensory cortex (sensory homunculus).

Adapted from G.J. Tortora and S.R. Grobowski, 1993, *Principles of anatomy and physiology*, 7th ed. (New York: Harper Collin's College Publishers), 453. Copyright © 1993, John Wiley & Sons, Inc. This material is used by permission of John Wiley & Sons, Inc.

referred to as *somatotopy*. Somatotopic organization of the primary somatosensory cortex is commonly depicted as the *sensory homunculus* (figure 4.12).

Transmission of Pain Impulses

Current concepts of pain management hold that pain impulses can be modulated at various levels of the ascending neural pathways to the cerebral cortex, including the spinal cord and the brain stem, as well as through descending neural pathways from the brain stem to the spinal cord. Pain control in the management of acute musculoskeletal injuries is typically approached through the use of pharmacologic agents, physical agents (e.g., electrical stimulation), or both. Rationale for use of these therapeutic agents stems from an understanding of the neural mechanisms associated with transmission of pain impulses in the central nervous system, including the role of chemical neurotransmitters.

Somatosensory pain impulses arising from nociceptor stimulation are conducted to the cerebral cortex through the first order, second order, and third order neurons of the anterolateral system. Conduction of impulses along these neural pathways involves transmission across a functional junction between neurons called a *synapse*, or *synaptic junction*. Although nerve impulses can be transmitted directly from one neuron to the next at an *electrical synapse*, most synapses in the human nervous system rely on chemical *neurotransmitters* for transmission. These interneuronal junctions are referred to as *chemical synapses* (see figure 4.8). A chemical synapse consists of a *presynaptic membrane* at the terminal of one neuron, an intervening space called the *synaptic cleft*, and a *postsynaptic membrane* that represents the receptor of the next neuron. When a nerve impulse reaches the terminal of a presynaptic neuron, chemical neurotransmitters are released from *synaptic bulbs* into the synaptic cleft. These chemicals diffuse across the synaptic cleft and bind to receptor sites on the postsynaptic membrane, initiating electrochemical changes that produce an *action potential*, or *nerve impulse*, in the postsynaptic neuron (Ganong 1995).

Chemical neurotransmitters may be *excitatory* or *inhibitory*. Chemicals that activate a nerve impulse in the postsynaptic neuron are called *excitatory neurotransmitters*, whereas those that prevent activation of a nerve impulse are referred to as *inhibitory neurotransmitters*. Although neurotransmitters are generally classified as excitatory or inhibitory, some neurotransmitters may be excitatory in one location and inhibitory in another (Tortora and Grabowski 1993). Two important examples of chemical neurotransmitters associated with transmission of noxious impulses are *substance P*, which acts as an excitatory neurotransmitter in the dorsal horn of the spinal cord (see figure 4.8), and *serotonin*, which functions as an inhibitory neurotransmitter in descending pain inhibitory systems. The clinical significance of specific chemical neurotransmitters, as related to the analgesic effect of pharmacologic and physical agents, is discussed in subsequent sections of this chapter.

Pain-Spasm-Pain Cycle

When mechanical deformation of nociceptive nerve endings occurs at the time of injury, pain impulses are transmitted by afferent neurons to the spinal cord, through the ascending spinal cord pathways to the thalamus, and finally to the primary somatosensory cortex where pain is perceived. Noxious stimulation of the fast-conducting A-delta fibers at the time of injury is thought to account for the initial, "sharp," comparatively intense fast pain (first pain) that is associated with sudden tissue disruption (Hargreaves 1990). Thus, the initial pain associated with acute sports injuries results from rapidly applied mechanical forces to body tissues that house nociceptive nerve endings. Continuation of pain, however, is influenced by factors associated with subsequent inflammatory responses. Obviously, because fast pain occurs at the time of injury, it cannot be modified by therapeutic intervention. Hence, initial therapeutic measures are directed to sources of pain associated with the early inflammatory responses to tissue damage.

Although nociceptors may continue to be stimulated by increased interstitial pressure as edema develops in an acute injury, they are also excited by chemical mediators associated with the inflammatory response (e.g., prostaglandins, bradykinin). The terminal ends of both A-delta fibers and C pain fibers can become highly sensitized by noxious chemicals and thus more readily irritated, although their vulnerability appears to differ. Chemical irritation of nociceptive nerve endings can be a source of slow pain (second pain) that presents implications for therapeutic intervention. Due to continued chemical irritation, a state of secondary *hyperalgesia*, or increased sensitivity to painful stimuli, may result (DePace and Newton 1996). Hyperalgesia has been described as spontaneous pain characterized by an increased magnitude of perceived pain that is out of proportion to a given stimulus (Hargreaves 1990). This increased pain sensation has been attributed to a lowered threshold of firing, or sensitization, of C fiber nociceptors when these nerve endings are subjected to subsequent stimulation following initial activation (Fine 1993). Thus, even mild tissue loading (e.g., stretching), in the presence of hyperalgesia, may provoke an intensified pain response that otherwise would not occur. Prolonged chemically derived pain indicates that the responsible chemical mediators are still being released in inflamed tissues. As acute inflammation subsides, chemical irritation of nociceptors diminishes and stronger mechanical stimuli can be tolerated. Given these considerations, it is understandable that pain is an important guide to appropriate levels of tissue loading during therapeutic exercise.

Increased sensitivity of nociceptors with hyperalgesia is a prime stimulus for involuntary muscle spasm (DePace and Newton 1996). When related to tissue trauma, muscle spasm is typically manifested as a tonic, or sustained, state of *hypertonus* (i.e., increased tension). Hypertonus results from continual noxious stimuli that cause the contractile elements of muscle fibers (i.e., muscle spindles) to maintain a state of partial tension beyond that considered normal muscle tone, or *tonus*. Externally applied stress to a spasmodic muscle (e.g., stretch) provides a noxious mechanical stimulus to nociceptive nerve endings and causes pain, especially in the presence of hyperalgesia. Thus, the "vicious cycle" of pain and muscle spasm is completed. Because pain is a signal that loaded tissues have reached a point of potential failure, regional muscle spasm represents an inherent mechanism through which damaged tissues are protected from further injury.

Like nociceptors, proprioceptors play an integral role in the pain-spasm-pain cycle. Proprioceptors, the sensory receptors that provide information about joint position and movement, are located in musculotendinous tissues, joint capsules and ligaments, and the skin. Most relevant to an understanding of muscle spasm is the *muscle spindle*, a mechanoreceptor consisting of small, specialized muscle fibers (i.e., intrafusal fibers) that lie between the extrafusal muscle fibers (figure 4.13). A sudden stretch stimulus applied to the central portion of intrafusal fibers elicits a dynamic stretch reflex with resulting muscle contraction. Normal muscle tone, on the other hand, is a steady state of muscle contraction that depends on continual efferent impulses reaching the ends of intrafusal fibers in the muscle spindles via small motor fibers called *gamma motor (efferent) neurons* (Tortora and Grabowski 1993). When gamma motor firing and muscle spindle activity is exceedingly high, however, a state of increased tension (hypertonus), or muscle spasm, occurs. The neuroanatomy

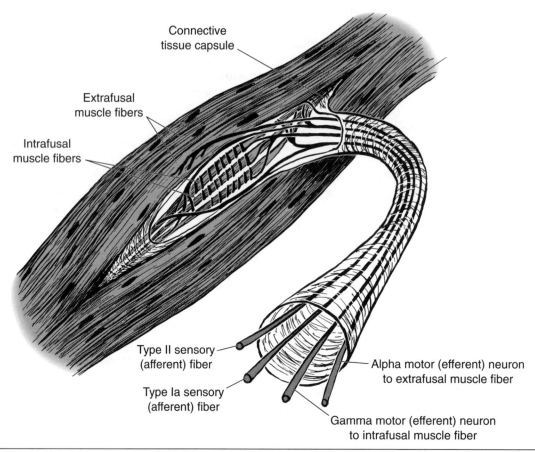

Figure 4.13   Neuroanatomy of a muscle spindle.

Adapted from G.J. Tortora and S.R. Grobowski, 1993, *Principles of anatomy and physiology*, 7th ed. (New York: Harper Collin's College Publishers), 450. Copyright © 1993, John Wiley & Sons, Inc. This material is used by permission of John Wiley & Sons, Inc.

and neurophysiology of the muscle spindle is discussed in greater depth in chapter 8. Various therapeutic agents directed to modulation of muscle spindle activity and reduction of muscle spasm are discussed in a following section of this chapter.

Theoretical Bases of Pain

As noted by Feuerstein (1994), the International Association for the Study of Pain (IASP) has proposed one of the most widely accepted definitions of pain. This definition characterizes pain as "an unpleasant sensory and emotional experience associated with actual or potential tissue damage, or described in terms of such damage." According to the IASP, pain is always a subjective psychological experience, even though it most often results from a physical cause. For many years, investigators have diligently searched for more precise explanations for pain experiences. Contemporary pain theories tend to fall into three general categories, which collectively present indications for a multifaceted approach to pain management. As summarized by Hanegan (1992), current theoretical bases for pain include those that focus on (1) neurophysiological mechanisms and associated neuroanatomical structures, (2) motivational and behavioral factors, and (3) psychiatric considerations. Because psychological considerations in pain management are addressed briefly in a subsequent section of this chapter, discussion in this section is focused on those theories associated with the neurophysiological mechanisms of pain. Theoretical concepts associated with the neuroanatomy and neurophysiology of pain provide rationale that is most relevant to the use of pharmacologic and physical agents in the management of musculoskeletal pain.

Over the years, several neural mechanisms have been proposed to explain the transmission of pain impulses and the perception of pain. Two early theories that emerged in the 1800s are the *specificity theory* and the *pattern theory* (DePace and Newton 1996). Some concepts in these pain theories have withstood the rigor of scientific inquiry, whereas others have been refuted, modified, or judged incomplete. A third, more recent pain theory, the *gate control theory* proposed by Melzack and Wall (1965), has received comparatively widespread attention as a basis for therapeutic intervention in disorders of the musculoskeletal system. Related theories of pain modulation, involving descending neural pathways from the brain stem to the spinal cord, have also been proposed (Martin 1996). In this regard, Martin (1996) refers to a *descending pain inhibitory system*. Collectively, the neural mechanisms inherent in these pain theories provide reasonable rationale for use of a wide range of pharmacologic and physical agents in pain management.

Early Pain Theories

The specificity theory holds that stimulation of a specific system of pain receptors always elicits the same sensation (i.e., pain), regardless of the type of stimulus (DePace and Newton 1996). According to the specificity theory, excitation of nociceptive A-delta and C fiber nerve endings by a stimulus of sufficient intensity will elicit a pain response, regardless of whether the stimulus is mechanical, thermal, or chemical (Hanegan 1992). In more recent years, nociceptors that respond to several types of noxious stimuli have been termed *polymodal nociceptors*, whereas those that respond only to one type of noxious stimuli are called *specific nociceptors* (DePace and Newton 1996). The specificity theory of pain is derived from the *doctrine of specific nerve energies*, which embraces the principle of receptor specificity (DePace and Newton 1996). Although this doctrine has been questioned since first proposed by Johannes Muller in 1826, it remains as an accepted principle of sensory physiology (Ganong 1995). Nevertheless, the specificity theory has been questioned in view of the observation that one type of nerve ending (e.g., free nerve ending) can transmit various sensations (Weisberg 1994).

In contrast to the specificity theory of pain, the pattern theory discounts the association of specific pain receptors with pain sensations. Initially proposed in 1894, the *pattern theory*, also referred to as the *intensity theory*, suggests that a pain pattern is produced by excessive noxious stimulation of nonspecific sensory receptors (DePace and Newton 1996; Hanegan 1992). As proposed, pain is the perceived sensation if a particular stimulus is of sufficient intensity and frequency, regardless of the energy source (mechanical, thermal, etc.). Thus, the pattern theory of pain is based on the neurological concept of *summation*, which refers to an increase in the concentration of a neurotransmitter at a chemical synapse resulting from an increase in the frequency of afferent impulses in a nerve fiber (temporal summation) or the number of afferent fibers stimulated (spatial summation). As related to the pattern theory of pain, excessive stimulation of nonspecific sensory receptors results in temporal and spatial summation of pain impulses, excitatory synaptic transmission, and increased conduction of pain impulses to higher centers of the central nervous system (Hanegan 1992). As discussed by DePace and Newton (1996), a particular fallacy of the pattern theory lies in its failure to recognize the existence of specialized sensory receptors (e.g., nociceptors) that have been demonstrated histologically. It is significant to note, however, that Melzack and Wall (1965) acknowledged the concept of spatiotemporal summation and proposed that large-diameter A fiber input normally acts to prevent summation of noxious impulses conducted by small-diameter A-delta and C fibers.

Gate Control Theory

Perceived deficiencies in the specificity theory and the pattern theory as singular, uni-dimensional pain mechanisms led to development of the gate control theory, first reported by Melzack and Wall (1965). The gate control theory embraces certain principles inherent in earlier pain theories (e.g., sensory receptor specificity, spatiotemporal summation) but proposes additional, multidimensional mechanisms of pain modulation. Although the gate control theory has attracted widespread attention as a basis for pain management, it has not been universally accepted as a complete, technically correct pain theory. As noted by Kelly (1985), several experimental studies have failed to substantiate some of its claims. Nevertheless, the gate control theory is credited for its recognition of pain as a multidimensional cognitive, emotional, and behavioral experience rather than a purely sensory phenomenon. Despite considerable scientific scrutiny and historical debate, the central tenets of the gate control theory remain among the most frequently cited explanations for the efficacy of physical agents in pain management, especially electrical stimulation (e.g., transcutaneous electrical nerve stimulation). The neural structures depicted in figure 4.14 provide the basis for explanation of the gate control theory.

Hanegan (1992) noted that the primary neuroanatomy of the gate control mechanism includes the *substantia gelatinosa* located in the dorsal horn of the spinal cord and *transmission cells* (T cells) that conduct pain impulses to higher centers of the central nervous system. The substantia gelatinosa has been identified as Rexed's lamina II of the dorsal horn (Martin 1996), although some authors have implicated lamina I (DePace and Newton 1996) (see figure 4.7). A central tenet of the original gate control theory is that the substantia gelatinosa is the site of excitatory or inhibitory synaptic transmission of nerve impulses conducted by afferent nerve fibers (first order neurons) to ascending second order neurons in the spinal cord. The transmission cells, or T cells, referred to by Melzack and Wall (1965) represent second order neurons (i.e., the spinothalamic tracts) (DePace and Newton 1996). According to the gate control theory, transmission of pain impulses is determined by the balance of neural input from large-diameter A afferent nerve fibers on one hand and small-diameter A-delta and C afferent nerve fibers on the other hand. Input from large-diameter A fibers, in effect, inhibits synaptic transmission from small-diameter A-delta and C fibers, thus "closing the gate" to pain impulses. As depicted in figure 4.14, synaptic inhibition of nerve impulses from A-delta and C afferent pain fibers occurs through a small intervening interneuron in the dorsal horn. Synaptic inhibition at this level blocks

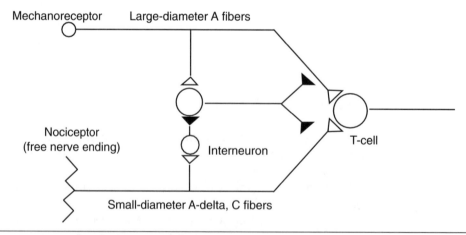

Figure 4.14   Theoretical basis of the gate control theory. The solid block triangles represent inhibitory synapses. Excitatory synapses are represented by the open triangles.

Adapted, by permission, from J.L. Hanegan, 1992, Principles of nociception. In *Electrotherapy in rehabilitation*, edited by M.R. Gersh (Philadelphia: F.A. Davis), 27.

transmission to second order neurons (spinothalamic tracts) that otherwise would relay pain impulses to the brain. Excitatory synaptic transmission from the large-diameter A fibers, however, permits conduction of nonnoxious nerve impulses through ascending spinal cord pathways (Hanegan 1992). Whereas the gate control theory implicates the substantia gelatinosa as the primary site of inhibitory synaptic transmission of pain impulses to ascending spinal cord tracts, it has been suggested that similar "gating" mechanisms may operate in other layers of the dorsal horn (DePace and Newton 1996).

In simplistic terms, the central tenet of the gate control theory is that a nonpainful stimulus can block the transmission of a noxious stimulus. Thus, the clinical significance of this concept lies in the use of various physical agents (e.g., heat, electricity) to apply a nonnoxious stimulus to large-diameter A fibers. Hence, nonnoxious nerve impulses are conducted rapidly to the spinal cord where they stimulate the inhibitory interneuron in the dorsal horn. Clinical stimulation of the inhibitory interneuron, in turn, decreases neural input to the transmission cells (T cells), thus overriding or blocking transmission of pain stimuli (Donley and Denegar 1990). Without this inhibitory mechanism, noxious impulses reaching the spinal cord via small-diameter A-delta and C fibers would be allowed to ascend through the spinal cord to the thalamus and, subsequently, to the primary somatosensory cortex where pain perception occurs.

Descending Pain Inhibitory Systems

Discussion in previous sections of this chapter has focused on pain control through inhibition of neural impulses conducted by afferent nerve fibers and ascending spinal cord pathways. Neurophysiological rationale for pain management also incorporates concepts involving descending pain inhibitory pathways that originate in the brain stem and project to the spinal cord. In this regard, Martin (1996) refers to a *descending pain inhibitory system*. Because the neural pathways in this system originate from a central anatomical region (i.e., the brain stem), pain control through descending inhibitory systems has also been referred to as *centrifugal pain control* (DePace and Newton 1996). It is significant to note that the gate control theory proposed by Melzack and Wall (1965) allows for pain modulation through descending, as well as ascending, spinal cord pathways (see figure 4.6). These investigators proposed the existence of a "central control trigger" that activates selective brain processes to exert control over afferent sensory input. Modification of the original gate control theory proposed that central biasing mechanisms operating at higher levels of the central nervous system inhibit conduction of pain impulses when these mechanisms are activated by intense somatosensory stimulation (Gaupp, Flinn, and Weddige 1994).

Although descending pain inhibitory pathways also originate from higher regions of the brain, those that descend from the brain stem are most relevant to the use of physical agents in pain management. Clinical intervention for pain control that focuses on the descending pain inhibitory system necessitates an understanding of two primary brain stem structures. These two structures are the *periaqueductal gray matter* (PAG), which surrounds the central aqueduct (canal) of the midbrain, and the *raphe nuclei*, specialized groups of nerve cells in the pons and medulla. Figure 4.15 represents a schematic illustration of the descending pain inhibitory pathways from the PAG and the raphe nuclei. Experimental investigations and clinical observation have demonstrated pain control through electrical stimulation of the PAG directly (i.e., by surgical electrode implantation) or indirectly through stimulation of peripheral afferent nerve fibers with surface electrodes (North 1994). Although the spinothalamic tract is a significant pain pathway in the anterolateral system, not all components of the anterolateral system project directly to the thalamus. Projection of the spinomesencephalic tract to the PAG in the midbrain provides an ascending neural pathway through which the PAG can be stimulated by afferent (sensory) nerve stimulation, thereby providing a mechanism through which descending pain inhibitory systems can be activated (Martin 1996).

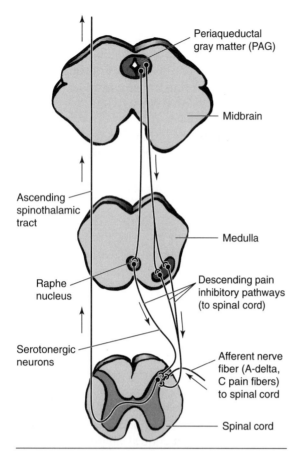

Figure 4.15   Descending pain inhibitory pathways.

Adapted from S.G. Waxman and J. deGroot, 1995, *Correlative neuroanatomy*, 22nd ed. (Norwalk, Connecticut: Appleton & Lange), 209. Reproduced with the permission of The McGraw-Hill Companies.

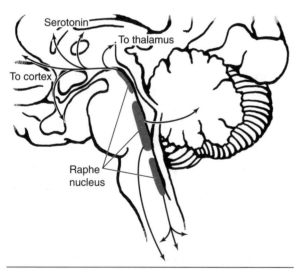

Figure 4.16   Anatomical location of the raphe nuclei in the brain stem. Note the release of serotonin, an inhibitory neurotransmitter.

Adapted from J.H. Martin, 1996, *Neuroanatomy*, 2nd ed. (Stamford, Connecticut: Appleton & Lange), 87. Reproduced with the permission of The McGraw-Hill Companies.

In the descending pain inhibitory system, stimulation of the PAG is commonly thought to suppress synaptic transmission of afferent pain impulses in the dorsal horn of the spinal cord through two primary mechanisms. These mechanisms include (1) release of inhibitory neurotransmitters from the raphe nuclei (e.g., serotonin) and (2) release of endogenous drug-like opioids (Ganong 1995; Martin 1996). Discussion of these mechanisms as separate entities is not meant to imply the existence of unrelated descending pain inhibitory systems. On the contrary, they most likely coexist as integrated, complementary systems.

In the first mechanism, stimulation of the PAG, which projects neurons to the raphe nuclei, activates the release of *serotonin*, an inhibitory neurotransmitter (figure 4.16). Descending serotonergic neurons from the raphe nuclei, in turn, project to the dorsal horn of the spinal cord (see figure 4.15). As noted by Waxman and deGroot (1995), these descending serotonergic neurons terminate in laminae I and V, which also represent the termination sites of afferent nociceptive nerve fibers (i.e., A-delta and C fibers). Thus, it has been proposed that serotonin inhibits synaptic transmission of pain impulses from these afferent pain fibers to ascending spinal cord pathways (i.e., spinothalamic tracts) (DePace and Newton 1996). Martin (1996) noted the role of descending serotonergic projections of the spinal cord in inhibition of nociceptive impulses originating from afferent nerve fibers. Although serotonin is widely recognized as an inhibitory neurotransmitter in descending pain control systems, gamma-aminobutyric acid (GABA) has also been identified as a major inhibitory neurotransmitter in the central nervous system (Hanegan 1992; Solomon 1994).

The second mechanism of descending pain control resulting from PAG stimulation involves the release of natural drug-like opioids (Martin 1996). These opioids, which represent a group of neuropeptides with known analgesic properties, have been found in many regions of the brain and spinal cord. Thus, they are referred to as *endogenous opioids*. As noted by Ganong (1995), at least 18 active opioid peptides have been identified. Endogenous opioids most commonly associated with descending pain inhibitory systems include *enkephalins* and *endorphins*, particularly *beta-endorphin*. When released, these morphine-like opioids bind to specific receptors found in high concentration in the dorsal horn of the spinal cord. Although the exact mechanisms are somewhat unclear, endogenous opioids are considered inhibitory neurotransmitters that function to suppress synaptic transmission of pain impulses in the dorsal horn. Evidence exists that activation of this mechanism occurs through descending neural projections from the PAG (Ganong 1995; Waxman and deGroot 1995). The analgesic effect of endogenous opioids has been attributed to their ability to inhibit release of substance P, an excitatory neurotransmitter, from the presynaptic membrane of afferent nociceptive C fibers in the dorsal horn of the spinal cord (Solomon 1994).

Therapeutic Strategies and Techniques

Authorities generally agree that perception of pain is a multifaceted experience that has emotional and psychological, as well as physical, dimensions. On this premise, effective pain control in the management of sports injuries may be most effectively accomplished through a multidimensional approach. Most commonly, sports health care clinicians are confronted by patients with acute, rather than chronic, pain. Traditionally, acute pain management in the sports population has been characterized by the use of physical agents and pharmacologic agents. More recently, however, the value of psychological intervention in acute pain management has been recognized. Given these considerations, a comprehensive approach to the management of pain and muscle spasm may include the complementary use of (1) physical agents, (2) pharmacologic agents, and (3) psychological intervention.

Physical Agents

Because pain and muscle spasm represent a reciprocal cycle of clinical manifestations, therapeutic intervention may rationally focus on relief of pain, alleviation of muscle spasm, or both. Recognized principles of musculoskeletal tissue innervation and prevailing pain theories provide rationale for the use of a wide range of physical agents in the management of pain and muscle spasm. Cryotherapy, thermotherapy, electrotherapy, massage, and therapeutic exercise have all been used with varying degrees of success.

Based on theories associated with the "gating" mechanisms of pain control, clinical application of a nonnoxious stimulus that is of greater intensity than the noxious stimulus is a primary consideration in the use of physical agents for pain management. Pain relief occurs because the stronger nonnoxious stimulus is preferentially selected for transmission to the brain via large-diameter A fibers (Griffen and Karselis 1979). Granting the validity of this premise, the key to effective intervention appears to be the judicious selection of appropriate therapeutic dosages, regardless of the specific physical agent. Application of appropriate therapeutic stimuli is consistent with the concept of counterirritation in which the stronger, nonnoxious effects of physical agents (i.e., thermal, electrical, mechanical agents) counteract the "irritant," or mild to moderate pain (Griffen and Karselis 1979; Starkey 1993). As indicated by Hall (1994), however, ordinarily nonnoxious stimuli can become noxious, pain-producing stimuli if the intensity surpasses a certain threshold (e.g., extremes of heat and cold). Thus, persistent use of physical agents that provoke a painful response is counterproductive and inconsistent with appropriate therapeutic management.

Another guide to selection of appropriate therapeutic dosages is discussed by Donley and Denegar (1990), who noted that receptor *adaptation* to repeated or prolonged stimuli may occur. For example, thermoreceptors may accommodate and become less sensitive to the application of superficial heating modalities during the treatment regimen, thus reducing transmission of nonnoxious thermal stimuli with less inhibition of noxious, painful stimuli. Although the clinician's seemingly logical response to this phenomenon might be to increase the intensity of the thermal stimuli to effect pain relief, care must be taken to avoid dosages that exceed the critical threshold of intensity and become noxious stimuli. Assurance of intact sensory pathways and the patient's perception of pain thus become essential guides to selection of appropriate therapeutic dosages.

Pain and muscle spasm are complications that typically overlap in time with the early vascular and cellular responses to tissue injury. Consequently, selection of physical agents that may have positive effects on control of pain and muscle spasm must be weighed against their potential adverse effects on vascular and cellular responses during the first three or four days after injury. For example, rationale exists for the use of superficial or deep heat for pain control and reduction of muscle spasm (Griffen and Karselis 1979). On the other hand, increased tissue temperature leads to increased capillary hydrostatic pressure, increased vascular permeability, and edema (Fischer and Solomon 1965). Given these considerations, selection of physical agents for pain control and reduction of muscle spasm is not only a matter of selecting appropriate therapeutic modalities and dosages but also a matter of judicious timing. Traditional approaches to the management of pain and muscle spasm include the use of cryotherapy, thermotherapy, and electrotherapy.

Cryotherapy

Although rationale for the use of physical agents in the management of pain and muscle spasm is commonly attributed to basic concepts inherent in the "gating" mechanisms of pain control, the effect of some modalities may also be explained by related mechanisms or other modes of action. For example, the efficacy of cold as an analgesic agent is commonly attributed to its ability to affect sensory or motor nerve conduction velocity (VonNieda and Michlovitz 1996). Clinical research has demonstrated the sensitivity of peripheral sensory receptors to cold, which, when applied in appropriate dosages, lowers nerve tissue temperature and decreases nerve conduction velocity. Hence, transmission of nociceptive impulses from peripheral sensory receptors via afferent neurons is inhibited or even blocked. Slowing of nerve conduction velocity also offers a reasonable explanation for relaxation of skeletal muscle spasm that results from excessive muscle spindle activity. As summarized by VonNieda and Michlovitz (1996), cold applications may reduce muscle spasm through two primary mechanisms: (1) decreased conduction velocity of Type Ia or Type II afferent (sensory) neurons that originate in the intrafusal fibers of the muscle spindle or (2) decreased conduction velocity of efferent gamma motor neurons that transmit motor impulses to the contractile portions of the intrafusal fibers (see figure 4.13). Either of these mechanisms disrupts the monosynaptic arc in the spinal cord that mediates reflex muscle contraction.

Thermotherapy

Although the exact mechanisms are somewhat unclear, the effectiveness of thermal agents in the management of pain and muscle spasm has been observed clinically. Stimulation of thermoreceptors by nonnoxious dosages of external heat that overrides the transmission of pain impulses is consistent with the gate control theory and the concept of counterirritation (Fischer and Solomon 1965). Thermal agents used in the management of somatic pain and muscle spasm include both superficial-heating modalities (e.g., hot packs) and deep-heating modalities (e.g., shortwave diathermy, microwave diathermy, ultrasound). Although superficial-heating modalities do not affect deep tissues directly, stimulation of thermoreceptors in the skin has been shown to be effective in the relief of pain and muscle spasm (Stillwell 1965). Shortwave diathermy, microwave diathermy, and ultrasound have been used to stimulate thermoreceptors in deep tissues (Prentice 1990; Santiesteban 1990).

In addition to stimulation of thermoreceptors, thermal agents may have a direct effect on reduction of muscle spasm through alteration of muscle spindle activity, thus further contributing to disruption of the pain-spasm-pain cycle. Muscle spindles are the mechanoreceptors responsible for normal muscle tone through continual efferent impulses to intrafusal muscle fibers via gamma motor neurons. Excessive muscle spindle activity, however, produces a state of hypertonus, or muscle spasm. As proposed by Fischer and Solomon (1965), increasing tissue temperature decreases gamma motor neuron firing, thereby decreasing muscle spindle activity. To the extent that externally applied heat has this effect, the sustained state of hypertonus, or increased tension, associated with muscle spasm is reduced. As explained by Rennie and Michlovitz (1996), tissue temperature elevation increases firing of Type Ib afferent (sensory) fibers from Golgi tendon organs (see chapter 8, figure 8.5), thereby initiating an inhibitory reflex arc in the spinal cord (see chapter 8, figure 8.6). As a result, efferent (motor) nerve conduction to the contractile fibers of the muscle spindle is reduced, thereby allowing relaxation of the spasmodic muscle (see figure 4.13).

Electrotherapy

As noted by North (1994), impetus to the use of electrical nerve stimulation for pain management was provided by publication of the gate control theory in 1965. During the late 1960s, the term *stimulation analgesia* emerged to describe the effect of electrical stimulation through surgical implantation of electrodes in the brain (e.g., the periaqueductal gray matter) or the spinal cord. Originally, externally applied devices that produced *transcutaneous electrical nerve stimulation* (TENS) were used to screen chronic pain patients as potential candidates for electrode implantation. As observed by practicing clinicians, however, pain was successfully controlled in a significant number of patients with the use of TENS alone (North 1994). Hence, TENS emerged as an effective approach to pain management, including the clinical management of acute and subacute pain associated with various sport-related musculoskeletal injuries.

Since the 1960s, a number of electrical devices and clinical approaches to pain management have been developed. Collectively, rationale for these techniques is based on prevailing theoretical models of pain modulation, notably the proposed "gating" mechanisms and descending pain inhibitory systems. As noted by DePace and Newton (1996), suppression of pain through descending neural tracts may be opiate mediated or nonopiate mediated. Several peripheral nerve electrical stimulation techniques have been used to activate the pain modulation mechanisms inherent in these pain theories, with various degrees of success. Snyder-Mackler (1995) noted that peripheral nerve stimulation techniques fall into four general categories. These categories, as depicted in figure 4.17, include (1) subsensory stimulation (i.e., microcurrent electrical nerve stimulation, or MENS), (2) sensory-level stimulation (i.e., conventional TENS), (3) motor-level stimulation (e.g., acupuncture-like TENS), and (4) noxious-level stimulation. Authorities commonly note an absence of clinical or scientific evidence to support the efficacy of electrical stimulation below sensory levels in pain management, such as that used in MENS (Snyder-Mackler 1995; Stralka 1992). The remaining three levels of peripheral nerve stimulation, however, have demonstrated effectiveness in the management of musculoskeletal pain.

Sensory-level stimulation, which involves electrical stimulation at or above the sensory level but below the motor threshold, is exemplified by the use of conventional TENS. Conventional TENS is the most widely used electrical stimulation technique for pain control in sport-related musculoskeletal injuries. Based primarily on neural mechanisms inherent in the gate control theory, conventional TENS employs low-frequency, nonnoxious electrical stimulation of large-diameter afferent A fibers (i.e., A-alpha and A-beta fibers) through the application of surface electrodes, either at the site of pain or on segmentally

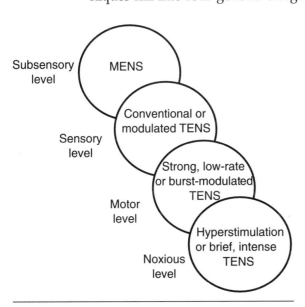

Figure 4.17 Electroanalgesic stimulation methods with corresponding intensity levels.

Adapted, by permission, from L. Snyder-Mackler, 1995, Electrical stimulation for pain modulation. In *Clinical electrophysiology: Electrotherapy and electrophysiologic testing*, 2nd ed. Edited by A.J. Robinson and L. Snyder-Mackler (Baltimore, MD: Lippincott, Williams and Wilkins), 292.

related dermatomes. As the result of afferent A fiber stimulation, analgesia is thought to result from synaptic inhibition, or "gating," of pain impulses in the dorsal horn of the spinal cord. Although other potential sites of synaptic inhibition exist, the substantia gelatinosa has traditionally been implicated as the site of pain modulation through the use of conventional TENS. Peripheral nerve stimulation through the use of conventional TENS produces a comfortable state of mild paresthesia during application. This effect usually does not extend for a significant period of time beyond the duration of the treatment session, however. Thus, conventional TENS units have been designed for prolonged application during activities of daily living. Accommodation of afferent (sensory) nerve fibers to prolonged stimulation is sometimes observed, but can be accounted for by manual or automatic adjustment of stimulation variables such as pulse width, frequency, or intensity (Santiesteban 1990).

The use of *noninvasive electroacupuncture*, or *acupuncture-like TENS*, represents motor-level electrical stimulation, which by definition is capable of evoking a visible muscle contraction as well as a sensory response (Snyder-Mackler 1995). In comparison to conventional TENS, acupuncture-like TENS is more directly associated with pain management through descending pain inhibitory systems. Modified TENS units equipped with small electrodes referred to as *point stimulators* are used to provide high-intensity stimulation of acupuncture points, trigger points, or localized painful areas. These techniques are thought to activate the release of endogenous opioids in the brain stem. As previously discussed, opioid-mediated pain modulation is theoretically associated with electrical stimulation of the periaqueductal gray matter (Gaupp, Flinn, and Weddige 1994). Some authors have suggested that transcutaneous electroanalgesia resulting from endogenous opioid release is best accomplished by intense electrical stimulation of acupuncture points, although trigger points are also used (Prentice 1990). In contrast to conventional TENS, the analgesic effect of acupuncture-like electrical stimulation typically lasts for an extended period of time following the treatment session, perhaps supporting endogenous opioid release as a prime mechanism of pain modulation (Snyder-Mackler 1995). In some clinical settings, electroacupuncture is used in conjunction with conventional TENS for relief of musculoskeletal pain (Santiesteban 1990).

Although infrequently used in the management of sports injuries, noxious-level stimulation represents a third approach to pain management. Also referred to as *brief intense TENS*, this technique involves painful point stimulation of small-diameter pain fibers, either at the site of pain or on acupuncture points, trigger points, or motor points. Commonly, these techniques produce pain modulation referred to as *hyperstimulation analgesia*. As noted by Snyder-Mackler (1995), analgesia produced by noxious-level, brief intense TENS is believed to be associated with systemic release of endogenous opioids. Thus, this type of electrotherapy is associated with descending pain inhibitory systems.

Pharmacologic Agents

Pharmacologic agents used to control the pain-spasm-pain cycle may focus on pain control, relief of muscle spasm, or both. The two basic categories of drugs used for control of pain and muscle spasm are (1) analgesics and (2) skeletal muscle relaxants. In some medications, drugs with analgesic and muscle-relaxation properties are combined to form a compound, a pharmaceutical product that contains the ingredients of both drug types.

Analgesic drugs

The array of drugs available for pain management have been classified generally as *opioid analgesics* and *nonopioid analgesics* (Ciccone 1990). Referred to historically as *narcotic analgesics*, exogenous opioid analgesics represent a group of morphine-like medications used to treat moderate or severe pain. Because of their potential to produce physical or psychological dependence and their propensity for abuse, these drugs are categorized as controlled substances in the United States. Although many opioid analgesics are available to the attending physician, propoxyphene hydrochloride (Darvon) is a familiar opioid analgesic sometimes used for control of mild to moderate pain in sports injury management. Codeine is another example of an opioid analgesic with mild to moderate strength (Ciccone 1990).

The effects of opioid analgesics is attributed to their ability to bind to a *drug receptor*, a nerve cell component that combines with a drug to alter cellular function, thereby inhibiting synaptic transmission of pain impulses. Drug receptors referred to as *opioid receptors* have been located in several areas of the central nervous system, including the periaqueductal gray matter in the brain stem and the dorsal horn of the spinal cord. As discussed in a previous section of this chapter, transmission of pain impulses across a chemical synapse is dependent on the presence of an excitatory neurotransmitter (e.g., substance P). Modification of synaptic transmission through the use of pharmacologic agents occurs as the result of alteration in the quantity of a neurotransmitter released from the presynaptic terminal, altered stimulation of the postsynaptic receptor, or both (Ciccone 1990). Pain relief associated with the use of opioid analgesics, for example, has been attributed to inhibited release of substance P from the presynaptic terminal of nociceptive afferent neurons in the spinal cord (Solomon 1994) as well as interactions that occur between opioid analgesics and opioid receptors on the postsynaptic membrane (Ciccone 1990). The inhibitory effect of opioid analgesics on synaptic transmission of pain impulses is depicted in figure 4.18.

Although opioid analgesics are sometimes indicated in the management of sports injuries, nonopioid analgesics, which include nonsteroidal anti-inflammatory drugs (NSAIDs) and acetaminophen, are more commonly used. The various categories of NSAIDs are summarized in table 4.1. Because nonopioid analgesics lack the narcotic side effects of opioid analgesics (e.g. sedation), their use is typically more compatible with other methods of therapeutic intervention in sports injury management. Control of vascular permeability due to inhibition of prostaglandin production represents an anti-inflammatory effect of NSAIDs. Certain prostaglandins also act to increase the sensitivity of nociceptors to other pain-producing chemicals (e.g., bradykinin). Consequently, decreased synthesis of prostaglandins provides rationale for the use of NSAIDs in the control of mild or moderate pain. Acetylsalicylic acid, or aspirin, is one of the most commonly used anti-inflammatory and analgesic drugs. Like other NSAIDs, aspirin inhibits synthesis of prostaglandins, thereby producing an analgesic effect (Ciccone 1990). Aspirin, however, has a prolonged anticoagulation effect. Consequently, the use of aspirin may be contraindicated until hemostasis has been established.

A simple analgesic sometimes substituted for NSAIDs, including aspirin, is acetaminophen (e.g., Tylenol). Acetaminophen has analgesic properties similar to those of NSAIDs and aspirin but lacks significant anti-inflammatory and anticoagulant effects. In contrast to NSAIDs, platelet aggregation, which is essential to formation of the temporary platelet plug in primary hemostasis, is thought to be unaffected by acetaminophen (Ciccone 1990). Consequently, the side effects commonly associated with

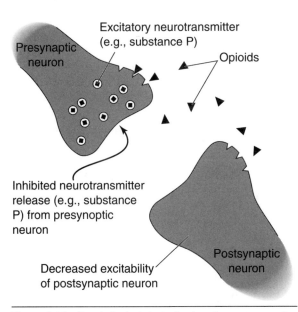

Figure 4.18 Psychological strategies in pain management.
Adapted, by permission, from C.D. Ciccone, 1990, *Pharmacology in rehabilitation* (Philadelphia: F.A. Davis), 184.

NSAIDs and aspirin (e.g., prolonged bleeding, gastrointestinal irritation) are avoided with the use of acetaminophen (Abramson 1990).

Skeletal muscle relaxants

Management of the pain-spasm-pain cycle has been approached through the use of drugs referred to collectively as *skeletal muscle relaxants*. Skeletal muscle relaxants are classified generally as centrally acting drugs that exert their primary effects at the spinal cord level or peripherally acting drugs that affect skeletal muscle cells directly (Ciccone 1990). Although muscle relaxants are also indicated in the treatment of spasticity, a condition characterized by an exaggerated stretch reflex resulting from central nervous system lesions, their use in the management of sports injuries is directed to relief of involuntary muscle spasm associated with the inflammatory response to tissue trauma. Most commonly, skeletal muscle relaxants used in sports injury management are centrally acting drugs. Some familiar examples of muscle relaxants are carisoprodol (e.g., Soma), chlorzoxazone (e.g., Paraflex), methocarbamol (e.g., Robaxin), and orphenadrine citrate (e.g., Norflex). In some cases, muscle relaxants are combined with analgesics such as aspirin (Norgesic Forte) and acetaminophen (Parafon Forte) to form compounds.

Although their specific mode of action is somewhat unclear, it has been suggested that centrally acting muscle relaxants inhibit reflex spinal cord activity that otherwise occurs in response to noxious stimuli, thereby decreasing excitation of efferent (motor) neurons and conduction of motor impulses to the muscle spindle (Ciccone 1990). The effect of these drugs on reduction of muscle spasm, however, is more commonly thought to be secondary to a depressant effect on the central nervous system, resulting in generalized sedation (Gallager 1994). The ability of skeletal muscle relaxants to relieve local muscle spasm without causing sedation and the potential side effects of drowsiness, dizziness, fatigue, and muscular weakness remains questionable (Ciccone 1990; Gallager 1994). Whereas generalized sedation is compatible with prescribed bed rest, its clinical manifestations may be unacceptable to an injured but otherwise healthy student athlete who must continue academic studies and maintain compliance with rehabilitation programs. Furthermore, the characteristic side effects associated with prolonged use of skeletal muscle relaxants are generally incompatible with optimal sports performance.

Psychological Intervention

Historically, research and psychological intervention in pain management have focused on the management of chronic pain. In more recent years, however, psychological intervention in the management of acute pain has received increased attention. For the most part, the comparatively short-term nature of most sports injuries presents a challenge of acute pain control, rather than chronic pain management. Typically, sports health care providers have relied on pharmacologic and physical agents to meet this challenge. With the emergence of sports psychologists, however, psychological intervention in the control of acute pain has added another dimension to the management of sports injuries. In selected cases, sports psychologists who have a special interest and training in acute pain control may be called upon for intervention. In other cases, the sports psychologist may function as a consultant to physicians, certified athletic trainers, and other sports health care clinicians who can effectively implement psychological approaches to acute pain management on a day-to-day basis.

Psychologists generally agree that the perception of pain is a subjective experience influenced not only by physical factors (i.e., the type and extent of tissue trauma) but also by a multitude of psychological and social variables (Hanegan 1992). Consequently, wide variations exist among athletes in the way they respond to pain experiences. Despite individual variations, however, reactions to acute pain commonly involve characteristic behavioral, cognitive, and emotional responses. All of these variables may be affected by the acute pain experience (Gill 1992). For example, the physically detrimental effects of behavioral responses including general inactivity, avoidance of certain body movements, and altered gait patterns are familiar to the experienced sports health care clinician. Acute pain experiences may also influence cognitive processes associated with concentration, memory, problem solving, and decision making. Alterations in these cognitive processes may have a significant detrimental affect on a student athlete's academic performance (Gill 1992). Although fear and anxiety are among the most common emotional responses to acute pain, other reactions may include frustration, anger, and depression (Diamond and Conian 1991; Gill 1992). Sports health care providers should realize that the characteristic emotional responses to pain may be intensified in a highly competitive athlete who perceives a loss of control due to forced inactivity, especially as related to his or her status as a team member.

Although this chapter is focused on the use of physical and pharmacologic agents for pain control, a brief review of psychological strategies should alert the sports health care clinician to the benefits of psychological intervention in acute pain management. A fundamental factor affecting a patient's response to pain, and thus the success of intervention techniques, is the individual's perception of control over his or her health status. Individuals who believe that they can exert control over their health status through their own behavior are said to have an "internal health locus of control." Most likely, a patient with an internal health locus of control will assume a comparatively active role in his or her pain management. In contrast, other individuals may become passive participants, believing that they have little or no personal control over their pain. For example, athletes who believe that their health status is controlled only by fate or by other individuals (e.g., the physician or certified athletic trainer) are described as having an "external health locus of control" (Gill 1992; Peck 1986).

Regardless of individual beliefs and attitudes toward pain, psychological intervention is designed to enhance a patient's sense of control over his or her pain (Peck 1986). Although several psychological strategies for pain management have been developed, those that appear to be most applicable to acute pain management in the sports setting include *psychological support* and *coping skills training* (Diamond and Conian 1991; Gill 1992). These approaches are summarized in figure 4.19. As described by Gill (1992), psychological support involves reassurance provided through the interaction of trained personnel with the patient. As applied to the sports scene, reassurance by trained personnel includes encouragement and support provided by team physicians, certified athletic trainers, and other sports health care clinicians. Peck (1986) noted that psychological support includes development of effective patient-therapist relationships that facilitate expression and reflection of the patient's feelings, reinforcement of coping efforts, and encouragement of the patient's active role in the recovery process.

Coping skills training refers to teaching patients specific techniques and behaviors to enable them to cope with their pain experience. For the most part, these techniques are taught by trained professionals in selected cases where pain is a major problem. Teaching

---

Psychological support

- Reflection of patient's feelings
- Reassurance that anxieties are normal
- Reinforcement of copying efforts
- Encouragement of active participation
  (in recovery process)

Coping skills training (cognitive therapy)

- Imagery
- Distraction
- Relaxation training

Figure 4.19 Psychological strategies in pain management.

coping strategies designed to alter the patient's appraisal of painful stimuli or to divert their attention away from pain is referred to as *cognitive therapy* (Peck 1986). Specific strategies commonly include *imagery*, *distraction*, and *relaxation training*. Imagery involves focusing attention on an image that is emotionally incompatible with pain (e.g., an enjoyable event in the patient's life or a pleasant sensation such as warm sunshine or a cool breeze). Distraction, or attention diversion, encourages patients to divert their attention away from pain to activities that demand their attention (e.g., hobbies, social activities). Some authorities consider imagery to be an attention-diversion technique (Peck 1986). Relaxation training includes activities designed to reduce the tension and anxiety commonly associated with a pain experience. One technique involves teaching the patient to consciously tense and relax large muscle groups in a systematic, sequential manner. Another method involves the use of controlled breathing exercises (Diamond and Conian 1991; Gill 1992). A third approach involves mentally induced relaxation through imagery. In recent years, biofeedback has been incorporated into relaxation training to provide electromyogram (EMG) monitoring of the physiological responses to relaxation techniques (Diamond and Conian 1991; Gill 1992).

Summary

Intervention during the acute inflammatory stage of connective tissue repair may provide the sports health care clinician with the most advantageous opportunity to influence subsequent tissue-healing mechanisms. During the first three or four days after injury, the overall objective of therapeutic intervention is to optimize a favorable environment for tissue repair without interfering with normal healing mechanisms. The specific therapeutic objectives during the acute inflammatory stage of connective tissue repair are to control hemorrhage and edema (i.e., the primary inflammatory responses) and to alleviate pain and muscle spasm (i.e., the secondary inflammatory responses). These objectives represent the first two primary areas of therapeutic intervention in the management of sports injuries.

Management of the primary inflammatory responses to tissue trauma is typically accomplished through the use of physical agents, pharmacologic agents, or both. These measures are used for the specific purposes of (1) controlling hemorrhagic effusion and edema, (2) limiting secondary hypoxic injury, and (3) protecting injured tissues from undue mechanical loading. Most commonly, control of the early vascular responses to tissue trauma is accomplished through the use of cold applications, external compression, and elevation of the affected body part. In addition, limitation of movement or immobilization of the involved body part is commonly indicated. The beneficial effects of these modalities are optimized if applied as early as possible after injury. When used judiciously, nonsteroidal anti-inflammatory drugs (NSAIDs) can be an effective complement to physical agents for control of excessive inflammatory responses to tissue injury.

Pain and muscle spasm, the secondary inflammatory responses to tissue trauma, are commonly primary causes of restricted movement and limited joint motion, which may lead to loss of function in the affected body part if prolonged. Consequently, pain and muscle spasm often necessitate specific therapeutic intervention. Therapeutic strategies for management of pain and muscle spasm are based on rationale associated with the transmission of pain impulses, the neuromuscular mechanisms of the pain-spasm-pain cycle, and prevailing theories of pain and pain control. Because pain is considered an emotional, psychological, and physical experience, pain management may be most effectively accomplished through a multidimensional approach that incorporates the use of physical agents, pharmacologic agents, and psychological intervention. Cryotherapy, thermotherapy, and electrotherapy represent typical therapeutic approaches to management of the pain-spasm-pain cycle. Pharmacological intervention for pain control most commonly includes the use of analgesics, although skeletal muscle relaxants have been used for pain-related muscle spasm. Psychological strategies applicable to pain management in the sports health care setting include psychological support and coping skills training. Certified athletic trainers and team physicians who interact with injured athletes on a daily basis are in an advantageous position to provide reinforcement of coping efforts, reassurance, and encouragement. Coping skills training including imagery, distraction, and relaxation may be initiated by trained personnel and reinforced by other members of the sports health care team.

Problem-Solving Scenario

During summer vacation, a 21-year-old female college basketball player sustained a severe inversion ankle sprain approximately four weeks prior to the beginning of classes for the fall semester. Because of her summer job as a camp counselor in a sparsely populated community, she did not have ready access to a sports medicine physician. Consequently, she did not seek medical attention. Shortly after returning to campus, she reports to the athletic treatment center for advice and treatment. According to the athlete, her ankle was initially very swollen and quite painful. She also reports that she "turned her ankle again" about a week ago. A clinical assessment of the athlete's condition reveals that she continues to walk with a painful antalgic gait. Further inspection indicates moderate residual swelling and ecchymosis in the lateral aspect of her ankle. Clinical inspection also reveals a limitation in active dorsiflexion and plantar flexion with increased pain during passive inversion and plantar flexion.

Problem-Solving Questions

- What are the most likely tissue-healing mechanisms operating at this stage of the patient's recovery?
- What mechanisms offer the most plausible explanation for the patient's ankle pain at this stage of tissue healing?
- What causative factors should be considered in determination of the reason(s) for limited joint motion at this stage of recovery?
- What are the most relevant short-term treatment goals during the next two weeks of the patient's recovery period?
- What specific physical and pharmacologic agents are most appropriate for use in achievement of the short-term goals at this stage of recovery? Why?

References

Abramson, S.B. 1990. Nonsteroidal anti-inflammatory drugs: Mechanisms of action and therapeutic considerations. In *Sports-induced inflammation*, edited by W.B. Leadbetter, J.A. Buckwalter, and S.L. Gordon. Park Ridge, Ill.: American Academy of Orthopaedic Surgeons.

Baker, R.J., and G.W. Bell. 1991. The effect of therapeutic modalities on blood flow in the human calf. *Journal of Orthopaedic and Sports Physical Therapy* 13:23-27.

Behrens, T.W., and J.S. Goodwin. 1990. Oral corticosteroids. In *Sports-induced inflammation*, edited by W.B. Leadbetter, J.A. Buckwalter, and S.L. Gordon. Park Ridge, Ill.: American Academy of Orthopaedic Surgeons.

Buchanan, W.W., and K.D. Rainsford. 1990. Aspirin and nonacetylated salicylates: Use in inflammatory injuries incurred during sporting activities. In *Sports-induced inflammation*, edited by W.B. Leadbetter, J.A. Buckwalter, and S.L. Gordon. Park Ridge, Ill.: American Academy of Orthopaedic Surgeons.

Ciccone, C.D. 1990. *Pharmacology in rehabilitation*. Philadelphia: Davis.

Cotran, R.S., V. Kumar, and S.L. Robbins. 1989. *Robbins pathologic basis of disease*, 4th ed. Philadelphia: W.B. Saunders.

DePace, D.M., and R.A. Newton. 1996. Anatomic and functional aspects of pain: Evaluation and management with thermal agents. In *Thermal agents in rehabilitation*, 3rd ed., edited by S.L. Michlovitz. Philadelphia: Davis.

Diamond, A.W., and S.W. Conian. 1991. *The management of chronic pain*. New York: Oxford University Press.

Donley, P.B., and C. Denegar. 1990. Pain and mechanisms of pain relief. In *Therapeutic modalities in sports medicine*, edited by W.E. Prentice. St. Louis: Mosby.

Feuerstein, M. 1994. Definitions of pain. In *Handbook of pain management*, 2nd ed., edited by C.D. Tollison, J.R. Satterthwaite, and J.W. Tollison. Baltimore: Williams and Wilkins.

Fine, P.G. 1993. The biology of pain. In *Psychology of sport injury*, edited by J. Heil. Champaign, Ill.: Human Kinetics.

Fischer, E., and S. Solomon. 1965. Physiological responses to heat and cold. In *Therapeutic heat and cold,* 2nd ed., edited by S. Licht. New Haven, Conn.: Elizabeth Licht.

Gallager, M.R. 1994. Muscle relaxant medications. In *Handbook of pain management*, 2nd ed., edited by C.D. Tollison, J.R. Satterthwaite, and J.W. Tollison. Baltimore: Williams and Wilkins.

Ganong, W.F. 1995. *Review of medical physiology*, 17th ed. Norwalk, Conn.: Appleton and Lange.

Gaupp, L.A., D.E. Flinn, and R.L. Weddige. 1994. Adjunct treatment techniques. In *Handbook of pain management*, 2nd ed., edited by C.D. Tollison, J.R. Satterthwaite, and J.W. Tollison. Baltimore: Williams and Wilkins.

Gill, K.M. 1992. Psychological aspects of acute pain. In *Acute pain, mechanisms and management*, edited by R.S. Sinatra, A.H. Hord, B. Ginsberg, and L.M. Preble. St. Louis: Mosby-Year Book.

Griffen, J.E., and T.C. Karselis. 1979. *Physical agents for physical therapists*. Springfield, Ill.: Charles C. Thomas.

Hall, J.L. 1994. Anatomy of pain. In *Handbook of pain management*, 2nd ed., edited by C.D. Tollison, J.R. Satterthwaite, and J.W. Tollison. Baltimore: Williams and Wilkins.

Hanegan, J.L. 1992. Principles of nociception. In *Electrotherapy in rehabilitation*, edited by M.R. Gersh. Philadelphia: Davis.

Hargreaves, K.M. 1990. Mechanism of pain sensation resulting from inflammation. In *Sports-induced inflammation*, edited by W.B. Leadbetter, J.A. Buckwalter, and S.L. Gordon. Park Ridge, Ill.: American Academy of Orthopaedic Surgeons.

Kandel, E.R., J.H. Schwartz, and T.M. Jessell, eds. 1995. *Essentials of neural science and behavior*. Norwalk, Conn.: Appleton and Lange.

Kellett, J. 1986. Acute soft tissue injuries—A review of the literature. *Medicine and Science in Sports and Exercise* 18:489-99.

Kelly, D.D. 1985. Central representations of pain and analgesia. In *Principles of neural science*, 2nd ed., edited by E.R. Kandel and J.H. Schwartz. New York: Elsevier Science Publishing Company.

Knight, K.L. 1990. Cold as a modifier of sports-induced inflammation. In *Sports-induced inflammation*, edited by W.B. Leadbetter, J.A. Buckwalter, and S.L. Gordon. Park Ridge, Ill.: American Academy of Orthopaedic Surgeons.

Koester, M.C. 1993. An overview of the physiology and pharmacology of aspirin and nonsteroidal anti-inflammatory drugs. *Journal of Athletic Training* 28:252-59.

Leadbetter, W.B. 1990. An introduction to sports-induced soft-tissue inflammation. In *Sports-induced inflammation*, edited by W.B. Leadbetter, J.A. Buckwalter, and S.L. Gordon. Park Ridge, Ill.: American Academy of Orthopaedic Surgeons.

Martin, J.H. 1996. *Neuroanatomy*, 2nd ed. Stamford, Conn.: Appleton and Lange.

Melzack, R., and P.D. Wall. 1965. Pain mechanisms: A new theory. *Science* 150:971-79.

North, R.B. 1994. Neural stimulation techniques for chronic pain. In *Handbook of pain management*, 2nd ed., edited by C.D. Tollison, J.R. Satterthwaite, and J.W. Tollison. Baltimore: Williams and Wilkins.

Peck, C.L. 1986. Physiological factors in acute pain management. In *Acute pain management*, edited by M.F. Cousins and G.D. Phillips. New York: Churchill Livingstone.

Prentice, W.E. 1990. *Therapeutic modalities in sports medicine*. St. Louis: Mosby.

Rennie, G.A., and S.L. Michlovitz. 1996. Biophysical principles of healing and superficial heating agents. In *Thermal agents in rehabilitation*, 3rd ed., edited by S.L. Michlovitz. Philadelphia: Davis.

Rowinski, M.J. 1997. Neurobiology for orthopedic and sports physical therapy. In *Orthopedic and sports physical therapy*, 3rd ed., edited by T.R. Malone, T.G. McPoil, and A.J. Nitz. St. Louis: Mosby-Year Book.

Rucinski, T.J., D.N. Hooker, W.E. Prentice, E.W. Shields, and D.J. Cote-Murray. 1991. The effects of intermittent compression on edema in postacute ankle sprains. *Journal of Sports Physical Therapy* 14:65-69.

Santiesteban, A.J. 1990. Physical agents and musculoskeletal pain. In *Orthopaedic and sports physical therapy*, 2nd ed., edited by J.A. Gould III. St. Louis: Mosby.

Snyder-Mackler, L. 1995. Electrical stimulation for pain modulation. In *Clinical electrophysiology: Electrotherapy and electrophysiologic testing*, 2nd ed., edited by A.J. Robinson and L. Snyder-Mackler. Baltimore: Williams and Wilkins.

Solomon, G.D. 1994. Analgesic medications. In *Handbook of pain management*, 2nd ed., edited by C.D. Tollison, J.R. Satterthwaite, and J.W. Tollison. Baltimore: Williams and Wilkins.

Stankus, S.J. 1993. Inflammation and the role of anti-inflammatory medications. In *Handbook of sports medicine*, edited by W.A. Lillegard and K.S. Rucker. Boston: Butterworth-Heineman.

Starkey, C. 1993. *Therapeutic modalities.* Philadelphia: Davis.

Stillwell, G.K. 1965. General principles of thermotherapy. In *Therapeutic heat and cold*, 2nd ed., edited by S. Licht. New Haven, Conn.: Elizabeth Licht.

Stralka, S.W. 1992. Application of therapeutic electrical currents in the management of the orthopedic patient. In *Electrotherapy in rehabilitation*, edited by M.R. Gersh. Philadelphia: Davis.

Tortora, G.J., and S.R. Grabowski. 1993. *Principles of anatomy and physiology*, 7th ed. New York: Harper Collins College Publishers.

VonNieda, K., and S.L. Michlovitz. 1996. Cryotherapy. In *Thermal agents in rehabilitation*, 3rd ed., edited by S.L. Michlovitz. Philadelphia: Davis.

Walder, G.I., and B. Hainline. 1989. *Drugs and the athlete.* Philadelphia: Davis.

Waxman, S.G., and J. deGroot. 1995. *Correlative neuroanatomy*, 22nd ed. Norwalk, Conn.: Appleton and Lange.

Weisberg, J. 1994. Pain. In *Physical agents*, edited by B. Hecox, T.A. Mehreteab, and J. Weisberg. Norwalk, Conn.: Appleton and Lange.

Wilkerson, G.B. 1991. Treatment of the inversion ankle sprain through synchronous application of focal compression and cold. *Athletic Training* 26:220-37.

Therapeutic Implications: Scar Formation and Maturation

CHAPTER 5

Enhancement of Connective Tissue Repair
- Pharmacologic Agents
- Thermotherapy
- Mechanical Ultrasound
  - *Mechanical Phenomena*
  - *Physiological Responses*
- Electrotherapy

Prevention of Contractures and Adhesions
- Connective Tissue Immobilization
  - *Contractures*
  - *Adhesions*
- Therapeutic Strategies
  - *Continuous Passive Motion*
  - *Modified Immobilization and Protected Mobilization*
  - *Functional Electrical Muscle Stimulation*

Enhancement of Scar Tissue Structure and Function
- Principles of Therapeutic Tensile Loading
- Tissue Immobilization and Tensile Loading
  - *Effects of Immobilization*
  - *Effects of Tensile Loading*
- Biomechanics of Tensile Loading and Plastic Stretch
- Therapeutic Strategies and Techniques
  - *Low-Load, Prolonged Stretching*
  - *Proprioceptive Neuromuscular Facilitation*
  - *Joint Mobilization*
  - *Functional Tissue Loading*

Summary

Learning Objectives

After completion of this chapter, the reader should be able to

1. identify the three primary therapeutic objectives associated with connective tissue scar formation and scar maturation,
2. identify appropriate therapeutic agents for enhancement of connective tissue repair and describe the therapeutic rationale for each,
3. describe the pathological basis for development of soft tissue contractures and adhesions,
4. identify appropriate therapeutic agents and strategies for prevention of soft tissue contractures and adhesions and relate the therapeutic rationale for each, and
5. identify appropriate therapeutic strategies for enhancement of the structural and functional properties of scar tissue and relate the therapeutic rationale for each.

87

Control of hemorrhage and edema and alleviation of pain and muscle spasm are the two primary therapeutic objectives during the acute inflammatory stage of tissue healing. As these early inflammatory responses are brought under control, the sports health care clinician's attention is typically directed to the use of physical agents to influence the vascular and cellular events of fibroplasia, the second stage of connective tissue repair during which fibrous scar tissue is formed. Strategies to prevent complications associated with the repair process (e.g., contractures, adhesions) also become a focus of therapeutic intervention in this stage. Finally, as scar formation and maturation progress, intervention to maximize the structural and functional properties of the scar matrix may be indicated. Thus, the three primary therapeutic objectives during scar formation and scar maturation, the second and third stages of connective tissue healing, are to (1) enhance the physiological mechanisms of connective tissue repair, (2) prevent contractures and adhesions, and (3) enhance the definitive structural and functional properties of the scar matrix (e.g., tensile strength, plasticity). Therapeutic strategies to achieve these objectives are the focus of discussion in this chapter.

Enhancement of Connective Tissue Repair

Although dependent on the type of tissues involved and the extent of tissue damage, connective tissue repair follows a fairly predictable timetable beginning within a few days after injury. While acceleration of the repair process is a commendable objective in view of the motivated sports participant's desire to return to activity as soon as possible, sports health care clinicians should be cognizant of the extent to which the rate of connective tissue repair can be influenced by therapeutic agents. Unreasonable expectations regarding the degree to which repair mechanisms can be accelerated may, in fact, lead to overly aggressive and potentially counterproductive treatment regimens. In a practical sense, this is an important consideration for sports health care clinicians in view of influences to permit the return of injured athletes to competition as soon as possible after injury. Nevertheless, within the parameters of good judgment, enhancement of the physiological mechanisms of connective tissue repair is a worthy therapeutic objective that represents the third major area of intervention in the management of sports injuries (see chapter 1, figure 1.2).

The array of therapeutic agents available to the sports health care clinician for intervention during the inflammatory stage of connective tissue repair includes pharmacologic agents (e.g., analgesics, anti-inflammatory drugs) and physical agents (e.g., cold applications, compression). In comparison, however, the scope of therapeutic agents with demonstrated effectiveness in acceleration of the physiological mechanisms of fibroplasia appears to be limited. The primary cellular responses during this stage of repair are collagen synthesis and fibrogenesis, with eventual formation of fibrous scar tissue (see chapter 3, figure 3.5). Thus, the potential for pharmacologic or physical agents to accelerate the mechanisms of fibroplasia should be assessed in terms of their ability to enhance proliferation of fibroblasts, collagen synthesis and fibrogenesis, or related physiological responses that facilitate these tissue repair processes.

Whereas the positive effect of pharmacologic agents on acceleration of tissue repair is questionable, physiological rationale and clinical observations suggest a therapeutic role for selected physical agents during fibrous tissue formation and wound contraction, the two primary characteristics of the second stage of connective tissue repair. Therapeutic protocols for the specific purpose of accelerating connective tissue repair in sport-related musculoskeletal injuries commonly include the use of various thermal agents (i.e., superficial- and deep-heating modalities) and the nonthermal, mechanical effects of ultrasound. Although electrotherapy is widely used for a variety of therapeutic purposes in sports injury management, the routine use of electrical currents to accelerate the mechanisms of soft connective tissue repair in musculoskeletal injuries is largely unsupported by scientific evidence. Following a brief review of the role of pharmacologic agents in tissue healing, the therapeutic effects of thermal agents, mechanical ultrasound, and electrotherapy are addressed in subsequent sections of this chapter.

Pharmacologic Agents

Although histological investigations have addressed the effect of nonsteroidal anti-inflammatory drugs (NSAIDs) on tissue healing in musculoskeletal injuries (Obremsky et al. 1994), the value of NSAIDs and other pharmacologic agents in acceleration of specific repair mechanisms (e.g., collagen synthesis and fibrous tissue formation) is largely unsubstantiated (Abramson 1990). At the current time, there are no known drugs that have the capability to accelerate healing of musculoskeletal injuries (Salter 1999). As discussed in chapter 4, the primary benefits of NSAIDs in connective tissue repair stem primarily from their ability to combat persistent inflammatory responses that complicate fibrous tissue formation. In contrast to NSAIDs, corticosteroids have been shown to inhibit protein metabolism and suppress collagen synthesis, thus impairing connective tissue repair (Behrens and Goodwin 1990). Although corticosteroids are powerful anti-inflammatory drugs, sports medicine physicians typically do not advocate their routine use in the management of sports injuries in view of these deleterious effects (Behrens and Goodwin 1990; Leadbetter, Buckwalter, and Gordon 1990). As noted by Behrens and Goodwin (1990), the use of oral corticosteroids in sports injury management is not common. If used, corticosteroids are prescribed in carefully controlled dosages.

Thermotherapy

Typically, the use of cold applications to assist in the control of acute inflammatory responses is advocated during the first three or four days following injury. Although cryotherapy is sometimes continued into the second stage of connective tissue repair for control of edema or intervention in the pain-spasm-pain cycle, the reduction of tissue temperature associated with cold applications cannot be expected to accelerate the cellular responses necessary for tissue repair, namely proliferation of fibroblasts and collagen synthesis. Once hemorrhage and edema have been brought under control during the inflammatory stage of connective tissue repair, external heat applications commonly become the treatment of choice. Because the rate of tissue repair is related, in part, to the extent of vascularity and blood flow in the affected tissues, the use of thermal agents to increase tissue temperature and stimulate local blood flow represents a rational approach to acceleration of the repair process. Nevertheless, the extent to which thermotherapy contributes to shortened recovery periods following sport-related musculoskeletal injuries remains somewhat speculative.

The primary physiological responses to elevated tissue temperature and increased blood flow include local proliferation of white blood cells with increased phagocytosis, increased oxygen supply and cellular metabolism, and an increased supply of nutrients (American Academy of Orthopaedic Surgeons 1991; Stillwell 1965). These physiological responses are essential components of connective tissue repair that, if enhanced through the use of therapeutic heat, can theoretically be expected to facilitate tissue-healing mechanisms. The vascular and cellular responses to increased local tissue temperature that are most directly related to connective tissue repair during inflammation, scar formation (fibroplasia), and scar maturation are summarized in table 5.1.

Because of differences in the depth of penetration between various superficial-heating modalities (e.g., hot packs, whirlpool) and deep-heating modalities (e.g., ultrasound, shortwave diathermy), care should be taken to select thermal agents with penetration capabilities that correspond to the depth of the affected tissues. Both safety and effectiveness are

Table 5.1   Local Physiological Responses to Increased Tissue Temperature During the Three Primary Stages of Connective Tissue Repair

Inflammation	Scar formation (fibroplasia)	Scar maturation
Vasodilation/ ↑ blood flow	Vasodilation/ ↑ blood flow	Vasodilation/ ↑ blood flow
↑ Vascular permeability/ ↑ exudation of fluids and edema	↑ O_2/nutrient supply	Destabilization of collagen cross-links
↑ WBCs/phagocytosis	↑ Cellular metabolism	

considerations in this selection. Regardless of the modality chosen, the primary physiological effects that contribute to connective tissue repair are increased tissue temperature and improved local blood flow. In order to effect therapeutic physiological responses, temperature in the affected tissues must be raised to between 40° and 45°C (104° to 113°F) (Rennie and Michlovitz 1996). Temperature above 45°C, however, may cause tissue damage (Baumert 1993). Although theoretically beneficial, application of thermal agents to hypovascular areas in which local heat dissipation may be impaired (e.g., rotator cuff muscles, Achilles tendon) must be approached with caution. Judicious selection of thermal agents necessitates consideration of contraindications common to all techniques of application (e.g., ischemia, impaired sensation for pain and temperature), as well as specific contraindications and precautions associated with particular modalities. For example, the application of ultrasound to open epiphyseal plates is commonly contraindicated, as is the use of shortwave diathermy for treatment of body tissues with metallic implants.

Mechanical Ultrasound

Although ultrasound is commonly classified as a deep-heating modality, pulsed ultrasound has nonthermal, mechanical effects that have the potential to enhance the mechanisms of connective tissue repair. Whereas high-intensity ultrasound may inhibit collagen synthesis, thus having a detrimental effect on the repair process, low-intensity pulsed ultrasound has been found to accelerate specific mechanisms of fibrous tissue formation during the early fibroplastic stage of connective tissue repair (Gieck and Saliba 1990). Although potential benefits of nonthermal, pulsed ultrasound during the acute stage of inflammation have been noted (e.g., release of chemotactic agents from mast cells), premature use of ultrasound may disrupt the blood-clotting mechanism and exacerbate hemorrhagic effusion. Furthermore, if used prematurely, pulsed ultrasound may stimulate the release of histamine from mast cells, thereby enhancing vascular permeability, exudation of fluids into interstitial spaces, and edema formation. Consequently, it has been recommended that the use of ultrasound be delayed until hemostasis is established and until tissue swelling has been brought under control (Gieck and Saliba 1990). Some clinicians have suggested that the initiation of low-intensity pulsed ultrasound be delayed until the beginning of the cellular proliferation stage of tissue healing, thus corresponding with the vascular and cellular events of granulation tissue formation and fibroplasia (McDiarmid, Ziskin, and Michlovitz 1996).

Mechanical Phenomena

The therapeutic effects of nonthermal, pulsed ultrasound are attributed to two primary mechanisms operating at the cellular level, thereby altering cellular activities in the target tissues. These two mechanisms are *cavitation* and *acoustic streaming* (McDiarmid, Ziskin, and Michlovitz 1996). *Cavitation* refers to the vibrational effects of an ultrasound beam on small gas pockets, or bubbles, in tissue fluids. Within therapeutic ranges, the cyclic pressure changes induced by pulsed ultrasound causes alternating expansion and compression of gas bubbles, resulting in rhythmic oscillation. This phenomenon is referred to as *stable cavitation* (Dyson 1990). Stable cavitation is thought to facilitate diffusion of ions and metabolites across cell membranes, thereby enhancing cellular activity. In contrast to the therapeutic effects of stable cavitation produced by low-intensity pulsed ultrasound, increased cellular stress associated with the use of high-intensity pulsed ultrasound may cause *unstable*, or *transient*, *cavitation*, a response involving rapid enlargement and collapse of gas bubbles in the tissue fluids with a corresponding potential for tissue damage (Dyson 1990).

The second mechanical effect of pulsed ultrasound, acoustic streaming, involves movement of fluids or other matter away from a source of energy (Cole and Eagleston 1994; Sweitzer 1994). Because fluid movement is microscopic, this response has also been referred to as *microstreaming*. Acoustic streaming, possibly in combination with stable cavitation, increases cell membrane permeability, thereby enhancing ion and metabolite diffusion with a corresponding increase in cellular activity (Dyson 1990). The therapeutic effect of phonophoresis, during which anti-inflammatory drugs (e.g., hydrocortisone) and other medications are driven into body tissues by ultrasound, is attributed to the mechanical phenomenon of acoustic streaming (Cole and Eagleston 1994).

Physiological Responses

Acceleration of connective tissue repair through the use of pulsed ultrasound has been attributed to its effect on three primary physiological mechanisms: collagen synthesis, angiogenesis, and wound contraction (see chapter 3). When used during fibroplasia, the second stage of connective tissue repair, the therapeutic benefits of low-intensity pulsed ultrasound are associated with stimulation of the cellular functions of macrophages, fibroblasts, myofibroblasts, and vascular endothelial cells. The contributions of pulsed ultrasound to connective tissue repair can be summarized by relating its mechanical effects to the functions of these cells. As tissue healing begins, the presence of macrophages characterizes the early phase of fibroplasia during which granulation tissue is formed. Macrophages not only provide phagocytic and immunological functions during the inflammatory stage of tissue repair, but they also release chemotactic agents that attract fibroblasts to the damaged tissues. In addition, macrophages release various growth factors, some of which stimulate the metabolic functions of fibroblasts (i.e., collagen synthesis) (Cotran, Kumar, and Robbins 1989). Exposure of macrophages to the mechanical effects of low-intensity pulsed ultrasound stimulates the release of these chemotactic agents and growth factors, which in turn enhance fibroblast activity (Gieck and Saliba 1990). Several clinicians have suggested that low-intensity pulsed ultrasound also has a direct positive effect on the cellular functions of fibroblasts, thereby enhancing collagen synthesis with a corresponding increase in the tensile strength of the developing tissue matrix (Dyson 1990; Gieck and Saliba 1990; McDiarmid, Ziskin, and Michlovitz 1996).

As granulation tissue develops during the early phase of fibroplasia, vascular endothelial cell budding and sprouting of new blood vessels (i.e., angiogenesis) may be enhanced by therapeutic dosages of pulsed ultrasound, thereby accelerating formation of a new vascular network in the affected tissues (i.e., neovascularization). As noted by Dyson (1990), stimulation of endothelial budding may be due to an accelerated release of angiogenic growth factors from macrophages, rather than a direct mechanical effect on endothelial cell membrane permeability. In addition to acceleration of collagen synthesis and angiogenesis, the mechanical effects of ultrasound are thought to stimulate the contractile functions of myofibroblasts, the specialized fibroblasts responsible for wound contraction. Although the ultimate extent of wound contraction does not appear to be increased through the use of ultrasound, the rate at which contraction occurs is accelerated (Dyson 1990).

Electrotherapy

Electrotherapy in the management of musculoskeletal injuries has been widely used for many years. Various electrical stimulation techniques have been advocated and used with varying degrees of success for pain control, reduction of edema, prevention of disuse atrophy, neuromuscular reeducation, and tissue healing (Gersh 1992). With specific regard to tissue healing, the most conclusive evidence indicates the benefits of electrotherapy in the treatment of chronic skin lesions and delayed union or nonunion fractures (Cummings 1992). Despite demonstrated acceleration of tissue repair mechanisms in skin lesions and fractures, the benefits of electrical currents in the repair of soft connective tissues (e.g., ligaments and joint capsules, tendons) remains largely speculative. Nevertheless, some studies have demonstrated accelerated fibrous tissue formation and increased tensile strength following ligament and tendon repairs (Stanish et al. 1985) and tenotomy of Achilles tendons in animals through the use of galvanic currents (Owoeye et al. 1987). These findings suggest a consistency with studies indicating the benefits of electrical stimulation in skin healing and bone regeneration. Although high-voltage, pulsed galvanic stimulation (HVPGS) is used in the management of sports injuries for a variety of therapeutic purposes, scientific evidence supporting its routine use for the specific purpose of accelerating soft connective tissue repair in musculoskeletal injuries is sparse (Quillen, Mohr, and Reed 1990).

Prevention of Contractures and Adhesions

Complications arising directly from persistent inflammatory responses, abnormal wound contraction, or other deviations in the normal mechanisms of connective tissue repair may be manifested during recovery from musculoskeletal injuries. Soft tissue contractures and adhesions are among the most common complications. The functional consequences of contractures and adhesions are loss of tissue mobility with restricted joint motion, decreased musculotendinous extensibility, or a combination of both, depending on the particular tissues involved. Although contributing factors (e.g., edema, pain, muscle spasm) are present during the inflammatory stage of connective tissue repair, contractures and adhesions are typically manifested during fibroplasia, the second stage of tissue repair, at which time the responsible mechanisms are activated. To the extent that contractures and adhesions represent potential complications during recovery from musculoskeletal injuries, therapeutic measures to prevent loss of tissue mobility become a fourth major area of therapeutic intervention in the continuum of connective tissue repair (see chapter 1, figure 1.2). Although contractures and adhesions may be a direct consequence of tissue-healing mechanisms, the propensity for these conditions to occur is increased by inappropriate or prolonged immobilization. Because the amount of tension placed on healing tissues is a major factor that influences their structural and biomechanical properties, and thus the likelihood of contractures and adhesions, the effects of connective tissue immobilization are reviewed in the following section prior to a discussion of specific therapeutic protocols.

Connective Tissue Immobilization

Historically, the decision to prescribe rest (e.g., immobilization) or movement in the management of musculoskeletal injuries has been somewhat controversial. Although the necessity of restricted activity to prevent exacerbation of soft tissue damage during the early stages of connective tissue repair is generally accepted, the detrimental effects of prolonged immobilization on body tissues is widely reported. In general, these effects include (1) decreased mobility of noncontractile articular structures (i.e., joint capsules) or contractile musculotendinous tissues and (2) impaired tensile strength in the immobilized tissues. The first of these two conditions, decreased tissue mobility, can be attributed to fibrotic connective tissue contractures or adhesions, both of which may be exacerbated by immobilization. Research has indicated that impairment in the development of connective tissue tensile strength is a concomitant consequence of immobilization. Several investigators have demonstrated that inactivity and immobilization are detrimental to the development of tensile strength in connective tissues, whereas movement promotes the physiological mechanisms that contribute to tensile strength (Laros, Tipton, and Cooper 1971; Vailas et al. 1981). Thus, the combined deleterious consequences of immobilization, decreased tissue mobility and impaired tensile strength, represent clinically significant considerations in the management of connective tissue injuries. The effect of immobilization on connective tissue plasticity and tensile strength is discussed further in a subsequent section of this chapter.

Contractures

Shortening of connective tissues may occur in either contractile tissues or noncontractile tissues. Whereas loss of muscular strength during immobilization is attributed to alterations in the contractile unit of muscle tissue (i.e., the myofiber), decreased musculotendinous extensibility, or muscle shortening, results from fibrotic changes in the noncontractile connective tissue sheaths that surround individual muscle fibers (i.e., the myofibers) or muscle fiber bundles (see chapter 3, figure 3.8). Fibrosis of connective tissues can also lead to contractures in joint capsules and ligaments. Thus, with specific regard to tissue shortening and loss of mobility, the effects of immobilization are most appropriately assessed in terms of alterations in connective tissue properties, regardless of whether the tissues are constituents of joint capsules, ligaments, or musculotendinous structures.

As discussed in chapter 3, normal wound contraction can significantly reduce the size of a tissue defect. Lack of tension in the affected or adjacent tissues, however, may lead to excessive wound contraction and, consequently, undue shortening of connective tissues. For example, prolonged immobilization with tissues in their shortened, relaxed range increases the propensity for development of contractures. The severity of connective tissue contractures, as well as the rate of development, is increased when immobilization is superimposed on traumatized tissues (Cummings and Tillman 1992). Numerous histological studies have led to similar conclusions regarding the effects of immobilization on the structural and biomechanical properties of both normal and traumatized connective tissues. As proposed by Andriacchi et al. (1988), for example, shortening of traumatized tissues is due to degradation of existing collagen fibers, wound contraction through the action of myofibroblasts, and deposition of new collagen at the shortened length. Similarly, it has been hypothesized that cross-linkage of newly formed, randomly oriented collagen fibers results in interfibril bonding that resists elongation and restricts tissue mobility. As illustrated in figure 5.1, cross-links between newly formed collagen fibrils and existing fibrils may also develop (Harrelson 1991). Excessive collagen cross-links have been attributed to loss of water and glycosaminoglycans (GAGs) from the ground substance of connective tissue during immobilization. Loss of these lubricating constituents leads to decreased space between collagen fibers (i.e., fibers become more closely packed),

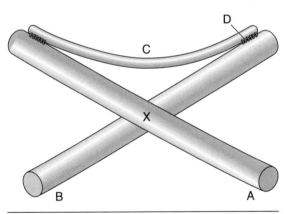

Figure 5.1 Mechanisms of connective tissue contracture. Note the contact point (X) of collagen fibrils (A and B) due to loss of intervening ground substance and cross-linking (D) of new collagen fibril (C).

Adapted, by permission, from G.L. Harrelson, 1991, Physiologic factors of rehabilitation. In *Physical rehabilitation of the injured athlete*, edited by J.R. Andrews and G.L. Harrelson (Philadelphia: W.B. Saunders), 23.

which permits random points of fixation, thereby impairing normal gliding functions (Akeson et al. 1977; Randall, Portney, and Harris 1992). As discussed shortly, early passive motion provides a means through which these adverse effects can be minimized or prevented.

Adhesions

In addition to connective tissue contractures, adhesions between adjacent tissues are generally recognized as a factor in loss of mobility. Injury that involves a particular type of tissue (e.g., a tendon) may also include adjacent structures (e.g., the synovial membrane). Because both types of adjacent tissues are incorporated within the same inflammatory response, subsequent fibrous scar formation leads to development of adhesions between the affected tissues. Although adhesions are directly related to fibrosis and scar formation, prolonged immobilization that restricts normal gliding movements between tissues enhances the likelihood that adhesions will develop. Controlled movement, on the other hand, maintains the normal gliding motion of adjacent tissue surfaces, thereby lessening the likelihood of adhesions. Because movement is a recognized deterrent to adhesions in contractile tissues, controlled motion is considered especially important to maintenance of normal gliding motions and prevention of adhesive tenosynovitis following surgical repair of tendinous lesions (Enwemeka 1991).

Therapeutic Strategies

To the extent that early therapeutic intervention (e.g., NSAIDs, cold applications) is successful in controlling excessive or prolonged inflammatory responses to acute tissue trauma, several factors contributing to development of connective tissue contractures and adhesions are minimized. Should contractures and adhesions be anticipated, however, additional therapeutic measures may be indicated. Initial therapeutic intervention, during the early stages of fibroplasia, is logically focused on prevention rather than resolution of existing contractures and adhesions. Cummings and Tillman (1992) noted that the tensile forces necessary to maintain connective tissue mobility are significantly less than the forces required to mobilize already shortened tissues. These authors used the term *therapeutic remodeling* to describe tissue loading that is of sufficient force and duration to reverse the processes of contracture and adhesion formation and to "guide" the development of desired collagen fiber size and alignment. In general, therapeutic measures to achieve these objectives include the use of (1) continuous passive motion, (2) modified immobilization or protected mobilization techniques, and (3) functional electrical muscle stimulation.

Continuous Passive Motion

Despite historical precedence that has favored immobilization in the management of musculoskeletal injuries, the trend toward early motion as an alternative treatment approach has increased over the years (Frank et al. 1984). One of the earliest proponents of early passive motion in the management of musculoskeletal injuries was Robert Salter, a noted orthopedic surgeon who expressed concern about the deleterious effects of immobilization on articular structures (Salter 1999). Consequently, Salter advocated the use of passive motion as an alternative to postsurgical immobilization and, in the early 1970s, pioneered the concept of *continuous passive motion* (CPM). Despite some controversy, the use of CPM in the management of postsurgical joint injuries has steadily increased since the early 1980s. Although CPM has been advocated for a variety of therapeutic purposes (e.g., articular cartilage nutrition, pain control), a review of the literature by O'Donoghue et al. (1991) indicated its increased use as a means of maintaining joint lubrication and minimizing joint stiffness following orthopedic surgery.

By definition, *passive joint motion* refers to movement of a joint produced by an external source, or a source other than intrinsic muscle contraction. Hence, the forces imparted to articular structures during passive joint motion are concentrated on ligamentous and capsular tissues. In a therapeutic context, the intensity and duration of passive joint motion may range from repetitive low-force manual movements to mobilize shortened tissues (e.g., joint mobilization) to a single high-force manual thrust to disrupt contracted tissues (i.e., manipulation). Whereas manual joint mobilization techniques are typically used to resolve existing joint contractures and adhesions, mechanical CPM devices provide a practical technique for early postsurgical intervention to prevent these complications. Use of CPM immediately following or within a few days after surgery is based on anticipation of joint contractures and adhesions associated with fibroplasia, the second stage of tissue healing that begins approximately five days after surgery. Thus, the emphasis is on the use of controlled CPM for prevention, rather than resolution of already formed contractures and adhesions.

Contemporary application of CPM involves the use of commercial mechanical devices that produce an external force and, thus, passive joint motion. Although commercial CPM devices have been developed for most major joints, the most common indication in the sports population appears to be postsurgical management of knee injuries. In recent years, lightweight portable CPM devices have been developed for home use following surgery of the knee, wrist, and fingers. Whereas some surgeons advocate immediate postoperative application, others prefer a two- or three-day delay in the use of CPM following surgery. Some studies, however, indicate the superiority of immediate postsurgical CPM application, as opposed to delayed mobilization, in maintenance of tissue mobility (O'Donoghue et al. 1991).

Presumably, the value of CPM in maintenance of joint motion after surgery is due to its effect on ligamentous and capsular structures. Some investigators, however, have demonstrated the benefits of controlled passive motion in maintenance of normal tendon gliding following experimental surgery. Using a canine flexor tendon model, Woo et al. (1981) observed that the postsurgical gliding function of the flexor digitorum profundus tendon was significantly greater in exercised tendons, as compared to immobilized tendons, at 6 and 12 weeks following surgery. Other investigators have reported decreased tendon adherence to adjacent tissues and maintenance of tendon excursion following the use of early passive mobilization (Gelberman et al. 1982). Although these studies involved the use of intermittent passive motion, rather than continuous motion, similar therapeutic effects on periarticular musculotendinous tissues can logically be expected from the use of mechanical CPM devices.

Modified Immobilization and Protected Mobilization

Historically, immobilization in rigid external devices (e.g., plaster casts) has been standard practice in the management of various types of musculoskeletal injuries. However, prolonged immobilization of injured connective tissues in their shortened state encourages excessive wound contraction, cross-linkage of randomly oriented collagen fibers, and formation of contractures. Over the years, several alternatives to prolonged, rigid immobilization at constant, fixed joint positions have evolved. Conceptual advancements in the early management of musculoskeletal injuries are exemplified by application of principles associated with *protected mobilization*, or protected motion (Cummings and Tillman 1992). Clinical application of protected mobilization concepts recognizes the necessity of protecting damaged tissues but at the same time acknowledges the therapeutic benefits of controlled motion during the early stages of connective tissue repair. In contrast to prolonged rigid immobilization, early introduction of protected mobilization promotes connective tissue repair, reduces the likelihood of contractures and adhesions, and enhances tissue tensile strength (Cummings and Tillman 1992).

Commercial response to trends in early musculoskeletal injury management, including postoperative treatment, has resulted in the development of a vast array of specialized protected mobilization devices for the upper and lower extremities. In general, these devices permit three primary therapeutic approaches to early injury management: (1) serial static immobilization, (2) static progressive splinting, and (3) dynamic splinting (Sadler and Koepfer 1992). Primary distinguishing features among these therapeutic approaches are the degree of joint motion allowed and the amount of tension applied to the affected tissues. The common therapeutic objective, however, is to protect damaged tissues while permitting or promoting appropriate tissue elongation and mobility.

Serial static immobilization

Compared to static progressive splinting and dynamic splinting, serial static immobilization represents one of the more traditional approaches to early musculoskeletal injury management in sports health care. Static immobilization involves the use of devices that have no movable parts, thus precluding joint motion and application of significant tension to the affected tissues (Sadler and Koepfer 1992). Serial static immobilization, involving the application of rigid splints or cast materials at periodically increased or decreased joint angles, nevertheless provides an alternative to prolonged immobilization of body parts in the same position. As tissue repair progresses and as the tensile strength of affected tissues permits, immobilization at varied joint angles allows continued healing with collagen fiber formation in the newly lengthened position. As a result, shortening of affected tissues during the recovery period is discouraged. Although newer concepts have evolved, initial postoperative immobilization of the ankle in plantar flexion after Achilles tendon repair, followed by immobilization in the neutral position, represents an example of serial static immobilization (Enwemeka 1991). Because static splints and casts have no movable components, unlike static progressive splints and dynamic splints, they require remodeling and reapplication to accommodate changes in joint position. Depending on the design of the protective device (e.g., cylinder casts or removable splints), static immobilization can be complemented by periodic removal of the protective device for intervening sessions of passive or active joint motion. For example, contemporary postoperative knee immobilizers permit splint removal and intervening sessions of continuous passive motion (CPM) after anterior cruciate ligament reconstruction. Removable splint wear with intervening mobilization sessions has also been used successfully in treatment of hand and finger injuries (Sadler and Koepfer 1992). These protocols represent additional attempts to prevent contractures and adhesions that are consistent with current concepts of protected immobilization.

Static progressive splinting

In contrast to serial static casts and splints, static progressive splints allow changes in joint position without the necessity of remodeling the splint device. A variety of inelastic components are used in commercial devices to facilitate static progressive splinting, including incorporation of hinges with adjustment controls (e.g., screws, rotating wheels). In comparison to rigid static casts and splints, static progressive splints allow convenient, timely changes in joint position and progressive introduction of controlled, low-force tensile loading. Thus, tension becomes a more prominent component of early connective tissue injury management with the use of these devices. Because static progressive splints lack the elastic components of dynamic splints, however, they function only to maintain tissues at their existing length without promoting continued lengthening. Nevertheless, static progressive splints provide opposing forces to excessive wound contraction, as well as tensile loading that encourages linear alignment of collagen fibers, provided that splint design allows application of forces in the appropriate line of pull. Adjustable hinged braces that facilitate protected postoperative mobilization of the knee exemplify the use of static progressive splinting in the sports health care setting. Static progressive splints have also been developed for the ankle, shoulder, elbow, wrist, and fingers.

Dynamic splinting

Unlike static casts and splints and static progressive splints, dynamic splints incorporate movable (i.e., dynamic) components such as rubber bands or adjustable coiled spring mechanisms. These features permit application of controlled, progressive tensile forces to shortened tissues over extended time periods. As compared to static progressive splints that are designed to maintain existing tissue length, dynamic splints permit application of low-load, prolonged tensile forces that promote desirable permanent, or plastic, tissue elongation. Dynamic splints were popularized in the 1940s as an approach to treatment of hand and finger injuries. Since this time, prefabricated or custom-fitted dynamic splints have been used to minimize development of contractures and tendinous adhesions in a variety of hand and finger injuries (Sadler and Koepfer 1992). Currently, commercial dynamic splints are available for the ankle, knee, elbow, wrist, and fingers. Despite occasional use in the management of sports injuries, early intervention to prevent contractures and adhesions has minimized the necessity of dynamic splinting in the sports health care setting. Typically, the use of dynamic splints in sports injury management is reserved for resolution of persistent contractures in large joints such as the knee and elbow.

Functional Electrical Muscle Stimulation

The use of electrical muscle stimulation (EMS) has been advocated as an approach to preventing tendinous adhesions and maintaining normal tendon excursion during periods of static immobilization or static progressive splinting. Electrical stimulation used for this purpose is referred to as *functional electrical muscle stimulation* (Sadler and Koepfer 1992). Functional electrical stimulation involves identification and stimulation of musculotendinous structures that, if restricted by adhesions, may lose their normal gliding function. Electrically induced muscle contractions brought about by motor point stimulation produces tendon movement, thus contributing to maintenance of normal tendon excursion. Functional electrical stimulation appears to be most effective in promoting tendon excursion in the distal extremities (e.g., wrist and fingers) where the motor points of flexor and extensor muscles can be readily stimulated by application of surface electrodes (DeVahl 1992; Stralka 1992). Motor point stimulation of the dorsiflexors, plantar flexors, and evertors of the ankle has also been advocated to prevent tendinous adhesions following acute ankle sprains.

Enhancement of Scar Tissue Structure and Function

Despite preventative measures during the early stages of musculoskeletal injury management, contractures and adhesions may result as a direct consequence of connective tissue repair and restricted activity. These complications frequently represent significant challenges to the sports health care clinician, commonly necessitating continued therapeutic intervention for satisfactory resolution. Even if actual tissue contractures and adhesions are prevented through early intervention, connective tissue repair inherently involves development of an abnormal fibrotic scar matrix that lacks the plasticity and tensile strength of normal tissues. Hence, the affected tissues may be more susceptible to recurrent injury during strenuous sports activities. The term *plasticity* refers to the ability of tissues to adapt, in form and behavior, to strain or tension without rupture (Thomas 1993). Similarly, *tensile strength* refers to the ability of body tissues to resist elongation, or *tensile strain*, without tearing (Whiting and Zernicke 1998). Tensile strength is calculated in terms of applied forces per a cross-sectional area of body tissues. The maximum amount of loading that can be tolerated by particular tissues without tearing determines their tensile strength.

Whereas decreased tissue plasticity and tensile strength may be comparatively inconsequential in a sedentary individual, loss of these connective tissue properties can represent a significant injury risk factor in a physically active sports participant. With resumption of sports activity after injury, damaged tissues are typically subjected to forces similar to those that produced the original traumatic overload. Consequently, sports health care clinicians are challenged to optimize the desired biomechanical properties of the scar tissue that forms during connective tissue repair. Thus, the use of modifiers to enhance scar tissue structure and function represents a fifth major category of therapeutic intervention in connective tissue repair (see chapter 1, figure 1.2). For discussion purposes, the scope of therapeutic objectives in this category of intervention ranges from resolution of contractures and adhesions to restoration of optimal connective tissue plasticity and tensile strength. Regardless of the challenge, the basic therapeutic principles underlying restoration of these tissue properties are essentially the same. Specific techniques and protocols, however, may differ in purpose and effectiveness, depending on the type of affected musculoskeletal tissues and the extent of involvement.

Principles of Therapeutic Tensile Loading

During scar formation and maturation, several events occur that determine the ultimate structure and functional properties of scar tissue (e.g., collagen deposition and degradation, wound contraction, collagen fiber realignment). Without therapeutic intervention, the definitive quality of the scar matrix is determined solely by these mechanisms. The usual result is formation of dense, fibrous scar tissue that lacks both the plasticity and tensile strength of normal connective tissue. With timely intervention, however, the quality of developing scar tissue can be enhanced. Most commonly, therapeutic measures to achieve this objective are introduced during the period of scar formation and continued into the tissue-remodeling phase. Tillman and Cummings (1992) suggested that therapeutic intervention to increase tissue mobility and joint motion is most effective during the period of fibroplasia and wound contraction (day 5 to day 21 after injury). As consolidation of the scar matrix occurs (day 21 to day 60), however, the ability of scar tissue to respond to treatment decreases. During the maturation stage of connective tissue repair (day 60 to day 360), scar tissue response to treatment continues to decrease.

The use of controlled tensile loading represents the primary approach to enhancement of the desired structural and biomechanical properties of scar tissue. Despite the benefits of early intervention during fibroplasia and wound contraction, the sports health care clinician must be mindful of the degree of tissue plasticity and tensile strength at each particular stage of repair, lest the premature introduction of harmful, overaggressive tissue loading. The deleterious effects of persistent inflammation, restricted activity, and immobilization are also important considerations in the selection of appropriate loading methods and dosages.

Tissue Immobilization and Tensile Loading

Therapeutic strategies to optimize connective tissue plasticity and tensile strength include the progressive application of controlled mechanical tensile forces, or tensile loading, as a fundamental approach. Decisions regarding initiation of tensile loading, as well as the intensity and duration of applied forces, can represent a significant challenge to the sports health care clinician. These decisions are facilitated by a fundamental understanding of tissue biomechanics and the response of connective tissues to immobilization and tensile loading. Safety considerations and rationale for selection of tissue-loading methods are most appropriately based on an awareness of the comparative effects of immobilization and tensile loading on connective tissue plasticity and tensile strength. These effects are reviewed prior to a discussion of therapeutic strategies and specific mobilization techniques.

Effects of Immobilization

The increased propensity for development of contractures and adhesions associated with prolonged immobilization was discussed in a previous section of this chapter. In essence, contractures and adhesions represent a significant loss of plasticity, the ability of tissues to adapt to tensile strain. Rationale for effective therapeutic management of musculoskeletal injuries is also based on an understanding of the effects of immobilization and restricted activity on the tensile strength of connective tissues. Andriacchi et al. (1988) noted that immobilization of surgically repaired ligaments may decrease both the quantity and quality of scar formation. Tipton et al. (1975) concluded that the physiological processes that determine tensile strength in surgically repaired ligaments are negatively affected by immobilization. In their study using animal models, these investigators found that knee ligaments in dogs subjected to experimental surgical repair without postsurgical immobilization had stronger ligaments than animals with repaired ligaments that were immobilized in plaster casts. In a subsequent study involving the comparative effect of progressive exercise and immobilization on surgically repaired medial collateral ligaments in rats, Vailas et al. (1981) noted that ligaments in exercised animals that were not immobilized were significantly heavier and stronger than in animals subjected to postsurgical immobilization and exercise and in animals subjected to prolonged immobilization without exercise. Similar detrimental effects of inactivity and immobilization on the tensile strength of connective tissues have been reported by other investigators (Enwemeka 1991; Frank et al. 1984; Laros, Tipton, and Cooper 1971). Inhibited development of tensile strength in immobilized connective tissues, as compared to tissues subjected to mechanical loading, is commonly attributed to a combination of factors, including decreased collagen synthesis and total collagen content, smaller collagen fiber size, random collagen fiber alignment, and a level of collagen degradation that exceeds collagen synthesis (Harrelson 1991). These primary determinants of connective tissue tensile strength during scar formation and maturation were discussed in chapter 3.

Effects of Tensile Loading

In general, continuous passive motion, protected mobilization, and functional electrical stimulation represent early therapeutic measures that apply tensile loading with forces sufficient only to prevent loss of tissue mobility. Nevertheless, because some degree of tension is applied, they represent initial efforts to influence the desired structural and biomechanical qualities of scar tissue, namely tensile strength and plasticity. As tissue repair permits, however, increased tensile loading is necessary to further enhance these connective tissue properties. Therapeutic tensile loading can have a positive effect on both the tensile strength and the viscoelastic properties of connective tissues.

Connective tissue tensile strength

As discussed in chapter 3, the increase in tensile strength that occurs during scar formation and maturation is related to a transition from Type III to Type I collagen synthesis, an overall increase in collagen production, and linear realignment of collagen fibers. The therapeutic value of tissue loading in these remodeling processes is widely reported. Experimental evidence suggests that heavier, stronger ligaments and tendons in exercised subjects, as reported by Tipton et al. (1975) and Vailas et al. (1981), may be due to greater total collagen content (Booth and Gould 1975). Conversely, the rate of collagen degradation may exceed collagen synthesis in immobilized tissues, resulting in decreased tensile strength. Tissue loading has also been suggested as a stimulus for conversion of Type III to stronger Type I collagen fibers during scar formation, further enhancing tensile strength (Price 1990). Collagen fiber realignment is also a major factor contributing to increased tensile strength in connective tissues. In response to therapeutically applied tensile loading, the randomly organized collagen fibers that characterize granulation tissue and early scar formation progressively assume a linear orientation during scar maturation. Consequently, tensile strength increases in the direction of the applied forces (American Academy of Orthopaedic Surgeons 1991; Kellett 1986).

Connective tissue viscoelasticity

In addition to its positive effect on tensile strength, tensile loading elicits two primary types of biomechanical behavior in connective tissues. When subjected to tensile loading, connective tissues demonstrate *viscoelastic* behavior because of their inherent viscous and elastic properties. While the viscous properties provide resistance to elongation during tensile loading, the elastic properties allow extensibility with a return to the original tissue length when tensile loads are removed. The inherent viscoelasticity of various connective tissues is related primarily to the proportion of collagen fibers to elastic fibers in each tissue type (Carlstedt and Nordin 1989). For example, dense connective tissues (e.g., ligaments, joint capsules, tendons) contain an abundance of collagen fibers that contribute significantly to their tensile strength but permit only limited extensibility and elastic behavior. In contrast, other soft tissues (e.g., the skin) consist of a greater number of elastic fibers that allow greater tissue extensibility with a higher degree of elasticity, or recoverable deformation.

Biomechanics of Tensile Loading and Plastic Stretch

The fundamental therapeutic objective associated with mobilization of shortened connective tissues is the application of controlled tensile loading that results in permanent tissue elongation without undue structural weakening. Tensile loading that applies tension to connective tissues is called *stretch*, whereas the capability of tissues to be stretched is referred to as *extensibility*. Depending on the magnitude and duration of force, tensile loading applies tension to connective tissue elements that demonstrate extensibility as well as those that provide resistance to elongation. In an attempt to differentiate, Sapega et al. (1981) suggested the term *elastic stretch* to describe tension placed on the elastic elements that permit extensibility, whereas the term *plastic stretch* was suggested to identify tension placed on the viscous elements that resist elongation. Elastic stretch, which results in temporary, recoverable tissue deformation, is described as a spring-like biomechanical behavior that accounts for the return of connective tissues to their original length after tensile loading is discontinued. This characteristic is called *elasticity* (Whiting and Zernicke 1998). In contrast, plastic stretch involves permanent, unrecoverable deformation that is attributed to a putty-like behavioral response, resulting in retention of tissue elongation after removal of the tensile load. This response is referred to as *plasticity*, which describes the capacity of connective tissues to be molded (i.e., permanently elongated). Thus, connective tissues have the potential to be permanently lengthened (i.e., molded) by application of therapeutic tensile loading.

Because a permanent increase in tissue elongation is the usual therapeutic goal, stretching techniques are consequently focused on placement of tension on the viscous elements that provide resistance to elongation. As some clinicians have noted, however, some degree of mechanical weakening occurs when connective tissues are permanently lengthened (Sapega et al. 1981). Based on their review of the literature, Tillman and Cummings (1992) concluded that the dense collagen fibers in connective tissues cannot be permanently lengthened without structural weakening. Consequently, the sports health care clinician is challenged to select stretching techniques that effectively produce permanent elongation with minimal tissue weakening.

When connective tissues are subjected to constant tension (i.e., tensile loading), their biomechanical properties allow for two primary behavioral responses that are related to permanent tissue elongation. These responses are referred to as *stress-relaxation* and *creep* (Whiting and Zernicke 1998). Stress-relaxation occurs when internal resistance to mechani-

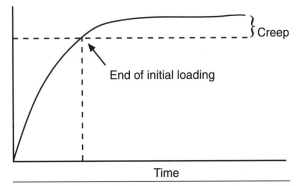

Figure 5.2 Connective tissue creep response to constant tensile load. Note the early rapid elongation and continued slow elongation (creep) at end of initial loading.

Adapted, by permission, from W.C. Whiting and R.F. Zernicke, 1998, Biomechanical concepts. In *Biomechanics of musculoskeletal injury* (Champaign, Ill.: Human Kinetics), 77.

cal loading (i.e., stress) decreases, or relaxes. Resistance to constant tensile loading is referred to as *tensile stress* (Whiting and Zernicke 1998). Hence, as tensile stress decreases, tissue elongation is permitted under continued constant loading. As stress-relaxation occurs, tissues deform rapidly as an initial response to a particular force level. Rather than maintain the initial level of deformation, however, tissues continue to elongate slowly, or creep, under constant tensile loading. As described by Carlstedt and Nordin (1989), the greatest amount of creep occurs during the first six to eight hours of tissue loading but continues at a slower rate over an extended period of time. Figure 5.2 illustrates these biomechanical behaviors. In their relaxed state, collagen fibers in dense regular connective tissues (e.g., tendons) typically demonstrate a wavy, or crimped, pattern (see chapter 1, figure 1.6).

When sufficient tensile forces are applied, collagen fibers straighten to their maximum elastic length. Beyond this limit, tropocollagen molecular stress occurs and intramolecular cross-links are disrupted (Cummings and Tillman 1992). These responses indicate that tension has been placed on the connective tissue components that resist elongation (i.e., the viscous elements). Although tissues stretched beyond their elastic limit shorten when tensile loads are removed, they do not return to their original length because their elastic limit has been exceeded. The remaining linear deformation reflects the amount of permanent tissue elongation (Whiting and Zernicke 1998). Disruption of the stabilizing cross-links that occur between tropocollagen molecules not only permits permanent tissue lengthening but also accounts for the accompanying structural weakness that is thought to occur.

Therapeutic Strategies and Techniques

Although several forms of therapeutic stretching have evolved over the years, three contemporary methods of connective tissue mobilization are widely used: (1) low-load, prolonged stretching, (2) proprioceptive neuromuscular facilitation (PNF), and (3) manual joint mobilization. Because differences exist among these methods with regard to primary target tissues and the manner in which tissue loading is applied, selection of appropriate therapeutic techniques depends on identification of the restricting tissues (i.e., articular structures, musculotendinous tissues) as well as an understanding of the effect of each technique on the structural and functional properties of connective tissues.

As the term implies, *low-load, prolonged stretching* describes the magnitude and duration of tensile forces used for connective tissue mobilization, rather than a specific method of application. Historically, low-load, prolonged stretching has been accomplished through the use of counterbalanced pulley systems, traction units, and similar tissue-loading devices. Some authors have referred to techniques that impart tensile forces for a period of 60 minutes or longer as *stress-relaxation therapy* (Cummings and Tillman 1992). Currently, stress-relaxation therapy is exemplified by the use of dynamic splinting for the resolution of persistent contractures and adhesions.

In contrast to continuous tensile loading devices, manual PNF and joint mobilization techniques represent specific loading methods that do not necessarily impart constant, prolonged tensile forces to the affected tissues. As manual therapies, these two techniques are designed to apply an intermittent passive stretch to particular musculoskeletal tissues. The primary target tissues during the use of PNF stretching methods are the connective tissue sheaths in musculotendinous structures, whereas joint capsules are the primary focus of joint mobilization techniques. Thus, these techniques differ both in purpose and method of application. Nevertheless, the common therapeutic objective in both techniques is connective tissue mobilization.

Low-Load, Prolonged Stretching

Because the usual therapeutic objective in connective stretching is to increase permanent, plastic elongation and lasting tissue mobility without further trauma, the most effective and safe protocols must be used. The extent to which tensile loading has a therapeutic effect on shortened connective tissues depends on three primary variables: (1) the magnitude of applied forces, (2) the duration of tensile loading, and (3) the temperature of the target tissues. These variables are related to the potential for tissue damage and structural weakening during tensile loading as well as the effect of loading on permanent tissue elongation.

Magnitude and duration of tensile forces

Compared to constant low-force loading, high-force tensile loading involves a greater risk of tissue damage and permanent structural weakening. During sudden application of high-force tensile loads, resistance to tissue elongation is comparatively high, due primarily to the viscous properties of connective tissues. Thus, tissue failure is more likely to occur before adaptation to the applied forces takes place (Whiting and Zernicke 1998). In contrast, gradually applied low-load tensile forces promote permanent linear deformation with a reduced risk of structural disruption (Sapega et al. 1981). During constant low-force tensile loading, stress-relaxation and creep occur in the affected tissues, which facilitate permanent tissue elongation over time. The time required to effect permanent elongation to a particular extent is inversely proportional to the magnitude of applied tensile forces. Thus, as compared to high-force tensile loading, low-force loading requires more time to produce the same amount of tissue elongation (Sapega et al. 1981). Nevertheless, to be effective, the magnitude of forces applied during prolonged low-force loading must be sufficient to challenge the resistance of tissue fibers that demonstrate viscous properties.

Effects of tissue temperature

Clinical research suggests that tissue temperature is a significant variable in the effectiveness of tensile loading in increasing flexibility and range of joint motion. Although several investigators have reported positive results from the use of thermal agents prior to application of tensile loading, general conclusions are difficult because of differences in methods of thermal application (e.g., superficial- or deep-heating modalities), tissue-loading protocols, and selected target tissues. Lentell et al. (1992) suggested that immediate increases in shoulder joint mobility (e.g., during a single treatment session) after the use of superficial-heating modalities (e.g., moist heat packs) and stretching may be due to inhibition of muscle spindle activity, reduced muscle tone, and decreased myofibril resistance to stretching. In contrast, Brodowicz, Welsh, and Wallis (1996) reported that static stretch of the hamstring muscles was enhanced in subjects when ice packs were applied during stretching compared to subjects who performed static stretching exercises with hot pack application or stretching without application of thermal agents. These investigators cited decreased muscle spindle activity resulting from cold applications as a plausible explanation for increased tissue extensibility. The use of cold applications to facilitate tissue stretching has been referred to as *cryostretching* (Sapega et al. 1981). Sapega et al. (1981) identified the use of cryotherapy to reduce pain and muscle spasm as a justifiable adjunct to stretching for the purpose of connective tissue elongation.

Notwithstanding the validity of research and clinical observations that attest to the value of thermal agents as adjuncts to soft tissue mobilization, claims that cold applications and superficial-heating modalities have a direct thermal effect on the plasticity of deep connective tissues should be interpreted with caution. It seems more plausible that these modalities function as "facilitators" of permanent plastic stretch because of their ability to reduce restrictive muscle tone and pain (Prentice 1982). Whereas superficial-heating modalities that promote muscle relaxation may facilitate concentration of tensile forces on shortened connective tissues, thermal agents that increase deep tissue temperatures directly may be especially beneficial adjuncts to therapeutic stretching. Tillman and Cummings (1992) noted that the viscoelastic behavior of tendons under tension can be altered by tissue temperatures between 37° and 40° C. At 37° C, stress-relaxation and slow tissue elongation (i.e., creep) occur. As the temperature increases to 40° C, tissues become more ductile without damage as long as tensile forces are low. Elevation of temperature above 40° C, however, increases tissue fragility and the likelihood of damage to dense connective tissues (Cummings and Tillman 1992). These observations suggest the importance of controlling both the temperature of shortened tissues and the tensile forces used during therapeutic stretching. Some clinicians contend that the use of heat as an adjunct to tensile loading is contraindicated when the integrity of shortened tissues must be preserved (Cummings and Tillman 1992).

The effect of increased tissue temperature on permanent elongation of connective tissues has been attributed to a partial disruption of the intermolecular cross-links of collagen fibers (McDiarmid, Ziskin, and Michlovitz 1996). The process through which the characteristic physical and chemical properties of protein (e.g., collagen) is altered in response to elevated temperature is referred to as *denaturation* (Thomas 1993). When the stabilizing hydrogen bonds formed during collagen synthesis and fibrogenesis are irreversibly disrupted, the collagen is said to be denatured (see chapter 3). Within therapeutic ranges, however, increased tissue temperature that destabilizes molecular bonding may allow elongation with a reduced risk of gross tissue damage, provided that superimposed tensile forces are kept at a low level (Sapega et al. 1981).

Alterations in connective tissue structure that result from elevated tissue temperature have been associated with the thermal effects of continuous ultrasound. As suggested by Gieck and Saliba (1990), the selective heating pattern of ultrasound appears to be of significant value as an adjunct to stretching of scar tissue in deep musculotendinous, ligamentous, and capsular structures. Wessling, DeVane, and Hylton (1987) reported that ultrasound applied to the triceps surae prior to static stretching, compared to stretching alone, produced a significantly greater immediate gain in ankle dorsiflexion. Permanent, residual tissue elongation was not assessed in this study, however. In a subsequent study, Draper et al. (1998) found that passive stretching of the triceps surae preceded by ultrasound to the musculotendinous junction increased ankle dorsiflexion significantly more than stretching alone during a single treatment session. After nine treatment sessions, however, these investigators found no significant difference in increased dorsiflexion between the two treatment groups, even though dorsiflexion increased significantly (11%) in both groups. In addition to the thermal effects of ultrasound, the mechanical effects of pulsed ultrasound have been shown to accelerate fibroblast activity and increase collagen production (Dyson 1990; Gieck and Saliba 1990). As noted by Dyson (1990), increased tensile strength of scar tissue is related to collagen content, whereas plasticity is associated with alterations in collagen fiber structure (i.e., reduction in cross-linkage). Thus, continuous ultrasound, involving both mechanical and thermal energy, may contribute to an increase in the tensile strength as well as the plasticity of scar tissue.

Effects of tissue cooling

A limited number of studies have attempted to determine the effect of cooling on permanent elongation of tissues during or following tensile loading. Some clinicians have suggested that the amount of permanent linear deformation that results from tensile loading can be enhanced if the forces are maintained while the tissues are cooling (Sapega et al. 1981). This effect has been attributed to restabilization of collagen microstructure at the newly established length. In their study on shoulder flexibility, however, Lentell et al. (1992)

failed to demonstrate that ice packs applied during tensile loading enhanced retention of plastic elongation. Instead, ice packs applied toward the end of stretching sessions diminished the cumulative gain in flexibility achieved by stretching of heated tissues. Although restabilization of collagen at lengthened tissue ranges may occur, evidence that cold applications facilitate this process is sparse. Whereas sound physiological rationale exists for the use of heat to facilitate connective tissue elongation, claims that cold applications enhance retention of linear deformation appear to be in need of further substantiation.

Research and clinical observations

Research conclusions regarding the effect of low-load, prolonged tensile loading on permanent elongation of soft tissues are somewhat hampered by discrepancies in interpretation of the terms *prolonged loading* and *permanent elongation*. Some investigators have reported positive results in studies involving as few as three treatment sessions over a five-day period with an actual stretch time of 15 minutes per session (Lentell et al. 1992). Other authors have reported success with clinical protocols involving tensile loading for 20 to 60 minutes (Sapega et al. 1981). Another study demonstrated significant increases in ankle dorsiflexion after nine sessions of static Achilles tendon stretching (two sessions per day, four minutes each) over a five-day period (Draper et al. 1998). Although studies have demonstrated positive effects of tensile loading on tissue mobility after periods of repeated treatment sessions (Gajdosik 1991; Lentell et al. 1992), most studies addressed relatively short-term cumulative effects of intermittent stretching rather than residual, long-term effects of constant prolonged tissue loading. Additional clinical studies that assess residual tissue elongation for extended time periods after discontinuation of intermittent stretching seem to be indicated before claims of permanent linear deformation can be substantiated or refuted.

Experimental protocols involving comparatively short periods of intermittent tissue loading are inconsistent with the basic concepts of low-load, prolonged tensile loading for the purpose of producing permanent, plastic tissue elongation. Repeated failure to resolve hip flexion contractures, contractures of the knee, and Achilles tendon shortening by manual stretching techniques led Kottke, Pauley, and Ptak (1966) to improvise counterbalanced pulley systems, weighted slings, and other devices to apply controlled, constant tissue loading. Compared to results obtained from manual methods, the repeated 20-minute sessions of constant tissue loading used by these clinicians were reported to be more effective for resolution of joint and musculotendinous contractures. Currently, more comfortable, convenient dynamic splints are available for application of low-load tensile forces for sustained periods of time. The typical, adjustable coiled spring mechanisms in these devices permit application of controlled tensile forces with progression to overnight wear (Hepburn and Crivelli 1984).

Proprioceptive Neuromuscular Facilitation

As the term implies, *proprioceptive neuromuscular facilitation* (PNF) is an approach to therapeutic exercise that employs mechanical stimulation of somatosensory receptors (i.e., proprioceptors) to promote a desired neuromuscular response (Voss, Ionta, and Myers 1985). Depending on the specific technique, PNF can be used to enhance one of two primary neuromuscular responses: (1) excitation of muscle spindle activity and stronger muscle contraction or (2) inhibition of muscle spindle activity and muscle relaxation. Thus, PNF techniques are designed to "facilitate" one or the other of these basic responses by virtue of their effect on muscle spindle activity, Golgi tendon organ responses, or both. Proprioceptive neuromuscular facilitation techniques that stimulate reflex muscle spindle activity (i.e., the stretch reflex) and stronger muscle contractions are referred to as *excitatory techniques*. In contrast, PNF techniques that promote muscle relaxation are considered *inhibitory*, or *relaxation, techniques*.

Whereas PNF excitatory techniques are designed for development of muscle strength and neuromuscular control in the rehabilitation of musculoskeletal injuries, relaxation techniques are used to enhance musculotendinous extensibility. Use of PNF relaxation techniques permits preliminary relaxation of the contractile elements in muscle tissues (i.e., the myofibers), thereby allowing greater concentration of tensile forces on shortened connective tissue sheaths (i.e., the endomysium, perimysium, epimysium) during therapeutic stretching. Scar tissue formation and shortening of connective tissue sheaths as a cause of decreased musculotendinous tissue mobility was discussed in chapter 3. As manual therapies, PNF relaxation techniques do not permit application of constant, prolonged tissue loading previously described as an effective method of enhancing permanent, plastic elongation. Nevertheless, these techniques provide the sports health care clinician with an effective means of promoting muscle relaxation as a prelude to application of intermittent tensile forces to restrictive connective tissue sheaths. In this regard, research and clinical experience have demonstrated the superiority of PNF relaxation techniques as compared to traditional static stretching.

Therapeutic principles and techniques

As described by Voss, Ionta, and Myers (1985), PNF relaxation techniques include (1) contract-relax, (2) hold-relax, and (3) slow reversal-hold-relax. Regardless of the specific technique used, the primary intent is to induce relaxation of the targeted muscle, or muscle group, prior to passive stretching. Muscle relaxation occurs when intramuscular tension is created by preliminary manual resistance to an isotonic contraction (contract-relax) or an isometric contraction (hold-relax). Protection from excessive muscle tension is a function of Golgi tendon organs, the somatosensory mechanoreceptors located near the musculotendinous junction. When Golgi tendon organs are stimulated by intramuscular tension, afferent (sensory) impulses are transmitted to the spinal cord where an inhibitory reflex arc is activated. As inhibitory impulses are conducted to the target muscles, relaxation occurs. Activation of inhibitory reflex mechanisms that elicits homonymous muscle relaxation is referred to as *autogenic* (i.e., self-generated) *inhibition* (Ganong 1995). During clinical application of PNF relaxation techniques, the target muscles are considered antagonistic to the desired direction of joint motion (i.e., the agonistic pattern of movement). Subsequent to a resisted isometric or isotonic contraction, the muscles to be stretched (e.g., the hamstring muscles) are permitted a momentary period of relaxation prior to passive movement of the extremity into the agonistic pattern (e.g., hip flexion). Thus, the relaxed muscles are stretched to their point of limitation. Because the point of limitation is largely determined by connective tissue sheaths, these structures become the specific target for tensile loading. As discussed in a previous section of this chapter, permanent elongation of restrictive connective tissue sheaths (i.e., plastic stretch) would require that these structures be stretched beyond their elastic limit. Typically, the stretch technique is repeated several times during a treatment session with a progression to a new point of tissue limitation as relaxation permits.

Whereas PNF contract-relax and hold-relax techniques are based on the concept of autogenic inhibition, other relaxation techniques incorporate the principle of *reciprocal inhibition*. These procedures involve an active or resisted concentric contraction, or a preliminary isometric contraction, of the muscle group responsible for producing the agonistic pattern of movement (e.g., hip flexion), rather than preliminary contraction of the muscle group targeted for stretching (e.g., the hamstrings). In this example, contraction of the hip flexors is accompanied by reflex inhibition and relaxation of the hamstring muscles, thus facilitating an effective stretch of connective tissue sheaths in the hamstring muscle group. Clinical experience and research has demonstrated that a greater degree of hip flexion is possible when the subject actively contracts the hip flexors with assistance into the agonistic movement pattern by the clinician (Gibbons 1980).

Hutton (1992) used the terms *contract relax*, *agonist contract* (CRAC) and *hold relax*, *agonist contract* (HRAC) to describe stretching techniques that combine the principles of autogenic inhibition and reciprocal inhibition. In these techniques, preliminary manual resistance is applied to an isotonic contraction (contract-relax) or an isometric contraction (hold-relax) of the muscle group to be stretched (i.e., the antagonists), thereby evoking autogenic inhibition and relaxation. Subsequently, with assistance by the clinician, the subject actively moves the extremity into the agonistic pattern, thus further facilitating relaxation of the antagonists (i.e., the muscles to be stretched) through the principle of reciprocal inhibition. Without incorporation of preliminary contract-relax or hold-relax techniques, Gibbons (1980) demonstrated that an "active-assisted" hamstring stretch involving concomitant concentric contraction of the agonists by the subject (i.e., the hip flexors) was more effective than passive manual stretching in producing short-term gains in hip flexion. Using a similar technique referred to as *agonist-contract-relax*, Osternig et al. (1990) also found a greater effect on hamstring extensibility as compared to traditional static stretching.

Research and clinical observations

Demonstrated clinical effectiveness has led to widespread use of PNF stretching techniques in the management of sports injuries. A survey of college and university certified athletic trainers by Surburg (1981) revealed that PNF contract-relax and hold-relax techniques are commonly used in the rehabilitation of injuries involving the neck, low back, and the upper and lower extremities. In a follow-up study in 1993, Surburg and Schrader (1997) reported continued widespread use of PNF stretching techniques by certified athletic trainers. Both the 1981 and 1993 studies revealed that contract-relax and hold-relax were the most frequently used PNF techniques (Surburg and Schrader 1997). Considering the popularity of PNF stretching techniques in sports health care, current research that addresses the effectiveness of these techniques in the management of sports injuries is surprisingly sparse. Nevertheless, during the 1970s and 1980s, several investigators compared the effects of PNF stretching techniques to the effects of traditional passive stretching (Ferreira 1978; Gibbons 1980; Prentice 1983; Tanigawa 1972). In general, these studies demonstrated the superiority of PNF stretching techniques. Tanigawa (1972) and Ferreira (1978), for example, found the hold-relax procedure to be more effective than passive mobilization for stretching of the hamstring muscle group. Superiority of the contract-relax method, compared to traditional passive stretching for hamstring mobilization, was demonstrated by Gibbons (1980). In a subsequent study, Prentice (1983) found the slow reversal-hold-relax technique to be more effective than static stretching for hamstring mobilization.

Most clinical research has addressed the cumulative effects of PNF stretching techniques during a series of treatment sessions over a relatively short time period. Some investigators, however, have attempted to assess retention of musculotendinous extensibility after discontinuation of PNF stretching techniques, presumably providing an assessment of permanent, plastic connective tissue elongation. Clinical studies indicating greater retention of hamstring extensibility for periods ranging from three weeks following cessation of treatment (Gibbons 1980) to 10 weeks (Prentice 1983) suggest that PNF stretching techniques are more effective than traditional passive stretching for increasing permanent elongation of connective tissues. Bristol and Holm (1998) assessed the residual effects of the hold-relax technique of hamstring stretching at six weeks following discontinuation of a three-week treatment period. After significant increases in hamstring extensibility during the treatment period, these investigators found no significant decrease in extensibility during the six-week period following the final treatment session. In a similar study, Weber and Wolff (1999) found that hamstring extensibility increased significantly during a three-week PNF contract-relax treatment period. Although decreases occurred during a six-week period after discontinuation of treatment, a residual increase in hamstring extensibility remained at six weeks when compared with pretreatment levels. As noted by Hutton (1992), the contract relax, agonist contract (CRAC) and the hold relax, agonist contract (HRAC) techniques have been shown to result in the greatest long-term gains in range of joint motion compared to traditional PNF techniques, static stretching, and ballistic stretching, although in the absence of statistical significance in some investigations.

Joint Mobilization

In general, the soft tissue mobilization techniques previously described (i.e., low-load, prolonged stretching and PNF) are directed primarily to restoration of physiological motions, the voluntary active movements produced by muscle contraction. Although passive joint structures (i.e., ligaments and joint capsules) are subjected to varying degrees of tension during physiological movements, therapeutic techniques that incorporate only physiological motion may be inadequate to address loss of *accessory joint motions* that result from joint contractures or adhesions. Accessory joint motions, also referred to as *arthrokinematic movements*, are those involuntary movements that must occur between joint surfaces to allow unrestricted physiological movements (Barak, Rosen, and Sofer 1990). Specific therapeutic techniques that concentrate forces on restricting joint capsules and ligaments may be necessary to restore the mobility necessary for accessory joint motions, and thus physiological movements, to occur. In cases where physiological joint motion is limited by periarticular musculotendinous structures as well as articular structures, joint mobilization techniques can be combined with PNF for effective therapeutic protocols (Voss, Ionta, and Myers 1985).

Accessory joint motions

Passive accessory joint motions that normally occur between joint surfaces during physiological movements of the limbs are described as *spin, roll, and slide* (Kisner and Colby 1990). In some instances, distractive forces (i.e., separation of joint surfaces) also occur in order to facilitate physiological movements. Spin occurs when a joint segment rotates around a stationary axis on an articulating segment. As illustrated in figure 5.3a, one point on a joint surface remains in contact with an unchanging point on the companion joint surface during spin (e.g., a merry-go-round). Roll, a second primary accessory joint motion, occurs when a new point on one joint surface comes in contact with a new point on the surface of a companion segment (e.g., a car tire rolling on pavement) (figure 5.3b). The third accessory joint motion, slide (i.e., glide), involves movement during which a point on the surface of one joint segment is always in contact with a new point on a companion surface (e.g., a car tire sliding on ice) (figure 5.3c). As illustrated during extension of the knee (figure 5.4), spin, roll, and slide typically occur in combination in order to allow an unrestricted physiological movement. In another example, abduction of the arm in the standing position not only requires roll of the head

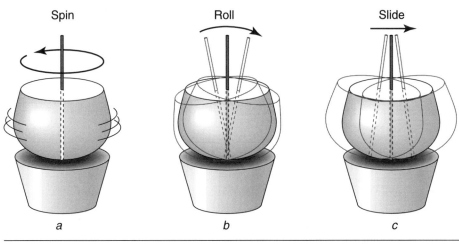

Figure 5.3   Primary accessory joint motions (arthrokinematic movements) in a synovial joint. *(a)* Spin. *(b)* Roll. *(c)* Slide (glide).

Adapted, by permission, from T. Barak, E.R. Rosen, and R. Sofer, 1990, Basic concepts of orthopaedic manual therapy. In *Orthopaedic and sports physical therapy*, 2nd ed., edited by J.A. Gould III (St. Louis: C.V. Mosby), 201.

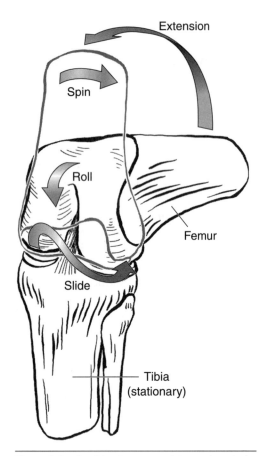

Figure 5.4   Combined accessory joint motions (spin, roll, slide) during extension of the knee.

Adapted, by permission, from T. Barak, E.R. Rosen, and R. Sofer, 1990, Basic concepts of orthopaedic manual therapy. In *Orthopaedic and sports physical therapy*, 2nd ed., edited by J.A. Gould III (St. Louis: C.V. Mosby), 203.

of the humerus on the surface of the glenoid fossa but also necessitates inferior glide (i.e., depression) of the humeral head in relation to the fossa. If the humerus is externally rotated during abduction, spin of the humeral head in the glenoid fossa is also required. Specific joint mobilization techniques, as developed by Maitland (1977), for example, address restoration of these accessory joint motions if restricted by articular tissue contractures or adhesions.

Joint mobilization techniques

Whereas restoration of joint mobility is a generic concept, the term *joint mobilization* commonly refers to the use of specific manual oscillatory movements to alleviate pain or to restore normal accessory joint motions. With regard to restoration of accessory joint motions, selection from among several manual maneuvers allows the sports health care clinician to target specific articular tissues, thereby directing forces to portions of the joint capsule or other structures that limit a particular accessory motion (i.e., spin, roll, slide). Joint mobilization protocols developed by Maitland (1977), for example, include grades of oscillatory movements categorized according to the amplitude of movement and the range of accessory joint motion in which the movements are performed. As summarized in table 5.2, the numerical grades of movement developed by Maitland include (1) Grade 1 (small amplitude movements performed at the beginning of the range of motion), (2) Grade II (large amplitude movements performed within the joint range but not reaching the limit of the range), (3) Grade III (large amplitude movements performed up to the limit of the joint range), and (4) Grade IV (small amplitude movements performed at the limit of the available range). Figure 5.5 illustrates the four grades of oscillatory movements used in the clinical setting for pain control and restoration of accessory joint motions. Because Grade I and II movements are not performed at the limit of available joint motion, they create minimal tension in the affected tissues. These grades are used primarily for reduction of joint pain. Grade III and IV movements apply tension up to, or at the limit of, existing ligament or capsular length. Thus, they are intended to apply sufficient force to stretch shortened tissues. A Grade V movement involves *manipulation*, a high-velocity manual thrust designed to tear shortened tissues. This maneuver lies largely within the domain of

Table 5.2   Maitland's Grades of Oscillatory Movement

Grade	Description of movement
I	Small amplitude movement at the beginning of the range
II	Large amplitude movement within the range, but not reaching either limit of the range
III	Large amplitude movement up to the limit of the range
IV	Small amplitude movement at the limit of the range

From Maitland, 1977.

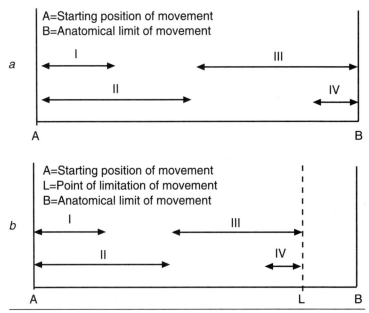

Figure 5.5 Grades of oscillatory movements in joint mobilization in a joint with *(a)* normal anatomical limits, and *(b)* limited joint motion.

Reprinted, by permission, from T. Barak, E.R. Rosen, and R. Sofer, 1990, Basic concepts of orthopaedic manual therapy. In *Orthopaedic and sports physical therapy*, 2nd ed., edited by J.A. Gould III (St. Louis: C.V. Mosby), 198.

the attending physician or specially trained clinicians and is typically reserved for treatment of persistent joint contractures and adhesions.

Research and clinical observations

In addition to the joint mobilization techniques developed by Maitland (1977), other specific methods and protocols for restoration of joint mobility have been developed by Cyriax (1974) and Kaltenborn (1980). Despite the availability and widespread use of these techniques since the 1970s, surprisingly little clinical research has been done to determine their effectiveness as compared to traditional passive mobilization methods. Difficulty in quantifying the magnitude and duration of tissue loading has hampered the design of controlled studies regarding the efficacy of manual joint mobilization techniques. Studies by Nicholson (1985) and Randall, Portney, and Harris (1992) are among the few reported investigations that have attempted to quantify the effect of manual oscillatory movements on restoration of joint motion. Using oscillatory techniques developed by Maitland (1977), Nicholson (1985) found these techniques effective in the management of adhesive capsulitis of the shoulder. Randall, Portney, and Harris (1992) applied longitudinal traction and gliding movements to previously immobilized metacarpophalangeal joints in subjects who had experienced metacarpal fractures. Following a series of three treatment sessions over a one-week period, these investigators found significantly greater increases in joint mobility in the treated subjects compared to subjects who received no mobilization treatments.

Despite the paucity of quantitative data, joint mobilization techniques that employ manual oscillatory movements have enjoyed widespread acceptance based on observed clinical effectiveness. To the extent that tensile forces of sufficient magnitude and duration are applied to joint capsules and ligaments, increases in permanent tissue elongation can be expected. It should be noted, however, that joint mobilization techniques, as described above, do not involve the application of prolonged tensile loading, which is generally recognized as an effective method of promoting permanent connective tissue elongation. Nevertheless, a particular therapeutic benefit is derived from the use of these techniques to localize tension forces to restrictive articular tissues, thereby addressing loss of accessory joint motions.

Functional Tissue Loading

Although clinical experience has demonstrated the benefits of prolonged tensile loading, proprioceptive neuromuscular facilitation, and manual joint mobilization techniques in connective tissue mobilization, these techniques are typically inadequate to address loss of tensile strength in immobilized or surgically repaired ligaments and joint capsules. Furthermore, traditional one-plane resistance exercises for development of muscular strength typically fail to simulate the functional physiological joint movements that occur during sports activity. Consequently, the mechanical loads imposed on ligaments and joint capsules during these therapeutic protocols may be insufficient to produce optimal tensile strength. Optimal collagen fiber size, alignment, and tensile strength may not occur until ligaments and joint capsules are subjected to the mechanical loads inherent in a particular sports activity. These considerations suggest the need for controlled, sport-specific functional activities that impart progressively increased tensile forces to ligaments and joint capsules. Lateral movements and cutting maneuvers, for example, may be necessary to impart adequate multidirectional loads to articular structures of the knee and other weight-bearing joints during later stages of rehabilitation. In a similar sense, progressive functional loading of musculotendinous structures may also be necessary for restoration of optimal tendon tensile strength. In general, these observations suggest that functional rehabilitation, commonly considered the final phase of sports injury management, be designed to incorporate progressive tissue loading that contributes to development of connective tissue tensile strength, as well as activities that promote the traditional components of physical fitness and motor skill performance. For example, as discussed further in chapter 9, activities such as carioca crossover maneuvers, figure eight running, and shuttle runs have been developed as tests of functional performance during recovery from lower extremity injuries, primarily as tests of dynamic joint stabilization. When incorporated as components of functional rehabilitation programs, these types of activities may also provide the mechanical loading necessary for optimal capsuloligamentous tensile strength. The results of studies demonstrating the positive effect of physical activity on the tensile strength of intact ligaments and tendons appear to support this contention (Enwemeka 1991; Tipton et al. 1975; Vailas et al. 1981).

Summary

As acute inflammatory responses to tissue trauma are brought under control during the first stage of connective tissue repair, therapeutic intervention during scar formation and scar maturation, the second and third stages of connective tissue repair, is directed to achievement of three primary objectives: (1) enhancement of the physiological mechanisms of connective tissue repair, (2) prevention of contractures and adhesions, and (3) enhancement of the definitive structure and functional properties of the scar matrix.

Although the rate of connective tissue repair is determined largely by natural physiological responses, rationale exists for the use of selected physical agents to enhance fibrous scar formation and wound contraction, the two primary repair mechanisms that characterize the second stage of tissue healing. These physical agents include various thermal agents and the nonthermal, mechanical effects of ultrasound. Physiological rationale supports the use of thermal agents to increase local tissue temperature and blood flow, thereby contributing to proliferation of white blood cells and increased phagocytosis, increased oxygen supply and cellular metabolism, and an increased supply of nutrients. The therapeutic effects of nonthermal, pulsed ultrasound are attributed to two primary mechanical phenomena, cavitation and acoustic streaming, both of which alter the physiological activities of cells involved in connective tissue repair. Stimulation of macrophages, fibroblasts, myofibroblasts, and vascular endothelial cells by low-intensity pulsed ultrasound is thought to enhance collagen synthesis, angiogenesis, and wound contraction. Although electrotherapy has been used extensively in the management of sports injuries for a variety of therapeutic purposes, the beneficial effect of electrical currents on acceleration of soft connective tissue repair in common sport-related musculoskeletal injuries is largely speculative.

Prevention of soft tissue contractures and adhesions, two complications that may be manifested during recovery from musculoskeletal injuries, represents an additional therapeutic objective during fibroplasia, the second primary stage of connective tissue repair. Although contractures and adhesions may arise as a direct result of persistent inflammation, abnormal wound contraction, or other deviations in normal connective tissue repair, the propensity for these conditions to occur is increased by inappropriate or prolonged immobilization. Therapeutic strategies to prevent contractures and adhesions include the use of continuous passive motion (CPM), modified immobilization or protected mobilization devices, and functional electrical muscle stimulation. Protected mobilization is the contemporary approach to musculoskeletal injury management. It acknowledges the necessity of protecting damaged tissues but also recognizes the therapeutic benefits of controlled motion during early connective tissue repair. Three primary approaches to protected mobilization include the use of serial static immobilization, static progressive splinting, and dynamic splinting.

Although therapeutic measures introduced during the inflammatory and fibroplastic stages of connective tissue repair can contribute significantly to the desired structural and functional properties of developing scar tissue, intervention during scar maturation, the third stage of connective tissue repair, is commonly more specific. Even though debilitating contractures and adhesions may be prevented through early intervention, connective tissue repair inherently involves development of an abnormal fibrotic scar matrix that lacks the plasticity and tensile strength of normal tissues, thereby representing a potential risk factor during return to strenuous sports activities. Restricted activity and immobilization typically exacerbate loss of these connective tissue properties. Therapeutic strategies to enhance connective tissue plasticity include the use of low-load, prolonged stretching; proprioceptive neuromuscular facilitation (PNF); and manual joint mobilization techniques. Whereas these techniques may contribute significantly to connective tissue plasticity and mobility, they may be inadequate for development of optimal tensile strength in injured tissues. Thus, sport-specific functional activities that provide multidirectional tissue loading may be necessary to maximize capsuloligamentous tensile strength. Similarly, progressive mechanical loading of musculotendinous structures during physical activity may also be necessary for restoration of optimal tendon tensile strength.

Problem-Solving Scenario

On referral from a high school team physician, a 16-year-old male sprinter reports to the sports medicine clinic for treatment of a pulled hamstring muscle. During an initial clinical assessment, the athlete indicates that he injured his left hamstring during track practice approximately six weeks earlier. Following initial cold applications, the athlete's treatment during the next three weeks was limited to rest and application of heat packs. Thereafter, relief of symptoms allowed him to resume track practice during which he reinjured his hamstrings approximately one week later. Consequently, he rested for an additional two weeks but received no treatment. During the initial clinical assessment, passive straight leg raising reveals considerable "tightness" and moderate discomfort in the athlete's proximal hamstring muscle group. Bilateral comparison indicates a notable limitation in hip flexion.

Problem-Solving Questions

• Considering the apparent severity of injury and the type of tissues involved, what is the most likely mechanism of tissue healing in this case?

• Given the patient's recent history, what structural and functional alterations have most likely taken place in the affected tissues?

• What specific factors offer the most plausible explanation for the "tightness" and limited extensibility in the hamstring muscle group at this stage of recovery?

• What additional treatment methods, if any, would have been appropriate for use during the first three to four weeks following the patient's original injury? Why?

• Based on the initial clinical assessment, what are the most appropriate short-term treatment goals during the next three weeks of the patient's recovery period?

• What specific mobilization techniques would be most effective for alleviation of the muscle "tightness" and limited extensibility in this case? Why?

References

Abramson, S.B. 1990. Nonsteroidal anti-inflammatory drugs: Mechanisms of action and therapeutic considerations. In *Sports-induced inflammation*, edited by W.B. Leadbetter, J.A. Buckwalter, and S.L. Gordon. Park Ridge, Ill.: American Academy of Orthopaedic Surgeons.

Akeson, W.H., D. Amiel, G.L. Mechanic, S.L.-Y. Woo, F.L. Harwood, and M.L. Hamer. 1977. Collagen cross-linking alterations in joint contractures: Changes in the reducible cross-links in periarticular connective tissue collagen after nine weeks of immobilization. *Connective Tissue Research* 5:15-19.

American Academy of Orthopaedic Surgeons. 1991. *Athletic training and sports medicine*, 2nd ed. Park Ridge, Ill.: American Academy of Orthopaedic Surgeons.

Andriacchi, T., P. Sabiston, K. DeHaven, L. Dahners, S.L.-Y. Woo, C. Frank, B. Oakes, R. Brand, and J. Lewis. 1988. Ligament: Injury and repair. In *Injury and repair of the musculoskeletal soft tissues*, edited by S.L.-Y. Woo and J.A. Buckwalter. Park Ridge, Ill.: American Academy of Orthopaedic Surgeons.

Barak, T., E.R. Rosen, and R. Sofer. 1990. Basic concepts of orthopaedic manual therapy. In *Orthopaedic and sports physical therapy*, 2nd ed., edited by J.A. Gould III. St. Louis: Mosby.

Baumert, P.W. 1993. Modalities in rehabilitation. In *Handbook of sports medicine*, edited by W.A. Lillegard and K.S. Rucker. Boston: Butterworth-Heineman.

Behrens, T.W., and J.S. Goodwin. 1990. Oral corticosteroids. In *Sports-induced inflammation*, edited by W.B. Leadbetter, J.A. Buckwalter, and S.L. Gordon. Park Ridge, Ill.: American Academy of Orthopaedic Surgeons.

Booth, F.W., and E.W. Gould. 1975. Effects of training and disease on connective tissue. In *Exercise and sport science reviews*, edited by J.H. Wilmore and J.F. Keogh. New York: Academic Press.

Bristol, H., and G. Holm. 1998. Residual effects of the hold-relax technique on hamstring flexibility. Unpublished research project. Arizona School of Health Sciences, Phoenix.

Brodowicz, G.R., R. Welsh, and J. Wallis. 1996. Comparison of stretching with ice, stretching with heat, or stretching alone on hamstring flexibility. *Journal of Athletic Training* 31:324-27.

Carlstedt, C.A., and M. Nordin. 1989. Biomechanics of tendons and ligaments. In *Basic biomechanics of the musculoskeletal system*, 2nd ed., edited by M. Nordin and V.H. Frankel. Philadelphia: Lea and Febiger.

Cole, A.J., and R.A. Eagleston. 1994. The benefits of deep heat. *The Physician and Sportsmedicine* 22:77-87.

Cotran, R.S., V. Kumar, and S.L. Robbins. 1989. *Robbins pathologic basis of disease*, 4th ed. Philadelphia: W.B. Saunders.

Cummings, G.S., and L.J. Tillman. 1992. Remodeling of dense connective tissue in normal adult tissues. In *Dynamics of human biologic tissues*, edited by D.P. Currier and R.M. Nelson. Philadelphia: Davis.

Cummings, J.P. 1992. Additional therapeutic uses of electricity. In *Electrotherapy in rehabilitation*, edited by M.R. Gersh. Philadelphia: Davis.

Cyriax, J. 1974. *Textbook of orthopedic medicine—Treatment by manipulation, massage, and injection*, vol. 2. Baltimore: Williams and Wilkins.

DeVahl, J. 1992. Neuromuscular electrical stimulation in rehabilitation. In *Electrotherapy in rehabilitation*, edited by M.R. Gersh. Philadelphia: Davis.

Draper, D.O., C. Anderson, S.S. Schulthies, and M.D. Ricard. 1998. Immediate and residual changes in dorsiflexion range of motion using an ultrasound heat and stretch routine. *Journal of Athletic Training* 33:141-44.

Dyson, M. 1990. Role of ultrasound in wound healing. In *Wound healing: Alternatives in management*, edited by L.C. Kloth, J.M. McCulloch, and J.A. Feedar. Philadelphia: Davis.

Enwemeka, C.S. 1991. Connective tissue plasticity: Ultrastructural, biomechanical, and morphometric effects of physical factors on intact and regenerating tendons. *Journal of Sports Physical Therapy* 14:198-212.

Ferreira, E. 1978. A comparison of hold-relax and passive stretch techniques to increase flexibility. Unpublished master's thesis. Hayward State University, Hayward, Calif.

Frank, C., W.H. Akeson, S.L.-Y. Woo, D. Amiel, and R.D. Coutts. 1984. Physiology and therapeutic value of passive joint motion. *Clinical Orthopaedics and Related Research* 185:113-25.

Gajdosik, R.L. 1991. Effects of static stretching on the maximal length and resistance to passive stretch of short hamstring muscles. *Journal of Sports Physical Therapy* 14:250-55.

Ganong, W.F. 1995. *Review of medical physiology*, 17th ed. Norwalk, Conn.: Appleton and Lange.

Gelberman, R.H., S.L-Y. Woo, K. Lothringer, W.H. Akeson, and D. Ameil. 1982. Effects of early intermittent passive mobilization on healing canine flexor tendons. *Journal of Hand Surgery* 7:170-75.

Gersh, M.R. 1992. *Electrotherapy in rehabilitation*. Philadelphia: Davis.

Gibbons, K.T. 1980. A comparison of three mobilization methods to increase and retain flexibility of hip joint extensors. Unpublished master's thesis. The University of Arizona, Tucson.

Gieck, J.H., and E.N. Saliba. 1990. Therapeutic ultrasound: Influence on inflammation and healing. In *Sports-induced inflammation*, edited by W.B. Leadbetter, J.A. Buckwalter, and S.L. Gordon. Park Ridge, Ill.: American Academy of Orthopaedic Surgeons.

Harrelson, G.L. 1991. Physiologic factors of rehabilitation. In *Physical rehabilitation of the injured athlete*, edited by J.R. Andrews and G.L. Harrelson. Philadelphia: W.B. Saunders.

Hepburn, G.R., and K.J. Crivelli. 1984. Use of elbow Dynasplint for reduction of elbow flexion contractures: A case study. *The Journal of Orthopaedic and Sports Physical Therapy* 5:269-74.

Hutton, R.S. 1992. Neuromuscular basis of stretching exercises. In *Strength and power in sport*, edited by P.V. Komi. Cambridge, Mass.: Blackwell Science.

Kaltenborn, F. 1980. *Manual mobilization of the extremity joints: Examination and basic treatment techniques*. Universitetagaten: Olaf Norlis Bokhandel.

Kellett, J. 1986. Acute soft tissue injuries—A review of the literature. *Medicine and Science in Sports and Exercise* 18:489-99.

Kisner, C., and L.A. Colby. 1990. *Therapeutic exercise: Foundations and techniques*, 2nd ed. Philadelphia: Davis.

Kottke, F.J., D.L. Pauley, and R.A. Ptak. 1966. The rationale for prolonged stretching for correction of shortening of connective tissue. *Archives of Physical Medicine and Rehabilitation* 47:345-52.

Laros, G.S., C.M. Tipton, and R.R. Cooper. 1971. Influence of physical activity on ligament insertions in the knees of dogs. *The Journal of Bone and Joint Surgery* 53-A:275-86.

Leadbetter, W.B., J.A. Buckwalter, and S.L. Gordon, eds. 1990. *Sports-induced inflammation*. Park Ridge, Ill.: American Academy of Orthopaedic Surgeons.

Lentell, G., T. Hetherington, J. Eagan, and M. Morgan. 1992. The use of thermal agents to influence the effectiveness of a low-load prolonged stretch. *Journal of Sports Physical Therapy* 16:200-207.

Maitland, G.D. 1977. *Peripheral manipulation*, 2nd ed. Boston: Butterworth and Company.

McDiarmid, T., M.C. Ziskin, and S.L. Michlovitz. 1996. Therapeutic ultrasound. In *Thermal agents in rehabilitation*, 3rd ed., edited by S.L. Michlovitz. Philadelphia: Davis.

Nicholson, G. 1985. The effects of passive joint mobilization on pain and hypomobility associated with adhesive capsulitis of the shoulder. *The Journal of Orthopaedic and Sports Physical Therapy* 6:238-46.

Obremsky, W.T., A.V. Seaber, B.M. Ribbeck, and W.E. Garrett. 1994. Biomechanical and histological assessment of a controlled muscle strain injury treated with piroxicam. *The American Journal of Sports Medicine* 22:558-61.

O'Donoghue, P.C., M.R. McCarthy, J.H. Gieck, and C.K. Yates. 1991. Clinical use of continuous passive motion in athletic training. *Athletic Training* 26:201-8.

Osternig, L.R., R.N. Robertson, R.K. Troxel, and P. Hansen. 1990. Differential responses to proprioceptive neuromuscular facilitation (PNF) stretch techniques. *Medicine and Science in Sports and Exercise* 22:106-11.

Owoeye, I., N.I. Spielholz, J. Fetto, and A.J. Nelson. 1987. Low-intensity pulsed galvanic current and the healing of tenotomized rat Achilles tendons: Preliminary report using load-to-breaking measurements. *Archives of Physical Medicine and Rehabilitation* 68:415-18.

Prentice, W.E. 1982. An electromyographic analysis of the effectiveness of heat or cold and stretching for inducing relaxation in injured muscle. *The Journal of Orthopaedic and Sports Physical Therapy* 3:133-40.

Prentice, W.E. 1983. A comparison of static stretching and PNF stretching for improving hip joint flexibility. *Athletic Training* 8:56-59.

Price, H. 1990. Connective tissue in wound healing. In *Wound healing: Alternatives in management*, edited by L.C. Kloth, J.M. McCulloch, and J.A. Feeder. Philadelphia: Davis.

Quillen, W.S., T.M. Mohr, and B.V. Reed. 1990. High-voltage pulsed galvanic stimulation as a modifier of sports-induced inflammation. In *Sports-induced inflammation*, edited by W.B. Leadbetter, J.A. Buckwalter, and S.L. Gordon. Park Ridge, Ill.: American Academy of Orthopaedic Surgeons.

Randall, T., L. Portney, and B.A. Harris. 1992. Effects of joint mobilization on joint stiffness and active motion of the metacarpal-phalangeal joint. *Journal of Sports Physical Therapy* 16:30-36.

Rennie, G.A., and S.L. Michlovitz. 1996. Biophysical principles of heating and superficial heating agents. In *Thermal agents in rehabilitation*, 3rd ed., edited by S.L. Michlovitz. Philadelphia: Davis.

Sadler, J.A., and J.M. Koepfer. 1992. Rehabilitation and splinting of the injured hand. In *Hand injuries in athletes*, edited by J.W. Strickland and A.C. Rettig. Philadelphia: W.B. Saunders.

Salter, R.B. 1999. *Textbook of disorders and injuries of the musculoskeletal system*, 3rd ed. Baltimore: Williams and Wilkins.

Sapega, A.A., T.C. Quedenfeld, R.A. Moyer, and R.A. Butler. 1981. Biophysical factors in range-of-motion exercise. *The Physician and Sportsmedicine* 9:57-65.

Stanish, W.D., M. Rubinovich, J. Kozey, and G. MacGillvary. 1985. The use of electricity in ligament and tendon repair. *The Physician and Sportsmedicine* 13:109-16.

Stillwell, G.K. 1965. General principles of thermotherapy. In *Therapeutic heat and cold*, 2nd ed., edited by S. Licht. New Haven, Conn.: Elizabeth Licht.

Stralka, S.W. 1992. Application of therapeutic electrical currents in the management of the orthopedic patient. In *Electrotherapy in rehabilitation*, edited by M.R. Gersh. Philadelphia: Davis.

Surburg, P.R. 1981. Neuromuscular facilitation techniques in sports medicine. *The Physician and Sportsmedicine* 9:115-27.

Surburg, P.R., and J.W. Schrader. 1997. Proprioceptive neuromuscular facilitation techniques in sports medicine: A reassessment. *Journal of Athletic Training* 32:34-39.

Sweitzer, R.W. 1994. Ultrasound. In *Physical agents: A comprehensive text for physical therapists*, edited by B. Hecox, T.A. Mehreteab, and J. Weisberg. Norwalk, Conn.: Appleton and Lange.

Tanigawa, M.C. 1972. Comparison of the hold-relax procedure and passive mobilization on increasing muscle length. *Physical Therapy* 52:725-35.

Thomas, C.L., ed. 1993. *Taber's cyclopedic medical dictionary*, 17th ed. Philadelphia: Davis.

Tillman, L.J., and G.S. Cummings. 1992. Biologic mechanisms of connective tissue mutability. In *Dynamics of human biologic tissues*, edited by D.P. Currier and R.M. Nelson. Philadelphia: Davis.

Tipton, C.M., R.D. Matthes, J.A. Maynard, and R.A. Carey. 1975. The influence of physical activity on ligaments and tendons. *Medicine and Science in Sports* 7:165-75.

Vailas, A.C., C.M. Tipton, R.D. Matthes, and M. Gart. 1981. Physical activity and its influence on the repair process of medical collateral ligaments. *Connective Tissue Research* 9:25-31.

Voss, D.E., M.K. Ionta, and B.J. Myers. 1985. *Proprioceptive neuromuscular facilitation: Patterns and techniques*, 3rd ed. Philadelphia: Harper and Row.

Weber, C., and R. Wolff. 1999. Residual effects of a contract-relax PNF stretching program. Unpublished research project. Arizona School of Health Sciences, Phoenix.

Wessling, K.C., D.A. DeVane, and C.R. Hylton. 1987. Effects of static stretch versus static stretch and ultrasound combined on triceps surae muscle extensibility in healthy women. *Physical Therapy* 67:674-79.

Whiting, W.C., and R.F. Zernicke. 1998. *Biomechanics of musculoskeletal injury*. Champaign, Ill.: Human Kinetics.

Woo, S.L-Y., R.H. Gelberman, N.G. Cobb, D. Amiel, K. Lothringer, and W.H. Akeson. 1981. The importance of controlled passive mobilization on flexor tendon healing: A biomechanical study. *Acta Orthop. Scand* 52:615-22.

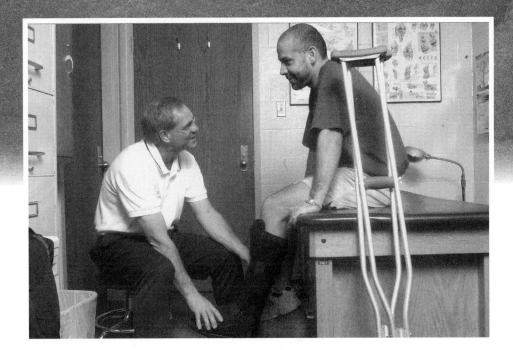

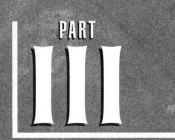

Fracture Healing and Therapeutic Management

Fractures that occur in the sports population commonly involve the upper and lower extremities. Consequently, management of fractures that occur in the long bones of the skeletal system is the primary focus of discussion in this part. Bone healing occurs throughout the three primary stages of hematoma formation and inflammation, cellular proliferation and callus formation, and remodeling. This part includes a review of fracture-healing mechanisms, a discussion of basic principles and concepts in fracture management, and presentation of implications for resumption of sports activity following a fracture. Chapter 6, Fracture Healing, includes a review of normal bone morphology and histology as a basis for subsequent discussion of normal bone-healing mechanisms. Abnormal bone healing, including nonunion, delayed union, and malunion, is also discussed in this chapter. Chapter 7, Therapeutic Implications: Fracture Healing, includes a review of principles and techniques in the medical management of fractures, including fracture reduction, skeletal fixation, and fracture immobilization. Therapeutic implications for restoration of bone and soft tissue function following a fracture are also reviewed in this chapter.

Fracture Healing

CHAPTER 6

Morphology and Histology of Bone
Morphology of Long Bones
Histology of Long Bones
Microstructure of Cortical Bone
Blood Supply
Osteogenic Cells

Bone Regeneration and Repair
Hematoma Formation and Inflammation
Cellular Proliferation and Callus Formation
Early Repair Phase
Intermediate Repair Phase
Late Repair Phase
Remodeling

Abnormal Bone Healing
Nonunion
Delayed Union
Malunion

Summary

Learning Objectives

After completion of this chapter, the reader should be able to

1. describe the normal morphological and histological structure of the long bones of the musculoskeletal system,
2. differentiate between primary bone healing and secondary bone healing,
3. identify and describe the three primary stages of secondary bone healing, and
4. identify and describe the three primary manifestations of abnormal bone healing.

By definition, a *fracture* is a break in the structural continuity of a bone with a loss of structural integrity (Salter 1999). Depending on the traumatic forces involved and the extent of bone fragment displacement, however, fractures typically involve some degree of injury to adjacent soft tissues. Thus, the sports health care clinician's understanding of fracture healing necessitates an awareness of soft tissue repair as a concomitant process, especially during the early stages of fracture healing. The mechanisms of soft tissue repair were discussed in chapter 3. Whereas soft connective tissue injuries heal by scar formation, uncomplicated fracture healing occurs through a process of regeneration, which restores the normal structural and biomechanical properties of bone. Regeneration of osseous tissue during fracture healing follows patterns of bone formation that occur during embryonic development and skeletal growth. Because fractures associated with sports participation commonly involve the upper and lower extremities, patterns of bone regeneration that characterize healing of the long bones of the skeletal system are the primary focus of discussion in this chapter. After a review of the structural characteristics of healthy adult bone, normal bone healing is discussed as a prelude to consideration of fracture treatment and therapeutic management in chapter 7. An overview of deviations in normal bone healing is also presented in this chapter.

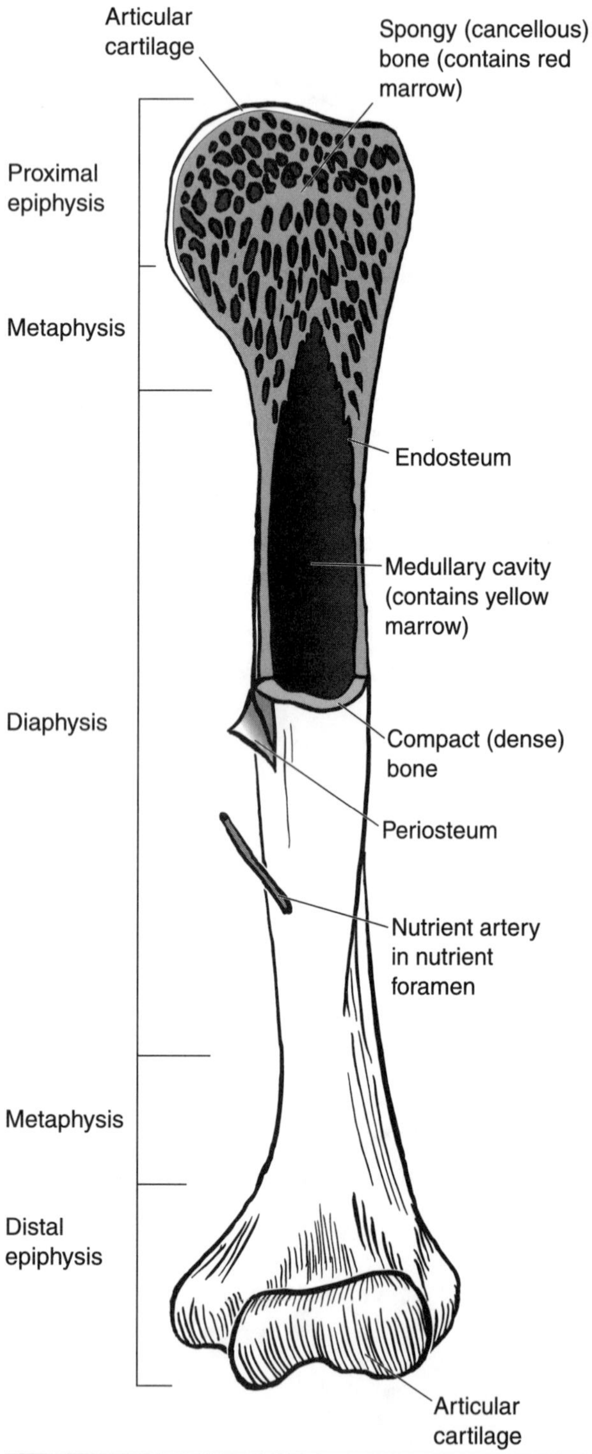

Morphology and Histology of Bone

Unless complications in bone regeneration arise during fracture healing (e.g., nonunion), restoration of the characteristic morphology (i.e., structure and form) and histology (i.e., microstructure) of osseous tissue is the normal outcome. Under favorable conditions, bone healing occurs on a continuum of interrelated vascular and cellular events that eventually restore the structural continuity and architectural integrity of osseous tissue. As a basis for understanding these physiological processes and the results of normal, uncomplicated fracture healing, the morphology and histology of the long bones of the skeletal system are reviewed prior to a discussion of fracture healing mechanisms.

Morphology of Long Bones

In contrast to short, flat, and irregular bones of the skeletal system (e.g., the carpals, tarsals, scapula), by definition, long bones have greater length than width (e.g., the humerus, femur). As illustrated in

Figure 6.1 Major parts of a long bone.

Adapted from G.J. Tortora and S.R. Grobowski, 1993, *Principles of anatomy and physiology*, 7th ed. (New York: Harper Collin's College Publishers), 148. Copyright © 1993, John Wiley & Sons, Inc. This material is used by permission of John Wiley & Sons, Inc.

Labels in figure: Articular cartilage; Spongy (cancellous) bone (contains red marrow); Proximal epiphysis; Metaphysis; Endosteum; Diaphysis; Medullary cavity (contains yellow marrow); Compact (dense) bone; Periosteum; Nutrient artery in nutrient foramen; Metaphysis; Distal epiphysis; Articular cartilage

figure 6.1, the primary structural components of mature long bones are the *diaphysis*, or shaft, and the proximal and distal ends referred to as *epiphyses*. A third major component of a mature long bone, the *metaphysis*, represents the region toward each end of the diaphysis that joins with the epiphysis. In immature growing bones, the metaphysis and the epiphysis are separated by the *epiphyseal plate* where longitudinal growth of the bone occurs.

The long bones of the skeletal system consist of both *cancellous* (spongy) *bone* and *compact* (dense) *bone*. Cancellous bone is characterized by a spongy network of *trabeculae*, or bony spicules, with large intervening spaces containing red marrow. Because of these structural characteristics, cancellous bone is also referred to as *trabecular bone*. A primary distinction between cancellous bone and compact bone is the comparative degree of *porosity*. Because cancellous bone contains a higher percentage of nonmineralized tissue (i.e., red marrow) in the spaces between trabeculae, it is more porous than compact bone (Nordin and Frankel 1989). In contrast to cancellous bone, which is most prominent in the epiphysis and the metaphysis of long bones, dense compact bone forms the outer layer, or *cortex*, of the diaphysis and is commonly referred to as *cortical bone*. In long bones, cortical bone is comparatively thick along the diaphysis where strength and stiffness are needed. The bone cortex encloses the *medullary cavity*, the cylindrical central portion of the diaphysis that contains fatty, yellow marrow. A dense, fibrous membrane called the *periosteum* covers the outer surface of the cortex except at the articulating surfaces, which are covered by a thin layer of hyaline cartilage. The periosteum consists of two layers, an outer *fibrous layer* composed of dense, irregular connective tissue and an inner osteogenic layer (i.e., the cambium layer) that contains osteoprogenitor cells and osteoblasts. A thinner, areolar membrane, the *endosteum*, lines the medullary cavity in the diaphysis and is also a source of osteogenic cells (Tortora and Grabowski 1993). As discussed shortly, osteogenic cells that originate from the periosteum and the endosteum are the connective tissue cells responsible for ossification and regeneration of bone tissue after a fracture.

Histology of Long Bones

Like other types of connective tissue, mature bone consists of three primary structural components including *cells*, *fibers*, and *ground substance* (see chapter 1). Collagen fibers, predominantly Type I fibers, and ground substance consisting of water, glycosaminoglycans (GAGs), and noncollagenous proteins that function as binding factors for calcium are the major components of the extracellular matrix (Schiller 1994). As a specialized form of dense connective tissue, the extracellular matrix of bone consists of solid, mineralized material rather than the amorphous, gelatinous substance that forms the ground substance of soft connective tissues. Inorganic minerals (e.g., calcium), which are deposited in the extracellular matrix and bound to collagen fibers during mineralization, provide bone density and stiffness, whereas the collagen fibers provide tensile strength. The mineral content of osseous tissue is a primary distinguishing feature between bone and other types of connective tissues (Whiting and Zernicke 1998). When the extracellular matrix becomes mineralized, the connective tissue is called *bone*.

Microstructure of Cortical Bone

In contrast to the irregular trabecular network of cancellous bone found in the epiphysis and the metaphysis of long bones, the dense compact bone that forms the outer layer of the diaphysis (i.e., the cortex) consists of organized structural units called *haversian systems*, or *osteons* (Tortora and Grabowski 1993). These cylindrical structures parallel the longitudinal axis of the bone (figure 6.2). A haversian system is composed of calcified rings, or *concentric lamellae*, that form a central canal referred to as a *haversian canal*. Additional components of a haversian system include *lacunae*, small cavities that contain bone cells called *osteocytes*, and *canaliculi*, tiny channels that radiate from the lacunae and contain

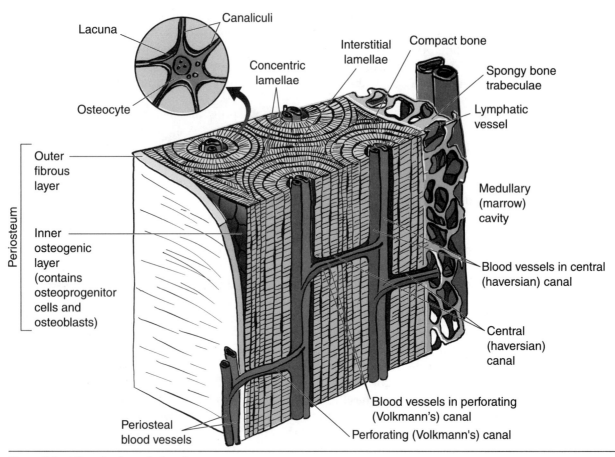

Figure 6.2   Microstructure of a long bone.

Adapted from G.J. Tortora and S.R. Grabowski, 1993, *Principles of anatomy and physiology*, 7th ed. (New York: Harper Collins), 150. Copyright © 1993, John Wiley & Sons, Inc. This material is used by permission of John Wiley & Sons, Inc.

cytoplasmic processes of the osteocytes. Like the osteons of compact bone, the trabeculae of cancellous bone also contain lacunae and canaliculi that house osteocytes and their extending cytoplasm. Osteocytes function to maintain bone as living tissue. In contrast to the concentric lamellae that form the haversian systems of compact bone, the intervening areas between osteons are composed of bony layers referred to as *interstitial lamellae*. The haversian canals formed by the concentric rings of an osteon are connected by *Volkmann's canals* that transverse the interstitial lamellae of the bone cortex (see figure 6.2). Together, these canals house the internal blood vessels, lymph vessels, and nerves of cortical bone.

Blood Supply

As illustrated in figure 6.3, blood supply to the diaphysis of long bones is provided by two main sources, branches of the *periosteal arteries* that penetrate the cortex and the *nutrient artery*, which enters the medullary cavity through an oblique opening referred to as the *nutrient foramen* (Tortora and Grabowski 1993). On entering the endosteum, branches of the nutrient artery extend longitudinally and reenter the cortex of the diaphysis (Whiting and Zernicke 1998). Branches of these arteries also provide blood supply to the metaphysis and the epiphysis. Blood supply to the epiphysis is also provided by a network of arterial branches that enter the epiphysis directly.

As previously noted, the haversian canals of the osteons and the transverse Volkmann's canals form a framework that houses the internal vascular system of cortical bone (see figure 6.2). As blood vessels enter the cortex through Volkmann's canals, they connect with blood vessels in the haversian canals and the medullary cavity to form a rich vascu-

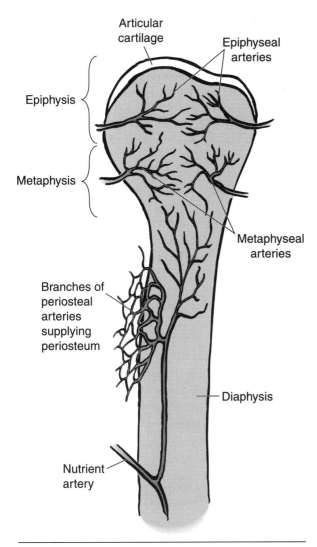

Figure 6.3 Blood supply of a long bone.

Reprinted, by permission, from D.H. Cormack, *Ham's histology*, 9th ed. (Philadelphia, PA: Lippincott, Williams, and Wilkins), 314.

lar network that supplies various portions of the diaphysis, metaphysis, and the epiphysis. Disruption of this vascular network is, in part, responsible for the hematoma that forms between bone fragments following fractures of long bones.

Osteogenic Cells

The cellular components of osseous tissue that lie within the bone matrix include *osteoprogenitor cells*, *osteoblasts*, *osteocytes*, and *osteoclasts* (Tortora and Grabowski 1993). By definition, osteoprogenitor cells are precursor cells that are derived from mesenchyme, the embryonic tissue from which mature connective tissue arises. These cells are capable of mitosis (i.e., division) and, thus, differentiation into osteoblasts, the osteogenic cells responsible for collagen synthesis and bone formation. Osteoprogenitor cells are found in the inner osteogenic layer of the periosteum and in the endosteum. As discussed shortly, disruption of the periosteum is a primary stimulus for proliferation of osteoblasts during the early stages of fracture healing. As osseous tissue forms during skeletal growth, osteoblasts become surrounded by components of the extracellular matrix and henceforth are referred to as *osteocytes*. Thus, osteocytes become residence cells of the small cavities (i.e., lacunae) in the lamellae of haversian systems of compact bone and the trabeculae of cancellous bone. Connection of osteocytes with neighboring osteocytes through their extending cytoplasmic processes in the canaliculi (i.e., the small interconnecting canals) form a network through which osseous tissue is supplied with nutrients from local blood vessels. Thus, osteocytes monitor the continual metabolic activities that maintain bone as living tissue (Loitz-Ramage and Zernicke 1996).

In contrast to osteoblasts, the osteogenic cells responsible for formation of the extracellular bone matrix, osteoclasts function to remove minerals and resorb unwanted osseous tissue from the bone matrix, a process referred to as *deossification* (Thomas 1993). These large, multinuclear cells, which are derived from hematopoietic cells in the bone marrow, are found in small depressions on the bone surface called *Howship's lacunae* (Schiller 1994). Howship's lacunae represent areas where bone resorption is occurring.

Through the combined processes of bone formation and bone resorption, growing bone assumes its ultimate structure. These two functions are also responsible for maintenance of the structural integrity of mature bone as continual "turnover" of osseous tissue occurs, a process that is analogous to collagen synthesis and collagen lysis in other connective tissues (Montoye 1987). After a fracture, the combined actions of osteoblasts and osteoclasts are essential to regeneration of osseous tissue and bone remodeling.

Bone Regeneration and Repair

The mechanisms responsible for development of osseous tissue are referred to collectively as *ossification*, or *osteogenesis*, the process through which other tissues are converted into bone. During embryonic development, two types of tissues, fibrous connective tissue membranes (i.e., mesenchyme) and cartilage, provide the supporting framework for ossification. The process through which fibrous connective tissue membranes are transformed into bone is referred to as *intramembranous ossification*, whereas conversion of cartilage into bone is called *endochondral ossification*. Although these two ossification models involve different patterns of bone formation, both processes involve the replacement of preexisting tissues with bone. Whereas certain flat bones of the skeletal system (e.g., skull, mandible) are formed by intramembranous ossification, formation of long bones occurs primarily through endochondral ossification. Healing of cortical bone after fractures of long bones involves gradual transformation of initially formed cartilage into bone, thereby following a pattern of endochondral, or intracartilaginous, ossification.

As is the case in soft connective tissue repair, normal fracture healing occurs through a sequence of overlapping stages of physiological events. The primary stages of fracture healing can be categorized as (1) hematoma formation and inflammation, (2) cellular proliferation and callus formation, and (3) remodeling. Although the specific mechanisms of bone regeneration and soft connective tissue repair differ in several respects, the primary stages of fracture healing are generally comparable to the three stages of soft tissue repair (i.e., inflammation, fibroplasia, and scar maturation). It is important to note that the stages of fracture healing described in this chapter characterize the type of fracture healing referred to as *secondary bone healing*, which occurs in the absence of rigid internal fixation of fracture fragments with metallic devices. Unlike *primary bone healing*, which occurs directly between approximated cortical bone fragments as the result of rigid internal fixation and interfragmental compression, secondary bone healing is characterized by development of an intervening fibrocartilaginous callus (Salter 1999). Primary bone healing associated with open fracture reduction and rigid internal fixation is discussed further in chapter 7.

Hematoma Formation and Inflammation

When diaphyseal fractures occur, hemorrhage results from a disruption of the periosteal arteries, the nutrient artery, or the blood vessel branches that form the internal vascular network of long bones (see figures 6.2 and 6.3). Although normal hemostatic mechanisms function to control intraosseous hemorrhage, a localized fracture hematoma develops around the bone ends at the fracture site (figure 6.4). Should more extensive bleeding result from significant periosteal disruption, displacement of fracture fragments, and damage to adjacent soft tissues, the resulting hematoma may extend into the surrounding soft tissues. Like the secondary hypoxic injury that occurs in acute soft connective tissue injuries, impairment of local blood supply associated with the fracture hematoma results in ischemic cellular necrosis. When fractures occur, blood supply to resident osteocytes is disrupted, resulting in necrosis of osseous tissue at the fracture site (Salter 1999). The absence of osteocytes from the lacunae of cortical bone is the hallmark of dead bone (Schiller 1994). During fracture healing, regenerative processes eventually replace bone tissue lost because of cellular necrosis, as well the osseous tissues that are disrupted by the acute traumatic incidence.

Although seemingly detrimental to subsequent bony union, the hematoma that forms during the first few hours after a fracture establishes the environment in which early bone regeneration occurs. Hence, the fracture hematoma, along with characteristic inflammatory responses, represents the normal initial stage of bone healing. As is the case in other connective tissue injuries, the initial fibrin network that forms in the traumatized tissues provides a structural framework for localization of the phagocytic white blood cells that are essential to resolution of acute inflammatory responses (see chapter 3). In addition, the fracture hematoma provides the medium for proliferation of the osteogenic cells necessary for collagen synthesis and new bone formation. During subsequent phases of fracture healing, the hematoma is resorbed to permit uncomplicated bone regeneration and solid bony union.

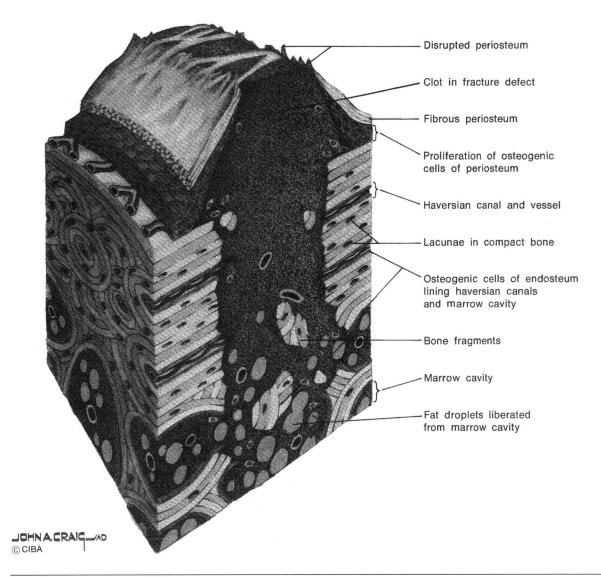

Disrupted periosteum

Clot in fracture defect

Fibrous periosteum

Proliferation of osteogenic cells of periosteum

Haversian canal and vessel

Lacunae in compact bone

Osteogenic cells of endosteum lining haversian canals and marrow cavity

Bone fragments

Marrow cavity

Fat droplets liberated from marrow cavity

Figure 6.4   Early phase of fracture healing (proliferation of osteogenic cells).

Cellular Proliferation and Callus Formation

Proliferation of osteogenic cells with subsequent callus formation and eventual bony union characterizes the second major stage of fracture healing. As is the case with the second stage of soft connective tissue repair (i.e., fibroplasia), cellular proliferation, collagen synthesis, and initial formation of an extracellular connective tissue matrix overlaps the inflammatory stage of secondary bone healing. As previously indicated, the fracture hematoma provides the medium for proliferation of osteogenic cells and granulation tissue formation. Subsequently, development of a fibrocartilaginous callus and eventual formation of a bony matrix occurs at the fracture site. The vascular and cellular mechanisms responsible for this sequence of events constitute the process of ossification, or new bone formation. Eventually, inorganic minerals are deposited in the bony matrix through the process of *mineralization*. For discussion purposes, bone regeneration and repair can be subdivided into an early, an intermediate, and a late phase (Bryant 1977).

Early Repair Phase

The early phase of fracture healing is characterized by proliferation of osteogenic cells of the periosteum and the endosteum (see figure 6.4). Within a few days after injury, osteoprogenitor cells originating from the damaged periosteum and the endosteum migrate to the fracture site and invade the fibrin network in the fracture hematoma. These ancestor cells differentiate into specialized osteogenic cells that function as *osteoblasts* to form new bone and *chondroblasts* that form cartilage. Disruption of the periosteum at the time of injury is a particularly strong stimulus to proliferation of osteoblasts, the osteogenic cells located in the inner periosteal layer (Raney and Brashear 1971). This periosteal response extends several millimeters beyond the immediate fracture site (Bryant 1977). It has also been suggested that osteoblasts arise from pluripotent cells (i.e., cells capable of forming different cell types) that migrate to the fracture site from the bone marrow or from surrounding soft tissues (Bryant 1977). The primary function of osteoblasts in fracture healing is collagen synthesis and formation of collagen fibers in the extracellular bone matrix. Collagen synthesis, development of collagen fibers (i.e., fibrogenesis), and formation of stabilizing collagen cross-links occur through the sequence of cellular events that characterize soft connective tissue repair (see chapter 3, figure 3.5). While osteoblasts produce bone, chondroblasts function to produce the cartilaginous callus that forms during early fracture healing. Resorption of necrotic bone tissue and bone fragments at the fracture site is a function of osteoclasts, whereas chondroclasts are responsible for resorption of calcified cartilage.

Intermediate Repair Phase

The intermediate phase of fracture healing is characterized by granulation tissue formation with subsequent development of a fibrocartilaginous callus at the fracture site (figure 6.5). As osteoblasts proliferate and synthesize collagen, a soft unorganized collagen fiber matrix develops around the fractured bone ends. Initially, weak granulation tissue, characterized by Type III collagen, is formed as endothelial budding (i.e., sprouting of new capillaries) occurs and new blood vessels invade the developing matrix, usually within two to three days after injury. This temporary fibrous bridge gradually replaces the previously formed hematoma within a few days after injury (Groner and Weeks 1992). Thereafter, the composition of the fibrous bridge progressively changes as the fibrocartilaginous callus is formed.

During the intermediate phase of diaphyseal fracture healing, both an *external callus* and an *internal callus* are formed as a primary characteristic of secondary bone healing (Salter 1999). The external callus, which develops in the cortex, is formed by cells originating from the deep osteogenic layer of the periosteum. As neovascularization of the external callus occurs through endothelial budding and development of new blood vessels, the early fibrocartilaginous callus is gradually replaced by new bone through the action of osteoblasts (see figure 6.5). Formation of osseous tissue in the external callus of cortical bone begins at a distance of several millimeters on each side of the fracture site where the periosteal blood supply has been preserved, proceeds toward the fracture site to replace the fibrocartilaginous callus, and eventually joins to form a bony callus that surrounds the bone ends (Schultz 1990). Histological evidence of new bone formation by osteogenic cells of the periosteum within two days after a fracture has been reported (Raney and Brashear 1971). As noted by Loitz-Ramage and Zernicke (1996), new bony trabeculae are typically formed within 3 to 14 days. Visible callus formation is typically evident on x-ray within 10 to 14 days after injury.

In contrast to the external callus, which is formed by osteogenic cells of the periosteum, the internal callus is formed by osteogenic cells of the endosteum. Formation of the internal callus typically lags behind external callus formation by several days. As new bone

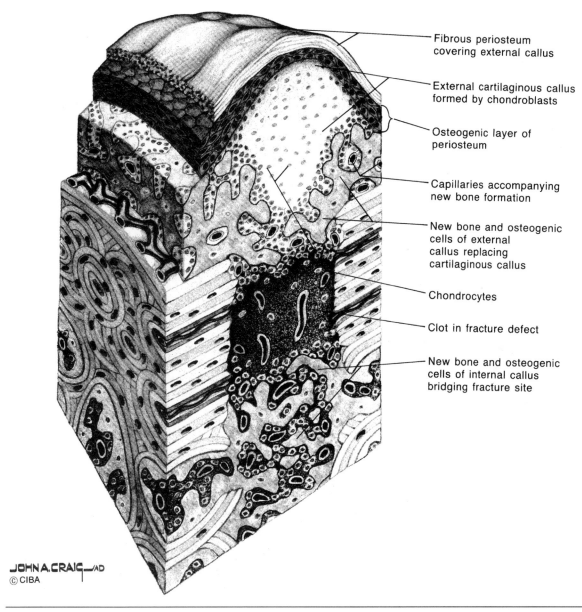

Fibrous periosteum covering external callus

External cartilaginous callus formed by chondroblasts

Osteogenic layer of periosteum

Capillaries accompanying new bone formation

New bone and osteogenic cells of external callus replacing cartilaginous callus

Chondrocytes

Clot in fracture defect

New bone and osteogenic cells of internal callus bridging fracture site

JOHN A. CRAIG—AD
© CIBA

Figure 6.5   Intermediate phase of fracture healing (formation of external and internal callus).

develops in the internal callus, an osseous bridge is formed between the fractured bone ends in the central portion of the diaphysis (see figure 6.5). Whereas fracture healing in both cortical bone and cancellous bone occurs through formation of an external callus and an internal callus, the principal healing mechanism in cancellous bone (e.g., the metaphysis) is formation of the internal callus.

The external and internal calluses that form during the intermediate phase of diaphyseal fracture healing consist of a comparatively weak mixture of cartilage and an irregular collagen fiber matrix. This temporary matrix has been referred to as a *provisional callus* (Schultz 1990). As cartilage is gradually replaced by bone, the callus hardens and stiffens so that movement no longer occurs at the fracture site. At this point, fracture healing is said to have progressed to *clinical union* (Salter 1999). Although new bone formation in the callus is evident on radiographic examination, the fracture line remains apparent. Solid bony union and optimal fracture stability have not yet been achieved.

Late Repair Phase

During the late phase of diaphyseal fracture healing, ossification continues, minerals are deposited in the bone matrix, and solid bony union occurs (figure 6.6). Union of bony spicules, or trabeculae, is characteristic of this phase. As the external and internal calluses develop, spicules of new bone project from each end of the fracture fragments and eventually unite. Bony spicules from the external and internal calluses also unite. Thus, the new bone of the external callus extends to join the new bone of the internal callus (see figure 6.6). The result is formation of *woven bone*, the initial type of bone formed during fracture healing (Schiller 1994). According to Loitz-Ramage and Zernicke (1996), the bony

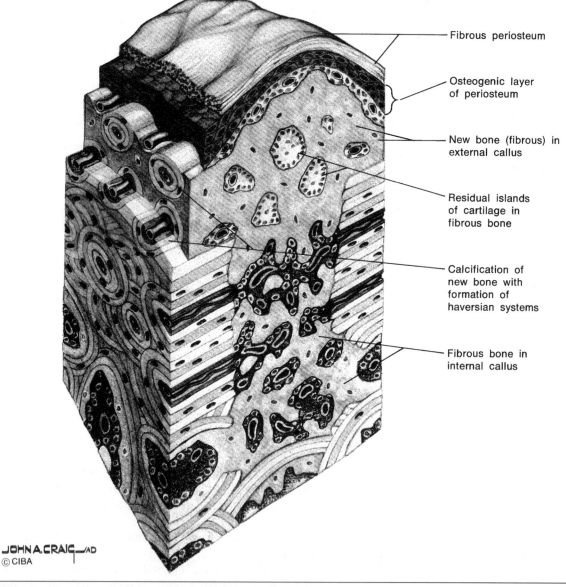

Fibrous periosteum

Osteogenic layer of periosteum

New bone (fibrous) in external callus

Residual islands of cartilage in fibrous bone

Calcification of new bone with formation of haversian systems

Fibrous bone in internal callus

JOHN A. CRAIG—AD
© CIBA

Figure 6.6   Late phase of fracture healing (formation of bony callus).

callus that bridges the fracture site develops within 14 to 40 days and provides good stability within six weeks. In comparison to the dense compact bone that eventually develops, however, the cancellous matrix of woven bone is structurally weak and capable of withstanding only limited tissue loading.

As the late phase of fracture healing continues, soft cancellous bone is gradually transformed into a hard bony callus that develops through the process of *mineralization* (Schultz 1990). Whereas *ossification* refers to new bone formation as the result of collagen synthesis by osteoblasts, *mineralization* involves deposition of inorganic minerals in the collagen matrix. As mineralization progresses, calcium and phosphorus, which are present in the blood plasma, are transported to the bone matrix where they enter the interstitial fluid and are deposited along the collagen fibers in the newly formed matrix (Raney and Brashear 1971). As a result, bone density increases. Hence, the interrelated but distinct processes of ossification and mineralization are both essential to solid bony union in fracture healing. With continued ossification and mineralization, the immature woven bone is systematically replaced by more mature *primary bone* (Loitz-Ramage and Zernicke 1996). During this transition, excess callus is resorbed, the medullary cavity of a long bone is gradually reestablished, and restoration of haversian systems in cortical bone occurs. At this point, solid bony union, or consolidation, has occurred and the fracture is said to have reached *radiographic union*. With continued ossification and remodeling, the fracture line is no longer visible on radiographic examination (Salter 1999).

The time frame in which a fracture is said to be healed is sometimes equated with solid bony union, a predictable physiological response in normal bone healing. Fracture-healing time depends on several factors. Among these factors are the amount of original bone damage, the extent of bone cell necrosis, and the degree of displacement (Raney and Brashear 1971). Healing time is also dependent on the size of the bone involved, the configuration of the fracture, and the local blood supply. With appropriate approximation of bone ends, smaller bones (e.g., radius and ulna) typically heal more rapidly than larger bones (e.g. the femur) (Raney and Brashear 1971). Generally, fractured bone ends with the greater surface area (e.g., oblique fractures) heal more rapidly than fractures with limited articulating surfaces (e.g., transverse fractures) (Schultz 1990). Fractures that occur in osseous tissues with a comparatively good blood supply heal faster than those in areas with poor vascularity (i.e., the scaphoid bone). Other factors being equal, fractures that occur in children prior to the age of puberty typically heal faster than fractures in adults (Salter 1999). In a practical sense, especially as related to resumption of sports activity, medical declaration of a healed fracture is appropriately relative to anticipated mechanical loading of weakened bone structures during sports participation. Although mechanical loading is necessary for restoration of optimal bone strength and stiffness, external forces must not be of such a magnitude to cause recurrent tissue failure.

Remodeling

Although processes contributing to the ultimate structure and functional properties of bone tissue begin during the intermediate and late stages of fracture healing, the process through which bones progressively resume their normal structure, size, and shape is called *remodeling*. Remodeling begins as stability of the fracture site is restored. Whereas the term *modeling* refers to deposition of new bone, as in skeletal growth, remodeling involves resorption of existing bone by osteoclasts and replacement with new bone by osteoblasts (Whiting and Zernicke 1998). Reorganization of the irregular trabecular structure is a primary characteristic of early bone remodeling. This process involves continual resorption of necrotic bone tissue and structurally ineffective components of the bone matrix by osteoclasts and deposition of new bone by osteoblasts. As new bone is deposited and as mineralization continues, the trabeculae gradually thicken. Thus, the intertrabecular spaces become smaller and the bone becomes increasingly dense. Resorption of trabecular bone in the internal callus restores the medullary cavity of long bones while new bone formation continues to restore the haversian systems (osteons) of cortical bone, including development of new lamellae, haversian canals, and Volkmann's canals (Bryant 1977). The type of bone that replaces primary bone formed during the earlier stages of bone healing has been referred to as *secondary bone* (Loitz-Ramage and Zernicke 1996). Secondary bone formation during remodeling is characterized by histological changes in cortical bone, primarily in the microstructure of the haversian systems, and is predicated on preliminary resorption of existing osseous tissues by osteoclasts. The sequence of bone remodeling has been summarized by the use of the acronym ARF, which involves activation of osteoclasts, resorption of existing bone, and formation of new bone by osteoblasts (Whiting and Zernicke 1998). During the remodeling process, deposition of new bone by osteoblasts occurs at a slower rate than resorption, usually involving a latent period of approximately one week between bone resorption and deposition (Loitz-Ramage and Zernicke 1996). Wolff's law, which holds that bone adapts in accordance with functional demands, is an important concept associated with the remodeling stage of fracture healing. The significance of Wolff's law, as related to remodeling and restoration of bone function, is discussed further in chapter 7.

Abnormal Bone Healing

Injury to adjacent soft tissues including musculotendinous structures, ligaments and joint capsules, blood vessels, and nerves may present initial complications directly associated with an acute fracture incident. Subsequently, early complications may include compartment syndromes, infection (i.e., osteomyelitis), and avascular necrosis. Post-traumatic osteoporosis, degenerative joint disease, and myositis ossificans are considered late complications (Salter 1999). Kilcoyne and Farrar (1991) categorized these conditions as *extrinsic complications* because they are not directly related to the mechanisms of fracture healing. Deviations from normal fracture healing that are directly associated with bone regeneration are referred to as *intrinsic complications*. These patterns of abnormal fracture healing include (1) nonunion, (2) delayed union, and (3) malunion (Salter 1999). In comparison with other segments of the population, abnormal fracture healing is less commonly associated with the types of sport-related fractures typically seen in the young, healthy sports participant. Delayed union or nonunion of scaphoid fractures of the wrist and Jones fractures of the 5th metatarsal may represent the most common exceptions. Despite the comparative low incidence of fracture complications in the sports population, the possibility of their occurrence should not be discounted. It is incumbent on sports health care clinicians to be cognizant of the factors that contribute to abnormal fracture healing. Whereas inherent contributing factors (e.g., vascular compromise) may be beyond the control of the clinician, potential complicating environmental factors such as inappropriate stabilization or interrupted immobilization, premature resumption of activity, and inadequate protective devices must be recognized and controlled.

Nonunion

Nonunion of fractures occurs when osteoblast activity and ossification have been interrupted and fracture fragments fail to unite. Although determination of a nonunion fracture is dependent on the bone involved, Raney and Brashear (1971) noted that nonunion should not be considered to have occurred in any fracture until at least six months after the date of injury because bony union has been known to occur beyond this time. Other authorities consider a diagnosis of nonunion to be valid at nine months after injury if no progressive signs of healing are noted for a minimum of three months (Thomas 1993). Although several factors may contribute to nonunion, fracture instability with excessive interfragmental movement and vascular compromise have been cited as two prime factors. Whereas a certain amount of movement at the fracture site is conducive to callus formation in secondary bone healing, excessive motion leads to vascular damage and interruption of osteogenesis (Brennwald 1996). Loitz-Ramage and Zernicke (1996) noted a prolonged presence of weak Type III collagen in unstable fractures. In uncomplicated bone healing, Type III collagen synthesis is subsequently replaced by synthesis of Type I collagen, the stronger constituent of healthy mature bone. Continued presence of Type III collagen in unstable fractures, however, suggests that the transition from Type III to Type I collagen synthesis has been interrupted, thus inhibiting solid bony union. The inability of Type III collagen to bind to minerals, thereby inhibiting mineralization of the newly formed tissue matrix, has been suggested as a related factor that interferes with bony union (Loitz-Ramage and Zernicke 1996).

When nonunion is present, the bone ends may become atrophic, sclerotic, and eburnated (i.e., dense and hard) with occlusion of the medullary cavity. In some cases, the opposing ends may be connected by unstable fibrous tissue, but without evidence of a bridging callus. In other cases, a *pseudarthrosis* (i.e., false joint) with formation of a synovial-like capsule may develop. Although avascular necrosis may occur in combination with nonunion fractures, the two conditions are not inherently coincident. Nonunion of fracture fragments may occur without avascular necrosis. Conversely, bony union may occur despite the presence of avascular necrosis (Schultz 1990). Avascular necrosis and nonunion are commonly associated with fractures of the scaphoid bone in the wrist, intracapsular fractures of the hip, and fractures of the talus. Diagnosed nonunion fractures commonly require surgical intervention with bone grafting for resolution (Raney and Brashear 1971). As discussed in chapter 7, however, electrical bone stimulation provides an alternative treatment approach to some types of nonunion fractures that have the potential for bony union.

Delayed Union

By definition, delayed union of fractured bones involves retardation, rather than complete failure, of the regeneration process. In cases of delayed union, the fractured bone eventually heals with solid bony union, but not within the typical or expected time frame for a particular bone or fracture type (Groner and Weeks 1992). The tibia, femur, and humerus are common sites of delayed union. Delayed union is differentiated from slow union. Whereas delayed union is considered a pathological condition, slow union involves the normal, but longer, healing time characteristically associated with certain fractures (Schultz 1990). A notable example encountered in the sports population is the slow healing time associated with scaphoid fractures of the wrist (Zemel 1992). Although fractures of the scaphoid bone characteristically heal slowly, the scaphoid may also be one of the more common sites of delayed union seen in the sports population.

Because normal bone-healing time varies with several factors, including the type of fracture and the particular bone involved, determination of delayed union is relative. For example, Raney and Brashear (1971) noted that delayed union is considered present if solid bony union does not occur in closed fractures of the tibia and femur in 20 weeks, and within 10 weeks in closed fractures of the humerus. Factors contributing to delayed union include those directly associated with the injury (e.g., severe tissue destruction, interposition of soft tissue, infection) as well as factors associated with initial medical treatment and follow-up care. Inadequate reduction, surgical complications (e.g., circulatory impairment), inappropriate internal fixation (i.e., metal plates, screws, etc.), distractive skeletal traction, and inadequate external immobilization (i.e., casts, splints) have been cited as potential complicating factors associated with initial fracture management (Schultz

1990). Poorly fitted casts, splints, or other external immobilization devices may permit disruptive movement at the fracture site or cause circulatory impairment due to excessive pressure, both of which may contribute to delayed union.

Malunion

Malunion is described as regeneration of bone with union of fracture fragments in a malaligned or imperfect position (Salter 1999). Inability to effect anatomical reduction and difficulty in maintaining appropriate stabilization are common causes of malunion (Raney and Brashear 1971). Although bony union occurs in malunion fractures, angular or rotatory deformities are the common results (Schultz 1990). A cubitus varus deformity of the elbow (i.e., "gunstock deformity") as a consequence of a supracondylar fracture of the humerus is an example of an angular deformity resulting from malunion (Kilcoyne and Farrar 1991). In some cases of malunion, the patient may be left with a disability that, if not correctable by surgery, may lead to necessary acceptance. In most cases, however, functionally significant malunion of fractures is preventable with satisfactory reduction and stabilization (Salter 1999). Minor residual deformities, although cosmetically undesirable, may have no functional consequences. Fractures of the middle one-third of the clavicle, for example, are common sport-related injuries that sometimes heal with irregularity in bony contours, but without functional loss.

Summary

Long bones of the skeletal system are composed of spongy cancellous bone found in the epiphysis and the metaphysis and dense compact bone that forms the bone cortex. The cortex of the diaphysis encloses the medullary cavity. In contrast to the irregular trabecular network of cancellous bone, cortical bone consists of structurally organized haversian systems, or osteons. Except at the articulating surfaces, the outer surface of the bone cortex is covered by the periosteum, whereas the medullary cavity is lined by the endosteum. Like other types of connective tissues, the structural components of osseous tissue include cells, fibers, and ground substance. Fracture healing occurs through the interrelated functions of osteoblasts, which form new bone, and osteoclasts that are responsible for bone resorption.

Fractures heal by regeneration, which restores the normal structural and functional properties of bone. The long bones of the skeletal system regenerate through the process of endochondral ossification during which cartilage is replaced by osseous tissue. Secondary bone healing occurs on a continuum of interrelated phases that include (1) hematoma formation and inflammation, (2) cellular proliferation and callus formation, and (3) remodeling. When fractures of long bones occur, disruption of blood vessels leads to formation of an interfragmentary hematoma, which provides the environment for subsequent bone healing. The characteristic inflammatory responses to acute soft tissue injury also occur in the initial stage of bone healing. During the second stage of bone healing, proliferation of osteogenic cells occurs with subsequent callus formation and bony union. Initially, granulation tissue forms at the fracture site that, as collagen synthesis continues, is gradually transformed into a soft fibrous bridge between the bone ends. With continued healing, an external callus develops in the bone cortex and an internal callus is formed in the central portion of the bone. The appearance of bony spicules, or trabeculae, marks the beginning of bony union, which occurs as spicules from the external and internal calluses unite. With continued bone deposition and mineralization, the initial woven bone is eventually transformed into dense compact bone.

Remodeling is the final stage of fracture healing during which the involved bone progressively resumes its normal structure, size, and shape. Reorganization of the irregular trabeculae is a primary characteristic of the early remodeling process. As remodeling progresses, the involved bone adapts and strengthens in response to mechanical loading in accordance with Wolff's law. Deviations from normal fracture healing include nonunion, delayed union, and malunion.

References

Brennwald, J. 1996. Fracture healing in the hand: A brief update. *Clinical Orthopaedics and Related Research* 327:9-11.

Bryant, W.M. *Wound healing.* 1977. Reading, Mass.: CIBA Pharmaceutical Co.

Groner, J.P., and P.M. Weeks. 1992. Healing of hard and soft tissues in the hand. In *Hand injuries in athletes*, edited by J.W. Strickland and A.C. Rettig. Philadelphia: W.B. Saunders.

Kilcoyne, R.F., and E.L. Farrar. 1991. *Handbook of orthopedic terminology.* Boca Raton, Fla.: CRC Press.

Loitz-Ramage, B.J., and R.F. Zernicke. 1996. Bone biology and mechanics. In *Athletic injuries and rehabilitation*, edited by J.E. Zachazewski, D.J. Magee, and W.S. Quillen. Philadelphia: W.B. Saunders.

Montoye, H.J. 1987. Better bones and biodynamics. *Research Quarterly for Exercise and Sport* 58:334-47.

Nordin, M., and V.H. Frankel. 1989. Biomechanics of bones. In *Basic biomechanics of the musculoskeletal system*, 2nd ed., edited by M. Nordin and V.H. Frankel. Philadelphia: Lea and Febiger.

Raney, R.B., Sr., and H.R. Brashear Jr. 1971. *Shand's handbook of orthopaedic surgery*, 8th ed. St. Louis: Mosby.

Salter, R.B. 1999. *Textbook of disorders and injuries of the musculoskeletal system*, 3rd ed. Baltimore: Williams and Wilkins.

Schiller, A.L. 1994. Bones and joints. In *Pathology*, 2nd ed., edited by E. Rubin and J.L. Farber. Philadelphia: J.B. Lippincott.

Schultz, R.J. 1990. *The language of fractures*, 2nd ed. Baltimore: Williams and Wilkins.

Thomas, C.L., ed. 1993. *Taber's cyclopedic medical dictionary*, 17th ed. Philadelphia: Davis.

Tortora, G.J., and S.R. Grabowski. 1993. *Principles of anatomy and physiology*, 7th ed. New York: Harper Collins College Publishers.

Whiting, W.C., and R.F. Zernicke. 1998. *Biomechanics of musculoskeletal injury.* Champaign, Ill.: Human Kinetics.

Zemel, N.P. 1992. Carpal fractures. In *Hand injuries in athletes*, edited by J.W. Strickland and A.C. Rettig. Philadelphia: W.B. Saunders.

Therapeutic Implications: Fracture Healing

Basic Concepts in Fracture Management

Principles of Fracture Treatment

Fracture Reduction

Fracture Fixation

Internal Skeletal Fixation

External Skeletal Fixation

External Immobilization
and Protected Mobilization

Rigid Casts and Splints

Functional Cast-Braces

Special Protective Devices

Electrotherapy in Fracture Management

Preservation and Restoration of Function

Restoration of Soft Tissue Function

Joint Mobility

Muscular Strength

Restoration of Bone Function

Wolff's Law

Mechanical Loading

Therapeutic Implications

Resumption of Sports Participation

Site-Specific Bone Hypertrophy

Bone Fatigue and Stress Fractures

Removal of Internal Fixation Devices

Summary

Learning Objectives

After completion of this chapter, the reader should be able to

❶ compare and contrast the AO/ASIF system and functional fracture bracing in the medical management of fractures,

❷ identify and describe common methods of fracture reduction, fixation, and immobilization in the medical management of fractures,

❸ identify the primary implications of contemporary medical practices in the therapeutic management and rehabilitation of fracture patients, and

❹ identify risk factors and formulate guidelines for resumption of sports activities after a fracture.

As is the case with soft tissue repair, fracture healing presents several implications for therapeutic management by the sports health care clinician. Although initial fracture treatment and early follow-up care lie primarily within the domain of medical personnel, subsequent rehabilitation and restoration of function necessitates the sports health care clinician's awareness of contemporary medical practices in fracture management. Appropriate clinical management not only necessitates a practical understanding of bone-healing processes but also requires familiarity with specific fracture treatment methods used by the attending physician.

The primary implications for clinical management of fractures can be summarized in four general categories. First, it is critical that sports health care clinicians recognize contraindications to the use of particular physical agents that result from implantation of metallic fixation devices (e.g., the diathermies), as well as the effects of internal fixation and external immobilization on fracture healing and the biomechanical properties of bone. Second, as fracture healing progresses through the stages of hematoma formation and inflammation, callus formation and bony union, and remodeling, it becomes important to consider the relative levels of fracture stability, bone strength, and resistance to extrinsic mechanical loading. Collectively, these factors establish the parameters for progressive tissue loading and resumption of physical activity. Third, it is incumbent on the sports health care clinician to minimize, or prevent if possible, the deleterious consequences of fracture immobilization and general disuse on affected body parts. In this regard, the extent of muscle atrophy and strength loss, joint stiffness, and disuse osteoporosis commonly varies with the method of fracture treatment used by the attending physician. Consequently, the clinician is challenged to become familiar with commonly used techniques of fracture fixation and stabilization, as well as the typical immobilization period associated with each treatment method. Finally, if resumption of physical activity and sports participation after a fracture is anticipated, the effects of exercise and sport-specific mechanical loading on recovering bone structures become important considerations.

Basic Concepts in Fracture Management

Over the years, two general treatment concepts have guided physicians in their approach to fracture management (Salter 1999). The first approach, referred to as the *AO/ASIF system*, is credited to the Association for Osteosynthesis (AO), an association of Swiss surgeons that subsequently became the Association for the Study of Internal Fixation (ASIF). This system is based on the premise that rigid internal fixation with interfragmentary compression at the fracture site precludes the necessity of prolonged external immobilization, thus minimizing functional losses associated with joint stiffness, muscle atrophy, and strength deficits. Conceptually, the use of open anatomical reduction and rigid internal fixation with interfragmentary compression permits *primary bone healing*, the type of healing that occurs directly between approximated, compressed cortical bone fragments without significant callus formation. In contrast, *secondary bone healing*, which occurs in the absence of rigid internal fixation, is characterized by formation of an internal and external callus, as described in chapter 6 (Brennwald 1996).

The second general approach to fracture treatment, referred to as *functional fracture bracing*, or *cast-bracing*, is exemplified by closed reduction if necessary, an initial period of immobilization, and subsequent application of a hinged cast or brace that facilitates changes in joint position (Salter 1999). This treatment method is based on the premise that rigid internal fixation with interfragmentary compression is not always necessary for satisfactory bone healing. Like the AO/ASIF system, functional fracture bracing represents an attempt to avoid the detrimental effects of prolonged, rigid immobilization by allowing increased joint motion as soon as satisfactory bone healing permits. Some authorities have noted that the controlled micromotion at the fracture site permitted by relative immobilization, including functional fracture bracing, may stimulate callus formation and related secondary bone-healing mechanisms (Salter 1999).

Although the AO/ASIF system and the functional bracing system of fracture management represent divergent treatment approaches, a common objective of these two methods is prevention of the deleterious effects of prolonged, rigid immobilization and preservation of function in the affected body part. Hence, both approaches have received general acceptance in the medical community. Nevertheless, the AO/ASIF and functional bracing systems of fracture management have comparative advantages and disadvantages that necessitate the physician's consideration of specific, individualized treatment protocols in particular cases. The array of specific fracture treatment methods available to the attending physician, as summarized by Salter (1999), is presented in figure 7.1. Although the sports health care clinician typically encounters specific fracture treatment methods with varying degrees of frequency, clinical experience indicates that several of the protocols identified in figure 7.1 are commonly used in the management of fracture types seen in the sports population.

- Protection (e.g., slings, crutch-walking) without reduction or immobilization.
- Immobilization (e.g., casts, splints) without reduction.
- Closed reduction by manipulation followed by immobilization (e.g., casts, splints).
- Closed reduction by continuous traction (e.g., skin traction, skeletal traction) followed by immobilization.
- Closed reduction (manipulation or continuous traction) followed by functional fracture bracing (e.g., hinged casts or braces).
- Closed redution by manipulation followed by external skeletal fixation.
- Closed reduction by manipulation followed by internal skeletal fixation (e.g., screws, bone plates, nails and rods).
- Open reduction followed by internal skeletal fixation (e.g., screws, bone plates, nails and rods).
- Excision of fracture fragments and replacement by an endoprosthesis (e.g., prosthetic joint).

Figure 7.1   Methods of fracture management.
Data from Salter 1999.

Principles of Fracture Treatment

Regardless of the particular treatment protocol, the four primary objectives of comprehensive fracture management are (1) fracture reduction, if necessary, and achievement of a satisfactory fracture fragment position, (2) maintenance of fracture fragment position and protection to permit solid bony union, (3) pain control, and (4) restoration of function in the affected body part (Raney and Brashear 1971). Basic principles and techniques of fracture reduction, internal and external skeletal fixation, and external immobilization are reviewed in the following sections of this chapter prior to consideration of therapeutic strategies for restoration of soft tissue and bone function. The principles of pain management discussed in chapter 4 are applicable to pain control in fracture management.

Fracture Reduction

Many types of fractures with little or no displacement do not require reduction. Nondisplaced fractures require only maintenance of the normal anatomical position with sufficient protection to allow uncomplicated bone healing (Salter 1999). Displaced fractures, however, require both reduction and stabilization. Raney and Brashear (1971) identified three types of fracture deformities that require reduction: (1) angulation, (2) shortening, and (3) rotation. Fracture deformities commonly result in one or both of two general types of anatomical deviations, *malalignment* or *displacement* (Schultz 1990). These terms are used to describe the abnormal position of fracture fragments, usually the position of the distal fragment in relationship to the proximal fragment. Malalignment involves angulation of the longitudinal axis of a long bone at the fracture site, producing a nonparallel relationship between the longitudinal axis of the proximal and distal fragments. Displacement, on the other hand, is a loss of opposition of bone ends, but without angulation. Loss of opposition and displacement may occur with or without overriding or rotation of bone fragments. Should displacement occur, a parallel relationship between the longitudinal axis of the fracture fragments is maintained unless angulation is also present. Nevertheless, displacement typically requires reduction.

After the attending physician's clinical assessment and radiographic confirmation of a fracture, the presence of malalignment or displacement and the need for reduction is determined. Should reduction be necessary, anatomical alignment and positioning of fracture fragments with adequate stabilization to permit uncomplicated bony union is the physician's ideal goal. Reduction of malaligned or displaced fractures is accomplished by one of two methods: *closed reduction* or *open reduction* (Schultz 1990). Closed reduction involves repositioning of fracture fragments by manual manipulation or continuous traction without surgical intervention. Although specific techniques vary with the type of malalignment or displacement, manual manipulation is the most commonly used method of closed fracture reduction. Another method of closed reduction, skeletal traction, involves transverse placement of wires or pins through the fractured bone with attachment to an external traction device (e.g., pulleys and weights). This method of reduction, most commonly used in the management of unstable cervical spine fractures and fractures of large long bones (e.g., the femoral shaft), also serves to maintain reduction and stabilization until a satisfactory level of fracture healing is achieved. In cases where lesser forces are required (e.g., selected fractures in young children), continuous traction through the use of adhesive tape applied to the skin (i.e., skin traction) is sometimes used (Salter 1999).

When the use of internal fixation devices (e.g., bone plates, screws) is contemplated, open operative reduction of malaligned or displaced fractures is commonly necessary. In some fractures, however, internal fixation is accomplished by percutaneous placement of fixation devices without actual opening of the fracture site. Open reduction involves alignment and positioning of fracture fragments through surgical exposure of the fracture site, thereby permitting direct visualization and application of internal fixation devices. The disadvantages of open reduction and internal fixation, as compared to closed reduction, include the risk of further disruption of the blood supply to fracture fragments and the possibility of surgical wound infection, both of which may interfere with normal bone healing (Salter 1999). In general, open reduction is indicated when closed reduction is not possible or in cases where a satisfactory fracture fragment position cannot be maintained after closed reduction.

Fracture Fixation

Whether reduced by closed or open methods, unstable fractures require maintenance of anatomical continuity until bony union is adequate to prevent displacement. As previously indicated, maintenance of anatomical continuity is considered a second major objective of fracture management. Stabilization of fractures is accomplished by internal or external skeletal fixation, external immobilization (e.g., casts, splints), or a combination of both. Regardless of the method used, the primary purposes of fixation and immobilization are to (1) prevent unacceptable angulation and displacement of fracture fragments, (2) prevent movement of fracture fragments that may interrupt bony union, and (3) alleviate pain (Kilcoyne and Farrar 1991; Raney and Brashear 1971). In general, fracture fixation is accomplished by one of two primary methods: (1) internal skeletal fixation with metal implants and (2) external skeletal fixation through the use of percutaneous pins or wires attached to an external metal frame (i.e., an external fixator).

Internal Skeletal Fixation

Rigid internal fixation of fracture fragments after open operative reduction involves the use of various metallic devices to secure and maintain bone fragment alignment and position. This technique has been referred to as *osteosynthesis* (Salter 1999). As advocated by proponents of the Swiss AO/ASIF system of fracture management, a primary objective of this treatment approach is rigid fixation that precludes the necessity of prolonged, debilitating external immobilization. An extensive variety of metallic devices, each of which are designed for particular purposes, has been developed for internal skeletal fixation. In general, these devices include (1) interfragmentary screws, (2) bone plates and screws, (3) intramedullary nails, and (4) metallic pins and wires. Although metallic fixation devices provide effective fracture stabilization, implantation of these devices can have clinically significant deleterious effects on osseous blood supply, bone density and mass, and tensile strength, thereby altering both the structural integrity and the biomechanical properties of normal bone. Consequently, familiarity with commonly used internal fixation devices and a fundamental understanding of their effects on osseous tissue, during implantation and after implant removal, are prerequisites to determination of appropriate follow-up care and rehabilitation.

Interfragmentary screws

Interfragmentary bone screws, typically in combination with metallic bone plates, are commonly used for internal fixation in fracture treatment. Two basic types of screws have been developed: *cortical screws* and *cancellous bone screws* (Kilcoyne and Farrar 1991). Designed for use in dense compact bone, cortical screws are commonly used in combination with various types of bone plates in the treatment of diaphyseal fractures of long bones. In contrast, the cancellous bone screw is specially designed to provide stabilization in fractures involving spongy cancellous bone. These screws are designed with comparatively wide threads that provide a greater fixation surface area, thereby facilitating fracture stability (Kilcoyne and Farrar 1991). Malleolar screws, for example, are a type of cancellous bone screw used for fixation of fractures involving the medial malleolus of the ankle.

The use of bone screws in fracture management has certain disadvantages related to the effect of the screw on bone strength at the site of insertion. Surgical insertion of bone screws creates a small defect referred to as a *stress riser*. The weakening effect of a stress riser, and thus the propensity for tissue failure, is attributed to concentration of mechanical loads at the site of the defect, as opposed to load distribution throughout the bone as would normally occur (Nordin and Frankel 1989). Bone screws not only represent a focal point for mechanical loads during the period of implantation but also create an area of residual bone weakness after removal. When bone screws are removed, the remaining screw holes represent a structural defect with an increased propensity for refracture (O'Sullivan, Chao, and Kelly 1989). Hence, a focal weakness exists until remodeling obliterates the screw holes, a process that may take several months. Radiographic evidence of screw holes for as long as one year after bone plate and screw removal has been observed (Gradisar 1990).

Bone plates and screws

Metallic bone plates represent a second type of rigid internal fixation device in fracture management. These devices, which transverse the fracture site in long bones, are attached to the cortical surface of the bone by screws. Various types of bone plates have been designed for fixation of fracture fragments in the diaphyseal and metaphyseal areas of long bones. These types of bone plates include (1) neutralization plates, (2) dynamic compression plates, and (3) buttress plates (Kilcoyne and Farrar 1991).

Neutralization plates, when used in combination with bone screws, neutralize and distribute torsion, shear, and bending forces that would otherwise be directed to the points of screw fixation, thus providing supportive stabilization. Neutralization plates are most commonly used to provide internal fixation in fractures of long bones. A second type of bone plate, a dynamic compression plate, is a specially designed, self-compressing fixation device. With this type of fixation, compression forces are applied by the tightening of screws placed in oval, beveled holes in the plate. The compression forces of a dynamic compression plate on a transverse diaphyseal fracture are illustrated in figure 7.2. This effect exemplifies the principles of compression and rigid internal fixation associated with the AO/ASIF system of fracture treatment. In contrast to neutralization plates and dynamic compression plates, which are used primarily to provide internal fixation in diaphyseal fractures, buttress plates are used to maintain fragment position in fractures of the metaphyseal region (Kilcoyne and Farrar 1991). For example, fractures involving the tibial plateau are commonly stabilized with a buttress plate and screws.

Facilitation of direct bony union is a purported benefit derived from the use of rigid metallic bone plates. Direct contact and firm compression between fractured bone ends is thought to facilitate direct bridging of osteogenic cells and blood vessels across the fracture line without significant callus formation (i.e., primary bone healing). Nevertheless, secondary bone healing with varying levels of callus formation has been observed in fractures treated with bone plates (O'Sullivan, Chao, and Kelly 1989). Notwithstanding the benefits of fracture treatment with rigid metal plates, these devices can have detrimental effects on osseous tissue that become clinically significant considerations. First, the pressure of metal plates, when attached to the surface of cortical bone, may compromise an already impaired periosteal blood supply, thus impeding osteogenic bone formation. This effect, in turn, may contribute to delayed union or nonunion (Raney and Brashear 1971; Salter 1999). A second concern related to satisfactory bone healing is maintenance of interfragmentary compression. Disruption of blood supply at the time of injury commonly results in ischemic necrosis of osseous tissue at the fracture site. Unless firm interfragmentary compression is maintained, the small gap created by bone necrosis and resorption may be maintained by some types of rigid metallic plates, leading to delayed bony union. This concern, however, has been alleviated by the use of dynamic compression plates that allow for adjustment of interfragmentary compression (Raney and Brashear 1971). A third consideration in the use of rigid bone plates is the observation that the interface between the ends of a metal plate and the underlying cortical bone represents a focal point for

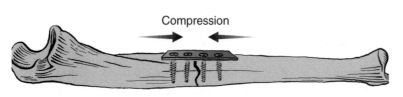

Figure 7.2   Internal fixation of a transverse ulna with dynamic compression plate.

mechanical loading, thereby creating an increased potential for a new fracture (Gradisar 1990). This risk factor, among others, has led to concern regarding the advisability of returning to strenuous sports activities during the period of bone plate implantation.

As noted by Strickland (1992), development of internal fixation devices that provide effective fracture stabilization has led to a temptation to permit premature resumption of sports participation, particularly by the highly competitive athlete. Strickland further cautioned that internal fixation devices are not designed to be exposed to the forces inherent in strenuous sports activities. Although somewhat controversial, removal of metal plates before resumption of sports activities is advised. Currently, AO/ASIF guidelines provide recommended periods of time before removal of internal fixation devices in various fractures. These time periods may range from one to three years, depending on the fracture type and location. Although prolonged absence from sports activities may be extremely frustrating to the competitive athlete and the serious recreation participant, physicians do not typically recommend compromise of established fracture treatment standards to allow sports participation.

As is the case with removal of interfragmentary bone screws, removal of rigid bone plates after fracture healing presents an additional concern, especially if a return to strenuous physical activity is anticipated. During the period of implantation, rigid metallic plates function effectively to provide "stress protection" to the underlying bone (Salter 1999). Stress protection occurs because mechanical loads that otherwise would be assumed by the bone are shared by the bone plate. In response, stress-protected bone atrophies and weakens, a condition referred to as *osteoporosis of disuse* (Thomas 1993). In the absence of normal mechanical loading, bone deposition decreases while bone resorption remains unchanged (Loitz-Ramage and Zernicke 1996). Hence, bone density and bone mass decrease. Structural alterations that occur in disuse osteoporosis include a decrease in cortical bone thickness, narrowing of the diaphysis, widening of the medullary cavity, and a general increase in bone porosity (Raney and Brashear 1971).

Intramedullary nails

Intramedullary nails are a third type of internal fixation device used in the management of diaphyseal fractures of selected long bones. These devices, which may be flexible or rigid, are inserted into the medullary cavity, thus transversing the fracture site and, in effect, functioning as an internal splint that shares mechanical loads with the bone (O'Sullivan, Chao, and Kelly 1989). Although intramedullary nails have been designed for use in various long bones (e.g., the tibia, humerus), they are most commonly used for management of fractures of the femoral shaft (Gradisar 1990). When intramedullary nails are used, fixation is typically secure enough to preclude the need for augmentative external support. Disruptive rotational and distractive forces, once considered a disadvantage of intramedullary nailing, are controlled by recent advances in the design of intramedullary devices (O'Sullivan, Chao, and Kelly 1989). In fractures of the femoral shaft, early partial weight bearing with the use of crutches is sometimes permitted and encouraged as a means of exerting compressive forces on the fracture site (Gradisar 1990). In some cases, depending on the fracture type, full weight bearing is permitted.

Pins and wires

In addition to interfragmentary screws, bone plates, and intramedullary nails, a variety of metallic pins and wires is commonly used for internal fixation in fracture management. Steinmann pins, Kirschner wires (K-wires), and wire tension bands are among the more familiar and versatile devices available for fixation of various fracture types. Various sizes of K-wires, for example, are used for transfixion or intramedullary fixation of several types of metacarpal and phalangeal fractures (Hastings 1992). Examples of internal fixa-

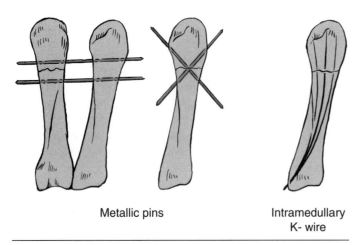

Metallic pins   Intramedullary
                                 K- wire

Figure 7.3   Methods of internal fixation of metacarpal neck fracture with metal pins and intramedullary wires (K-wires).

Adapted, by permission, from H. Hastings II, 1992, Management of extra-articular fractures of the phalanges and metacarpals. In *Hand injuries in athletes*, edited by J.W. Strickland and A.C. Rettig (Philadelphia: W.B. Saunders), 140.

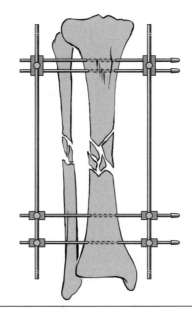

Figure 7.4   External skeletal fixation of a comminuted fracture of the tibia.

Reprinted, by permission, from R.B. Salter, 1983, *Textbook of disorders and injuries of the musculoskeletal system*, 2nd ed. (Baltimore: Lippincott, Williams & Wilkins), 383.

tion in metacarpal fracture management are illustrated in figure 7.3. In some cases, Steinmann pins are used individually or in combination with K-wires, wire tension bands, or other internal fixation devices (Salter 1999). In addition to their use for internal fixation, Steinmann pins and K-wires are also used for percutaneous insertion into bone as attachment sites for skeletal traction units (Thomas 1993).

External Skeletal Fixation

External skeletal fixation is a method of fracture stabilization commonly indicated for the treatment of unstable comminuted fractures of long bones (e.g., the tibia), especially open fractures that involve extensive soft tissue damage (Salter 1999). In this method, fixation is accomplished by percutaneous insertion of metal pins so that they transverse the bone above and below the fracture site. These pins serve as attachment sites for external metal frames (i.e., external fixator) that provide firm fragment fixation (figure 7.4). Medical experience has indicated that the healing response is related to the stiffness of the external fixator and, thus, the rigidity of bone fragment fixation. In general, the use of comparatively stiff metal fixators promotes primary bone healing without callus formation, whereas the use of less-rigid devices that allow micromovement at the fracture site is conducive to secondary bone healing with greater periosteal callus formation (O'Sullivan, Chao, and Kelly 1989). As is the case with internal skeletal fixation with rigid metal plates, the stress protection provided by stiff external fixators may promote osteoporosis.

External Immobilization and Protected Mobilization

In contrast to rigid internal fixation, external immobilization of fractures with casts, braces, or splints has been referred to as *relative immobilization* because, typically, some degree of motion can occur at the fracture site (Salter 1999). Hence, fractures treated by external immobilization without rigid internal fixation are repaired by secondary bone healing with callus formation rather than by primary bone healing that occurs directly between rigidly fixed, compressed bone fragments. In general, external immobilization is indicated to maintain fragment position in nondisplaced or reduced fractures that are unstable but do not require rigid internal fixation. In some cases, however, external immobilization with casts or splints is necessary for fracture protection after open operative procedures. Postoperative immobilization of scaphoid fractures of the wrist after a bone graft or internal fixation with metallic devices is an example (Zemel 1992).

Traditionally, external immobilization of fractures in long bones has been accomplished by the use of rigid casts or splints that incorporate at least one of the joints adjacent to the fracture site. In some cases, incorporation of adjacent joints both proximal and distal to the fracture site is deemed necessary to neutralize the forces of muscle contraction and joint motion on fracture fragments. This treatment approach, however, deviates from basic concepts of the AO/ASIF system of fracture treatment that emphasize rigid internal fixation, avoidance of prolonged external immobilization, and preservation of joint motion. Nevertheless, when open reduction and rigid internal skeletal fixation are contraindicated or determined unnecessary, external immobilization is the most commonly used method of fracture stabilization (Salter 1999).

Conceptual advances in fracture treatment have been accompanied by development of a variety of rigid cast and splint materials, hinged braces, and flexible soft splint materials. This array of commercial products permits judicious selection of prefabricated devices or fabrication materials that can be adapted to the various stages of fracture healing, the required degree of protection, and the permissible amount of joint motion. As discussed in chapter 5, proponents of protected mobilization, or protected motion, in musculoskeletal injury management acknowledge the necessity of restricted movement to protect damaged tissues, but they also advocate preservation of soft tissue function through the use of such techniques as serial static immobilization and static progressive splinting. The wide range of protective devices and materials currently available to the sports health care clinician permits application of protected mobilization concepts to fracture treatment as well as soft tissue injury management.

Rigid Casts and Splints

Historically, plaster of paris casts have been the mainstay of early fracture management. Because plaster casts offer certain advantages compared to other devices, they remain a commonly used method of fracture treatment. Plaster casting material is made of gauze impregnated with plaster of paris, a hemihydrated form of calcium sulfate (Thomas 1993). When soaked in water, the cast material becomes pliable and easily molded to the contours of the affected body part. Plaster of paris provides a means of rigid, reasonably durable support that can be adapted to a variety of anatomical areas. These features account for the long-standing popularity of plaster casts in early fracture management (Raney and Brashear 1971). Nevertheless, compared to more recently developed cast and splint materials, plaster of paris has a poor strength-to-weight ratio that may render it less desirable as a cast material in some cases.

Despite the positive features of plaster casts, newer commercial products provide several comparative advantages (Gradisar 1990). Low-temperature thermoplastic materials that can be rendered malleable by heat, for example, provide comparatively strong, lightweight cast or splint materials that are particularly adaptable to the management of sports injuries. Because the material used in these products is insoluble (i.e., waterproof), lightweight, and typically more durable than plaster of paris, exercise of unencumbered body parts during the immobilization period is facilitated. Comparatively, casts and splints made of thermoplastic materials are also better suited to withstand the rigors of an active patient's daily activities. Perusal of current commercial products reveals a considerable array of prefabricated rigid protective devices as well as a variety of thermoplastic materials that can be used for fabrication of specialized casts and splints.

Functional Cast-Braces

Initially, rigid immobilization with traditional cast or splint materials is commonly indicated for adequate protection in fracture management. As fracture healing progresses toward solid bony union, however, joint motion and increased tissue loading are not only tolerated but also therapeutically indicated in many cases. The use of hinged cast-braces that permit changes in joint position exemplifies the contemporary functional fracture-bracing approach to treatment. Cast-braces are modifications of traditional cylinder casts that are fitted with a hinge, which permits convenient adjustments in allowable joint motion. As fracture healing progresses, continued protection is afforded by the cast portion of the cast-brace while increments in joint motion are permitted by the hinged component, thus combating development of joint stiffness, muscle atrophy, and disuse osteoporosis. Additional rationale for the use of functional fracture bracing is based on the premise that rigid external immobilization is unnecessary in some cases and that secondary bone healing may be enhanced by controlled motion at the fracture site (O'Sullivan, Chao, and Kelly 1989; Salter 1999). Some authorities have cautioned, however, that excessive loading may lead to vascular compromise and nonunion (Brennwald 1996). Nevertheless, functional cast-bracing in fractures of the tibial shaft, the distal femur, and the humerus has been used successfully in adults after appropriate periods of rigid immobilization (Salter 1999).

Special Protective Devices

In addition to modification of cylinder casts as cast-braces, various commercial materials can be used by sports health care clinicians for creative fabrication of specialized splints and braces. Special protective devices can be designed to permit optimal, acceptable levels of joint motion, therapeutic exercise, and physical activity throughout the various stages of fracture healing. Removable splints and braces, for example, allow intervening sessions of functional electrical muscle stimulation, manual soft tissue mobilization, or muscle strengthening exercises (Sadler and Koepher 1992). Therapeutic strategies to preserve joint mobility and muscle strength during protective cast or splint wear are discussed in a following section of this chapter.

As fracture healing progresses to solid bony union and remodeling, progressive resumption of physical activity and sports participation may be permitted. Although rigid external immobilization is not ordinarily required at this stage of fracture healing, continued protection is frequently indicated in view of the extrinsic forces associated with strenuous sports activities, especially contact and collision sports. Provided that playing rules permit, the use of rigid, semirigid, or soft protective devices may be advisable for an extended period. In such cases, the athlete's resumption of sports participation frequently challenges the certified athletic trainer to fabricate effective, acceptable protective devices that pass the scrutiny of the attending physician and inspection by game officials who are charged with enforcement of playing rules. Although the certified athletic trainer is most commonly confronted with the necessity of fabricating splints for protection of wrist, hand, and finger fractures, special devices may also be required for protection of recent fractures in other bones of the skeletal system.

The sports health care clinician's familiarity with the composition and behavioral properties of contemporary commercial products is fundamental to selection of materials for fabrication of protective devices suitable for wear during sports participation. Material properties to be considered include the density, strength and rigidity, conformability, and durability of various products (Canelon 1995). Although low-temperature thermoplastic materials with varying plastic or rubberlike properties are available, flexible soft splints made of silicone rubber compounds may be particularly suitable for moderate protection of recent fractures during sports participation, particularly fractures of the distal radius or ulna, the carpal bones, and the metacarpals (Sadler and Koepfer 1992). Provided that adequate fracture healing precludes the necessity of rigid support, soft splints are usually acceptable protective devices during sports practice and competition. Regardless of the product used, however, selection of fabrication materials should be based on a realistic assessment of the required protection during any particular stage of fracture healing. The certified athletic trainer's expertise in assessing the extrinsic forces and mechanical loads associated with particular sports activities is also a major factor in determination of appropriate protective devices.

Electrotherapy in Fracture Management

Despite application of sound fracture management principles, delayed bony union and nonunion sometimes occur (see chapter 6). Although not commonly indicated in the routine treatment of sports injuries, the benefits of electrical bone stimulation in particular cases of delayed union and nonunion fractures are generally recognized. The use of electrical currents to enhance osteogenesis originated in the early 1950s when it was demonstrated that bone possesses piezoelectric properties and responds to external forces (e.g., bending) by development of bioelectric potentials (i.e., a state of tension or pressure). Subsequently, it was hypothesized that electrical currents might stimulate osteoblast activity, thereby enhancing osteogenesis and bone regeneration in fracture healing (Bryant 1977; Cummings 1992). A review of the literature by Cummings (1992) revealed several studies that demonstrated acceleration of bone growth in response to applied electric or electromagnetic fields. Since its early beginnings, electrical bone stimulation has emerged as an accepted approach to fracture management. To date, however, its use is typically limited to the treatment of selected delayed union or nonunion fractures, most commonly as an alternative to bone grafting. Traditionally, electrical stimulation has not been advocated for routine use in the treatment of fractures that demonstrate normal healing patterns (Gradisar 1990).

Three primary systems for electrical stimulation of osteogenesis in the treatment of delayed union and nonunion fractures have been developed. These methods include a noninvasive, a semi-invasive, and an invasive technique (Salter 1999). In the noninvasive method, an electrical coil surrounds the fracture site and generates an electromagnetic field that produces electrical currents within the tissues. The semi-invasive system involves insertion of percutaneous electrodes (e.g., Teflon-coated wires) into the fracture site with the power source (i.e., a battery) remaining external. In the invasive system, the entire bone-stimulating unit, including the electrodes and the power source, is surgically implanted within the tissues (Cummings 1992; Gradisar 1990). All three systems of electrical stimulation appear to be equally effective in enhancement of healing in delayed union or nonunion fractures with success rates ranging from 70 to 85% (Cummings 1992; Groner and Weeks 1992). Typically, treatments are continued for a three- to six-month period (Groner and Weeks 1992).

Because of the comparatively low incidence of delayed union or nonunion fractures in the sports population, the use of electrical bone stimulation in sport-related fractures is not widespread. Delayed union or nonunion fractures of the scaphoid sometimes seen in the competitive athlete may be the most notable indication. Although the role of the sports health care clinician in electrical bone stimulation appears to be limited, successful clinical treatment of nonunion fractures of the ulna, radius, and mandible with the use of noninvasive interferential current has been reported (Cummings 1992).

Preservation and Restoration of Function

Despite conceptual advances in fracture management that optimize preservation of function, current treatment methods are typically accompanied by varying degrees of functional loss. Hence, restoration of function is commonly identified as a third primary objective of comprehensive fracture treatment. Restoration of function in fracture management has traditionally been addressed as therapeutic intervention to restore joint motion and muscular strength in affected body parts after prolonged immobilization or restricted activity. In the absence of articular complications or significant periarticular soft tissue trauma, functional losses that develop during the recovery period can usually be attributed to the deleterious effects of restricted movement or immobilization on normal musculotendinous structures, joint capsules and ligaments, and other soft tissues. The detrimental effects of prolonged immobilization on the structural and biomechanical properties of soft connective tissues were discussed in chapter 5.

Although restoration of function in fracture management has traditionally implied reversal of deficits due to alterations in the biomechanics of soft tissues, the functional properties of osseous tissue may also be compromised by the stress protection capabilities of fixation and immobilization devices, general inactivity and disuse, or both. In a functional sense, bones provide the supporting framework for body organs and the lever system through which body movements are controlled by muscular contractions. Hence, if the unique structural and biomechanical properties of bone that permit these functions (i.e., strength and stiffness) are disrupted by injury and further compromised by immobilization and inactivity, a functional loss has occurred. Stress risers and disuse osteoporosis resulting from implantation of rigid internal fixation devices and generalized disuse atrophy associated with physical inactivity represent bony deficits that may affect the ability of bones to perform their normal functions without the risk of reinjury.

Notwithstanding the necessity of fixation and immobilization devices for satisfactory fracture stabilization, residual functional deficits may involve both bone and soft tissues. Consequently, a rational approach to fracture management includes therapeutic strategies to encourage uneventful restoration of normal bone structure and function as well as therapeutic measures to reverse functional losses due to soft tissue alterations. This conceptual framework is particularly applicable to sports injury rehabilitation during which sports activities expose recovering bone to potentially harmful mechanical loading. Nevertheless, controlled progressive mechanical loading of bone tissue during sports activities is a positive factor in bone remodeling and restoration of normal bone function.

Restoration of Soft Tissue Function

Therapeutic intervention to preserve or restore soft tissue function in fracture management necessitates close communication between the sports health care clinician and the attending physician. Regular consultation with the attending physician who relies on periodic radiographic examination to determine normal, timely fracture healing is necessary to establish appropriate parameters for therapeutic exercise. Although contemporary methods of fracture management encourage early joint motion, the extent of bony union and fracture stabilization are the prime determinants of appropriate therapeutic tissue loading. Within these parameters, the sports health care clinician is commonly confronted with challenges to preserve or restore joint mobility and muscular strength in the affected body part without disrupting normal bone-healing mechanisms.

Joint Mobility

Contemporary methods of fracture management emphasize preservation of joint mobility through encouragement of active motion in joints proximal and distal to the immobilization device (Raney and Brashear 1971), use of removable splints that permit intervening sessions of manual mobilization (Gradisar 1990), functional electrical muscle stimulation to preserve tendon excursion (Sadler and Koepfer 1992), and the use of hinged cast-braces that permit incremental changes in joint position (Salter 1999). Despite these preventative measures, limitations in joint motion may result from the use of fracture stabilization and protection methods.

Loss of soft tissue mobility and joint motion may be associated with articular trauma that results in contracture of capsular or ligamentous structures, adhesions between adjacent articular tissues, or a combination of both. Trauma to periarticular muscles with consequential fibrosis and formation of *fibrotic contractures* may also limit joint mobility (Thomas 1993). These complications are commonly attributed to the detrimental effects of persistent inflammatory responses, abnormal wound contraction, or fibrous scar formation during connective tissue repair. Despite an absence of soft tissue pathology, however, limitations in joint mobility may occur as the result of fracture treatment. Unless a fracture is accompanied by significant trauma to articular or periarticular soft tissues, it can reasonably be assumed that the joint "stiffness" and loss of joint motion associated with fracture management is related to the detrimental effects of immobilization and restricted movement. For example, as discussed in chapter 5, loss of tissue mobility during periods of immobilization is attributed to a loss of water and glycosaminoglycans (GAGs) from the ground substance of the extracellular connective tissue matrix and excessive cross-linkage of collagen fibers (see chapter 5, figure 5.1). In addition, adaptive shortening of periarticular muscle tissues in response to immobilization produces a nonpathological *myostatic contracture*, in contrast to a pathological fibrotic contracture that results from connective tissue repair (Thomas 1993).

The distinction between restricted tissue mobility associated with soft tissue repair and the joint stiffness that results from immobilization is clinically significant. Although uninjured soft tissues that have been immobilized as a necessary component of fracture management may shorten and lose tensile strength, they are not subject to the additional complicating effects of persistent inflammation, excessive wound contraction, and fibrous scar formation. Hence, as a general rule, they are able to tolerate greater amounts of therapeutic tensile loading (i.e., stretching). For example, immobilization of the elbow in the treatment of uncomplicated fractures of the radius or ulna can be expected to result in joint stiffness due to restricted joint motion rather than soft tissue trauma. Although the deleterious effects of immobilization on joint structures must be respected in this example, therapeutic efforts to restore joint mobility are not hampered by the consequences of articular pathology. Hence, the parameters for appropriate joint mobilization are determined primarily by the extent of bone healing and fracture stability.

If permitted by an acceptable level of bony union, selection of appropriate therapeutic techniques to restore joint motion can be based on typical clinical considerations, including identification of the specific restrictive tissues (i.e., articular structures or periarticular structures) and consideration of their structural and biomechanical integrity (e.g., tensile strength). Pending determination of the particular restricting tissues, restoration of joint mobility may be addressed through the use of traditional passive or active exercise to restore physiological joint motion, joint mobilization techniques to restore accessory joint motions, and proprioceptive neuromuscular facilitation (PNF) stretching techniques to mobilize shortened musculotendinous tissues (see chapter 5).

Muscular Strength

The detrimental effects of fracture immobilization on muscle tissues are widely recognized by attending physicians and sports health care clinicians. As is the case with other tissue types, prolonged immobilization leads to *disuse atrophy*. With disuse, selective atrophy of Type II fast twitch myofibers, the muscle fibers responsible for rapid, forceful muscle contractions, is thought to occur (Ambrustmacher 1994). Because muscle atrophy involves a decrease in the size of myofibers that contain the contractile elements of skeletal muscles, the ability of a muscle to contract with force is compromised. Disuse atrophy is thought to be related to decreased synthesis of myosin and actin, the contractile proteins that form the filaments, or *myofilaments*, within a muscle fiber (figure 7.5). As a result, the diameter of myofibers decreases and their ability to generate forceful contractions is diminished. In contrast to myofiber atrophy that results from immobilization and disuse, muscle fiber size increases with physical activity and muscle *hypertrophy* occurs in response to progressive resistive exercise. Muscle hypertrophy, in contrast to atrophy, is

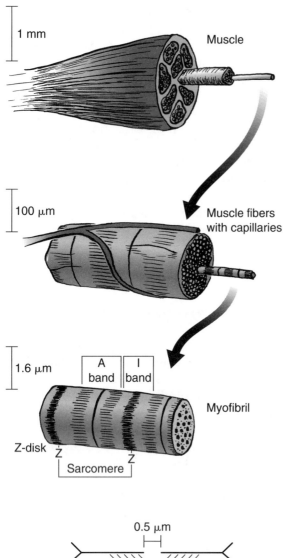

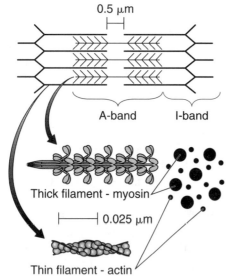

Figure 7.5 Structure and composition of skeletal muscle tissue.

Reprinted, by permission, from P.E. di Prampero, 1985, "Metabolic circulatory limitations to V̇O₂ max at the whole animal level," *Journal of Biologists Ltd.* 115:319-331.

attributed to increased synthesis of myosin (i.e., the thick filaments) and actin (i.e., thin filaments) and, thus, an increase in the diameter of myofibers. Correspondingly, the ability of muscle fibers to generate forceful contractions is increased (Tortora and Grabowski 1993; Whiting and Zernicke 1998). In addition to a dependence on muscle fiber size, muscle strength is also dependent on the integrity of efferent (motor) nerve innervation and recruitment of active motor units that provide the neural basis for muscle contraction. Whereas the term *contractility* refers to the ability of muscle fibers to contract, the capability of a muscle to contract with force, and thus resist or overcome external forces, is referred to as *strength* (Thomas 1993). Thus, muscle strength has a neurological component as well as a physiological component, both of which are addressed during restoration of neuromuscular function after fracture immobilization.

Whereas passive mobilization techniques may be effective for preservation or restoration of joint motion in fracture management, maintenance and restoration of muscular strength necessitates active isometric or isotonic muscle contractions. If permitted by an acceptable level of bone healing and fracture stabilization, early static "muscle setting" or isometric contractions are encouraged in an attempt to preserve neuromuscular function in immobilized muscle tissues. As fracture healing progresses, manually resisted isotonic muscle contractions involving movement of joints proximal and distal to the immobilization device are commonly indicated to enhance muscular strength. In some cases, immobilization of fractures in the distal extremities (e.g., the ankle) permits application of manual resistance proximal to a cast or splint and the use of proprioceptive neuromuscular facilitation (PNF) muscle-strengthening techniques (e.g., repeated contractions, slow reversal) to preserve or enhance neuromuscular function in the affected extremity.

Restoration of Bone Function

Monitoring of mechanical tissue loading after a fracture and progressive introduction of physical activity that promotes bone density, mass, and strength represent areas of therapeutic intervention that lie within the domain of the sports health care clinician. Loss of bone density and bone mass due to physical inactivity and disuse has been a consistent scientific observation for many years. Montoye (1987) cited numerous investigations demonstrating disuse atrophy in the bones of animals as well as humans.

Methods of imposed disuse in these studies included restricted exercise, immobilization, and weightlessness. Bone responds to removal of mechanical loading by a reduction in density, mass, and strength regardless of the reason for the reduced load. Conversely, bone responds to increased mechanical loading by an increase in these structural and functional properties. These adaptive responses, which exemplify the central tenet of Wolff's law, provide a basis for decision making regarding appropriate therapeutic tissue loading and resumption of physical activity after a fracture.

Wolff's Law

As formulated by Julius Wolff in 1868, Wolff's law holds that adaptive changes in the structure and biomechanical properties of bone occur in accordance with functional demands (Raney and Brashear 1971). For example, cortical bone in the epiphyseal and metaphyseal areas of long bones is comparatively thin. In contrast, cortical bone in the diaphyseal region is comparatively thick, in accordance with functional demands for strength and stiffness. The diaphysis of long bones has been found to respond to bending forces by deposition of new bone on the concave side and resorption of bone on the convex side. This adaptive behavior has been attributed to generation of electrical potentials in response to the application of pressure, a phenomenon referred to as *piezoelectricity* (Thomas 1993). Bassett and Becker (1962) demonstrated the piezoelectric effect in animal models through the application of electrodes to long bones. When bending forces were applied, the electrode on the concave side of the bone became negative whereas the electrode on the convex side became positive. Reversed polarity occurred when the bone was bent in the opposite direction. Thus, bone deposition occurs on the concave side as the result of a negative charge produced by pressure, or compression. Alternatively, the positive charge produced by tensile forces on the convex side of a long bone during bending favors bone resorption (Bryant 1977; Salter 1999).

Mechanical Loading

The central tenet of Wolff's law and the piezoelectric effect of mechanical forces on long bones provide rationale for progressive loading of osseous tissues at appropriate stages during recovery from a fracture. As discussed in chapter 6, remodeling of bone tissue after a fracture is the process through which the structure, size, and strength of a bone are eventually restored. Thus, remodeling is essential to restoration of normal bone function. Bone remodeling at the fracture site, as well as restoration of bone density and mass lost during immobilization and disuse, is enhanced by mechanical loading. As living, dynamic tissue, bone responds positively to weight bearing and physical activity. Muscular activity has been proposed as a primary source of osseous tissue loading that stimulates generation of bioelectric potentials, which in turn promote osteoblast activity and bone growth (Montoye 1987). Mechanical forces transferred to osseous tissues via the attachments of contracting muscles are thought to provide a stimulus to the piezoelectric effect. Thus, the functional demands placed on bones of the skeletal system during physical activity would be expected to promote adaptive increases in bone density, size, and strength in accordance with Wolff's law.

Numerous studies have substantiated the positive effect of physical activity on increased bone density and bone mass. Radiographic comparison of bone girth in the dominant and nondominant extremities of competitive athletes provides dramatic evidence of the effect of repetitive mechanical loading on osseous tissues. These comparisons have revealed greater bone girth in the dominant extremity of tennis players, including the humerus, radius, and ulna (Buskirk, Anderson, and Brozel 1956; Jones et al. 1977). In general, greater discrepancies in bone girth between dominant and nondominant limbs were noted in athletes than in nonathletes. Krahl et al. (1994) reported increased bone density and diameter in the distal ulna and the second metacarpal of the dominant extremity in nationally and internationally ranked tennis players. Bilateral discrepancies in bone girth of the distal humerus have been found in professional baseball pitchers (King, Brelsford, and Tullos 1969). These investigators reported consistent radiological evidence of bony hypertrophy in the distal humerus of the throwing arm.

Therapeutic Implications

Disuse atrophy of bone during immobilization can be profound and may occur rapidly within the first few weeks of immobilization (Loitz-Ramage and Zernicke 1996). The extent to which disuse atrophy can be reversed and the time factors involved, however, are somewhat speculative. Nevertheless, as noted by Whiting and Zernicke (1998), bone mineral loss is reversible to a certain extent. Restoration of bone mineral content, however, does not occur as rapidly as bone mineral loss. Furthermore, the extent of bone mineral loss and the potential for restoration appears to be related to the duration of immobilization. The longer the immobilization period, the greater the detrimental effects (Raney and Brashear 1971). Along with a concern for preservation of soft tissue function, these observations have prompted approaches to fracture treatment that focus on prevention of bone atrophy. In a clinical sense, progressive mechanical loading becomes an important therapeutic modality in fracture management as bone healing permits.

Current medical practices reflect incorporation of progressive mechanical loading in fracture treatment. Physicians generally recognize that immobilization should be continued only long enough for solid bony union to occur and discontinued as soon as mechanical loading can be safely assumed. In the event of necessary immobilization, however, static contraction of muscle groups included within a cast or splint is commonly recommended unless precluded by fracture-healing considerations. Additionally, active or resisted movement of joints adjacent to an immobilization device is typically encouraged. Although these measures are usually associated with maintenance of soft tissue function, they also represent rational early measures to combat disuse osteoporosis through controlled mechanical loading. As previously discussed, muscle contractions are thought to exert beneficial mechanical forces on bones that stimulate osteoblast activity and bone deposition (Loitz-Ramage and Zernicke 1996).

With satisfactory progression of bone healing, modifications of rigid casts and splints are sometimes made to allow greater freedom of movement and progressive weight bearing. For example, progression from an elbow immobilizer or splint to a forearm and wrist splint in the treatment of fractures of the radius or ulna permits increased mechanical loading of osseous tissues through active elbow motion. In a similar manner, progression from a rigid ankle cast with a non-weight-bearing crutch gait to walking cast or an "ankle walker" with a rocker sole allows for increased loading of bony structures in fractures of the ankle and leg. Nevertheless, optimal restoration of bone density, mass, and strength after fracture immobilization may not occur until bone tissues are subjected to sport-specific functional demands.

Resumption of Sports Participation

Considering the extended time period associated with bone remodeling after a fracture, it seems reasonable to presume that competitive athletes and serious sports participants return to some level of physical activity, if not full participation, before remodeling is complete. This overlapping transition, from relative inactivity to more strenuous activity, presents implications for progressive sport-specific mechanical loading as well as reinjury risk management. The examples of bone hypertrophy in the dominant extremities of competitive athletes previously cited in this chapter provide impressive evidence of adaptation to sport-related functional demands. It is important to note, however, that these changes are the result of high-intensity, repetitive mechanical loading of normal bone over extended time periods. Restoration of function in bone tissues weakened by fracture, structural defects resulting from rigid internal fixation, or immobilization and general dis-use necessitates a less intense, guarded approach to physical activity. These considerations suggest the necessity of graduated levels of functional loading, which stimulate bone depo-sition but do not impose excessive mechanical forces that subject weakened bones to re-fracture (Whiting and Zernicke 1998). Thus, the distinction among low-intensity, moderate-intensity, and high-intensity exercise, as related to bone biodynamics, is relative to the structural and biomechanical properties of bone (e.g., strength and stiffness) at any par-ticular time during the remodeling process. Controlled sport-specific activity and progres-sive mechanical loading are important factors in restoration of the normal structural and biomechanical properties of bone. In summarizing current knowledge regarding the ef-fects of exercise on bone structure, Whiting and Zernicke (1998) noted that the amount of bone mass increase that can be achieved through physical activity appears to depend on the initial bone mass. This observation suggests the potential for increased bone mass and reversal of bone atrophy resulting from fracture immobilization and general inactivity.

Site-Specific Bone Hypertrophy

Plentiful evidence exists that exercise places functional demands on the skeletal system that result in increased bone density, mass, and strength (Montoye 1987). As noted by Loitz-Ramage and Zernicke (1996), however, these adaptive changes are "site-specific" rather than generalized to all bones of the skeletal system. Increased bone density and mass that result from exercise is greatest in those bones, or particular areas of a bone, that are the focus of mechanical loading. This phenomenon is observed in previously cited examples of regional hypertrophy of the radius, ulna, and the metacarpal bones in the dominant extremity of tennis players and in the distal humerus of the throwing arm in baseball pitchers. These examples of site-specific adaptation in normal, uninjured bone may have implications for the type, intensity, and duration of exercise necessary to re-verse disuse atrophy and maximize the biomechanical properties of bone after a fracture.

Optimal restoration of bone structure and function after a fracture in a sports partici-pant may not occur until the affected bone is subjected to sport-specific functional de-mands. By comparison, the effects of relatively moderate exercise such as walking and jogging, sometimes prescribed for reversal of osteoporosis in certain populations (e.g., postmenopausal women, the aging), would be expected to be somewhat generalized, al-though concentrated in the weight-bearing bones of the lower extremities. In a contrast-ing example, however, greater specificity of mechanical loading may be required to maxi-mize bone function after a fracture of the throwing arm (e.g., the humerus) in a competitive baseball player. In this example, progressive resumption of overhand throwing with gradual increases in velocity and duration represents rational application of sport-related functional demands that result in site-specific increases in bone density, mass, and strength. This approach, which allows for progressive adaptive changes in the structural and bio-mechanical properties of bone, exemplifies application of Wolff's law to functional reha-bilitation of an athlete with a sport-related fracture.

Bone Fatigue and Stress Fractures

The potential traumatic effects of repetitive mechanical loading on weakened bone tissues present implications for uneventful resumption of physical activity after a fracture, espe-cially if the fracture involves bones of the skeletal system that are exposed to repeated cyclic mechanical forces (e.g., the lower extremities of a distance runner). Although refractures may occur as the result of a single, suddenly applied high-magnitude force (e.g., direct impact), excessive stress resulting from premature weight bearing and repeti-tive forces is a more likely cause. An understanding of the biomechanics associated with fractures resulting from cumulative stress provides the sports health care clinician with insight regarding appropriate levels of activity and mechanical loading during recovery from a fracture. Fractures resulting from repetitive loads of comparatively low intensity are commonly referred to as *fatigue fractures*, or *stress fractures* (Nordin and Frankel 1989; Whiting and Zernicke 1998). As defined by Whiting and Zernicke (1998), the term *fatigue*, as related to bone dynamics, is used to describe a loss of strength and stiffness that results from repeated cyclic loads. The load, or force, imparted to a bone per unit area as the result of external mechanical loading is referred to as *stress* (Nordin and Frankel 1989). Thus, excessive stress results in bone fatigue, which in turn increases the propensity for stress fractures to occur. Loss of bone strength and stiffness, or fatigue, has been attributed to development of microscopic cracks (i.e., microfractures) within and between the haversian systems, or osteons, of cortical bone (Whiting and Zernicke 1998). If these disruptions are minimal, normal bone remodeling, with bone resorption and deposition of new bone, repairs the defects, thereby arresting progression to a detectable fracture (Nordin and Frankel 1989). Bone remodeling in response to repetitive mechanical loading but without radiographic evidence of an actual fracture has been described as a *stress reaction* (Loitz-Ramage and Zernicke 1996). As noted by Whiting and Zernicke (1998), however, stress reactions are detectable through the use of bone scans and magnetic resonance imaging (MRI). In the presence of continued repetitive mechanical stress that exceeds the ability of bone remodeling to repair microscopic tissue deficits (i.e., bone fatigue), an accumulation of microfractures may result in a true stress fracture (Nordin and Frankel 1989; Schiller 1994). Stress fractures of the metatarsals, the tibia, and the femur in distance runners and dancers are familiar to the experienced sports health care clinician.

Repetitive mechanical stress that is sufficient to cause bone failure during exercise is a product not only of the magnitude of loading and the number of repetitions but also of the frequency of load application (i.e., the number of repetitions within a specific time frame). Although repetition of low-magnitude loads may be nontraumatic if applied gradually, the cumulative effect of repeated low loads over a short time period may exceed the ability of bone to adapt, thus predisposing the bone to fracture (Montoye 1987; Nordin and Frankel 1989). Along with a realistic assessment of bone strength and stiffness based on the sports health care clinician's knowledge of the remodeling process, these etiological factors are important considerations in interpretation of such terms as low-intensity and high-intensity exercise.

In addition to the frequency and duration of repetitive forces, muscle fatigue has also been noted as a contributing factor in stress fractures (Nordin and Frankel 1989). Although normal muscle contractions are thought to stimulate bone deposition by transmission of mechanical loads to bones via muscle and tendon attachments, they also diminish or neutralize forces on bones during physical activity. As muscles fatigue during strenuous activity, their ability to contract forcefully diminishes. Consequently, increased loading, altered distribution of mechanical forces, and greater stress concentration occur in bones of the skeletal system (figure 7.6). Should stress (i.e., load per unit area) be concentrated in bone tissues weakened by fracture, immobilization, or general disuse, the pro-

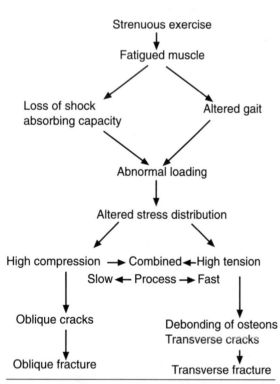

Figure 7.6 Theoretical mechanisms of a fatigue (stress) fracture of the lower extremity.

Reprinted, by permission, from M. Nordin and V.H. Frankel, 1989, Biomechanics of bones. In *Biomechanics of the musculoskeletal system*, 2nd ed., edited by M. Nordin and V.H. Frankel (Philadelphia: Lea and Febiger), 19.

pensity for tissue failure increases. Hence, restoration of neuromuscular function, muscle strength, and muscular endurance becomes an important component of sports injury rehabilitation as related to protection of bone tissues from traumatic forces.

Removal of Internal Fixation Devices

As discussed in chapter 6, removal of bone screws, metallic bone plates, and other internal fixation devices may be accompanied by residual bone deficits, including defects associated with vacant screw holes and disuse osteoporosis. If a return to sports activities after removal of internal fixation devices is anticipated, the relative risk factors must be considered until such time that bone deficiencies are resolved. It is generally accepted that, after removal of rigid metallic implants, loading mechanisms inherent in physical activity are conducive to reversal of disuse atrophy, in accordance with Wolff's law. As noted by Salter (1999), however, healed bones require protection from excessive mechanical loads during the few months following removal of metallic bone plates and screws. Should stress resulting from physical activity be concentrated in weakened osseous tissues, recurrent tissue failure may occur. Because of their knowledge of bone biodynamics and their familiarity with loading mechanisms inherent in various sports, the sports medicine physician and the certified athletic trainer are key personnel in decision making regarding resumption of sports participation after removal of bone plates and other internal fixation devices.

Summary

Rehabilitation and restoration of function after a fracture necessitates the sports health care clinician's familiarity with contemporary fracture treatment methods. Two basic approaches to fracture management, the Swiss AO/ASIF system and functional bracing, have evolved over the years. The primary approach to fracture treatment in the AO/ASIF system is through the use of rigid internal fixation and interfragmentary compression that favors primary bone healing without significant callus formation. In comparison, functional bracing makes use of hinged cast-braces that allow incremental changes in joint position as fracture stabilization permits. Secondary bone healing with callus formation is characteristically associated with fractures treated by the use of functional cast-braces. Despite differences in treatment approaches, prevention of the deleterious effects of prolonged, rigid external immobilization is the common objective of both the AO/ASIF system and functional fracture bracing.

Regardless of the particular treatment method, the primary objectives of fracture management include achievement of a satisfactory fracture fragment position, fracture stabilization and protection, pain control, and restoration of function in the affected body parts. Reduction and stabilization of displaced fracture fragments are most commonly accomplished by closed reduction and external immobilization, open surgical reduction with internal skeletal fixation, or closed reduction with internal fixation. Commonly used internal fixation devices include interfragmentary screws, metallic plates and screws, intramedullary nails, and metallic pins and wires. Disadvantages associated with the use of rigid metallic plates and screws include creation of stress risers and residual bone deficits, including disuse osteoporosis. Contemporary fracture treatment methods are facilitated by a variety of prefabricated protective devices and fabrication materials that can be used to provide required levels of fracture stabilization and protection throughout the recovery period. These devices include traditional rigid casts and splints, functional hinged cast-braces, and a variety of commercial materials for fabrication of protective devices suitable for wear during sports participation. Despite application of sound fracture management principles, nonunion and delayed union of fractures occasionally occur. In certain cases, electrical bone stimulation has been effective in resolution of nonunion fractures.

Although contemporary fracture treatment methods emphasize preservation of function, varying levels of joint stiffness, muscle atrophy and strength loss, and disuse osteoporosis typically result from immobilization and inactivity. Rational approaches to restoration of function in fracture management, as related to resumption of sports participation, address functional consequences associated with structural and biomechanical alterations in both bone and soft tissues. Preservation of joint mobility and muscular strength are commonly addressed through early active joint motion as fracture healing permits. If restricted joint motion occurs, restoration of soft tissue function is based on identification of restrictive tissues and use of traditional passive or active exercise, joint mobilization techniques, or proprioceptive neuromuscular facilitation (PNF) stretching techniques. Reversal of disuse muscle atrophy and restoration of muscle strength necessitates active exercise and resisted isotonic muscle contractions.

The skeletal system provides the supporting framework for body organs and the lever system through which active movement occurs. Alterations of the normal structural and biomechanical properties of osseous tissues may compromise the ability of bones to perform these functions without the risk of reinjury. Loss of bone density and bone mass, two primary manifestations of disuse atrophy, are recognized consequences of immobilization and restricted activity during which mechanical loads on bone structures are diminished. Conversely, in accordance with Wolff's law, bone adapts to increased mechanical loading and functional demands by an increase in bone density, mass, and strength. Thus, in a clinical sense, progressive mechanical loading is an important therapeutic factor. As related to resumption of physical activity, Wolff's law suggests that sport-specific functional demands with progressive mechanical loading of osseous tissues are necessary for optimal restoration of bone structure and function.

Uneventful resumption of physical activity and sports participation after a fracture

Problem-Solving Scenario

During an intercollegiate tennis match, a 22-year-old male athlete suffered a fracture of the distal fibula in his right leg. Because internal skeletal fixation was deemed unnecessary, the attending orthopedic surgeon's treatment of choice was application of a short-leg cast. The following day, the athlete reports to the athletic treatment center for follow-up care. Subsequently, after the immobilization period, cast removal allows therapeutic attention to the affected ankle and leg. Clinical assessment after cast removal reveals a pain-free but "stiff" ankle joint with moderate limitation in ankle dorsiflexion and plantar flexion. Further evaluation indicates minimal but noticeable atrophy in the calf muscles.

Problem-Solving Questions

- Considering the method of fracture stabilization in this case, what were the most likely mechanisms of bone healing?

- What are the most appropriate short-term rehabilitation goals during the immobilization period?

- What intrinsic bone-healing factors were most likely considered in the orthopedic surgeon's decision to remove the immobilization device?

- What specific factors offer the most plausible explanation for the joint stiffness and restricted range of ankle joint motion after cast removal in this case?

- Based on the clinical assessment after cast removal, what are the most appropriate short-term treatment goals during the next two to three weeks of the patient's recovery period?

- As the athlete's rehabilitation progresses, what factors should be considered in decisions regarding appropriate functional activities and resumption of competition?

necessitates exposure to functional loads that stimulate bone deposition and enhance remodeling but do not exceed levels of stress that cause tissue failure. Although refractures may occur as the result of a sudden mechanical force of high intensity, tissue failure commonly results from repetitive loads of lesser magnitude that cause bone fatigue and stress fractures. Thus, the pathomechanics of tissue failure due to repeated loading become important considerations in restoration of the structural and functional properties of bones that are weakened by disuse osteoporosis and other deficits associated with fracture fixation and stabilization.

References

Ambrustmacher, V.W. 1994. Skeletal muscle. In *Pathology,* 2nd ed., edited by E. Rubin and J. L. Farber. Philadelphia: J.B. Lippincott.

Bassett, C.A., and R.O. Becker. 1962. Generation of electric potentials by bone in response to mechanical stress. *Science* 137:1063-64.

Brennwald, J. 1996. Fracture healing in the hand: A brief update. In *Clinical Orthopaedics and Related Research* 327:9-11.

Bryant, W.M. 1977. *Wound healing*. Reading, Mass.: CIBA Pharmaceutical Co.

Buskirk, E.R., K.L. Anderson, and J. Brozel. 1956. Unilateral activity and bone and muscle development in the forearm. *Research Quarterly* 27:127-31.

Canelon, M.F. 1995. Material properties: A factor in the selection and application of splinting materials for athletic wrist and hand injuries. *Journal of Sports Physical Therapy* 22:164-72.

Cummings, J.P. 1992. Additional therapeutic uses of electricity. In *Electrotherapy in rehabilitation*, edited by M.R. Gersh. Philadelphia: Davis.

Gradisar, I.A. 1990. Fracture stabilization and healing. In *Orthopaedic and sports physical therapy*, 2nd ed., edited by J.A. Gould III. St. Louis: Mosby.

Groner, J.P., and P.M. Weeks. 1992. Healing of hard and soft tissues in the hand. In *Hand injuries in athletes*, edited by J.W. Strickland and A.C. Rettig. Philadelphia: W.B. Saunders.

Hastings, H., II. 1992. Management of extra-articular fractures of the phalanges and metacarpals. In *Hand injuries in athletes*, edited by J.W. Strickland and A.C. Rettig. Philadelphia: W.B. Saunders.

Jones, H.H., J.D. Priest, W.C. Hayes, C.C. Technor, and D.A. Nagel. 1977. Humeral hypertrophy in response to exercise. *Journal of Bone and Joint Surgery* 59A:204-8.

Kilcoyne, R.F., and E.L. Farrar. 1991. *Handbook of orthopedic terminology*. Boca Raton, Fla.: CRC Press.

King, J.W., H.S. Brelsford, and H.S. Tullos. 1969. Analysis of the pitching arm of the professional baseball pitcher. *Clinical Orthopedics and Related Research* 67:116-23.

Krahl, H., U. Michaels, H.G. Pieper, G. Quack, and M. Montag. 1994. Stimulation of bone growth through sports. *American Journal of Sports Medicine* 22:751-57.

Loitz-Ramage, B.J, and R.F. Zernicke. 1996. Bone biology and mechanics. In *Athletic injuries and rehabilitation*, edited by J.E. Zachazewski, D.J. Magee, and W.S. Quillen. Philadelphia: W.B. Saunders.

Montoye, H.J. 1987. Better bones and biodynamics. *Research Quarterly for Exercise and Sport* 58:334-47.

Nordin, M., and V.H. Frankel. 1989. Biomechanics of bones. In *Basic biomechanics of the musculoskeletal system*, 2nd ed., edited by M. Nordin and V.H. Frankel. Philadelphia: Lea and Febiger.

O'Sullivan, M.E., E.Y.S. Chao, and P.J. Kelly. 1989. Current concepts review: The effects of fixation on fracture-healing. *The Journal of Bone and Joint Surgery* 71A:306-10.

Raney, R.B., Sr., and H.R. Brashear Jr. 1971. *Shands' handbook of orthopaedic surgery*, 8th ed. St. Louis: Mosby.

Sadler, J.A., and J.M. Koepfer. 1992. Rehabilitation and splinting of the injured hand. In *Hand injuries in athletes*, edited by J.W. Strickland and A.C. Rettig. Philadelphia: W.B. Saunders.

Salter, R.B. 1999. *Textbook of disorders and injuries of the musculoskeletal system*, 3rd ed. Baltimore: Williams and Wilkins.

Schiller, A.L. 1994. Bones and joints. In *Pathology,* 2nd ed., edited by E. Rubin and J.L. Farber. Philadelphia: J.B. Lippincott.

Schultz, R.J. 1990. *The language of fractures*, 2nd ed. Baltimore: Williams and Wilkins.

Strickland, J.W. 1992. A philosophy for the management of athletic injuries of the hand and wrist. In *Hand injuries in athletes*, edited by J.W. Strickland and A.C. Rettig. Philadelphia: W.B. Saunders.

Thomas, C.L., ed. 1993. *Taber's cyclopedic medical dictionary*, 17th ed. Philadelphia: Davis.

Tortora, G.J., and S.R. Grabowski. 1993. *Principles of anatomy and physiology,* 7th ed. New York: Harper Collins College Publishers.

Whiting, W.C., and R.F. Zernicke. 1998. Biomechanics of musculoskeletal injury. Champaign, Ill.: Human Kinetics.

Zemel, N.P. 1992. Carpal fractures. In *Hand injuries in athletes*, edited by J.W. Strickland and A.C. Rettig. Philadelphia: W.B. Saunders.

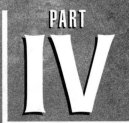

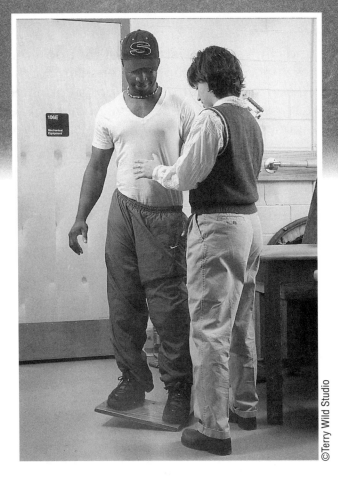

©Terry Wild Studio

Proprioceptive and Sensorimotor Deficits and Therapeutic Intervention

During the past several years, proprioceptive and sensorimotor deficits that accompany common musculoskeletal injuries have received increased attention in sports injury management. The primary purposes of this part are to review the neuroanatomy and neurophysiology of the sensorimotor systems of the body, describe the pathological basis of proprioceptive deficits, and present implications for restoration of proprioceptive and sensorimotor function. Chapter 8, Proprioception and Sensorimotor Function, includes a review of the relevant neuroanatomy and neurophysiology of the peripheral proprioceptive system, vestibular system, and visual system as a basis for development of therapeutic strategies. Chapter 9, Therapeutic Implications: Proprioceptive and Sensorimotor Deficits, is devoted to a discussion of the pathology and clinical manifestations of proprioceptive and sensorimotor deficits as well as a presentation of therapeutic considerations related to acute injury management, surgery, and sensorimotor training. The principles and concepts included in these two chapters provide a basis for development of sensorimotor training protocols as integral components of functional rehabilitation in sports injury management.

Proprioception and Sensorimotor Function

CHAPTER
8

The Peripheral Proprioceptive System
Peripheral Mechanoreceptors
Joint Receptors
Musculotendinous Receptors
Cutaneous Receptors
Neurophysiology of Mechanoreceptors
Receptive Fields
Electrophysiology of Mechanoreceptors
Receptor Adaptation
Integration of Mechanoreceptor Functions
The Dorsal Column-Medial Lemniscal System
Afferent (Sensory) Neurons
Ascending Spinal Cord Pathways
The Thalamus
Cerebral Cortex
Basal Ganglia and the Cerebellum
Basal Ganglia
The Cerebellum

Descending (Motor) Pathways
Direct (Pyramidal) Pathways
Indirect (Extrapyramidal) Pathways
The Vestibular System
Vestibular Receptors and Afferent (Sensory) Pathways
Vestibular Nuclei and Efferent (Motor) Projections
The Visual System
Visual Receptors and Afferent (Sensory) Pathways
The Superior Colliculus and Efferent (Motor) Projections
Summary

Learning Objectives

After completion of this chapter, the reader should be able to

1. describe joint position sense and kinesthesia as components of proprioception and differentiate between proprioception and sensorimotor function,

2. identify the relevant anatomical structures and neurophysiological functions of the peripheral proprioceptive system, vestibular system, and visual system in normal sensorimotor activity,

3. describe the proprioceptive functions of sensory receptors in ligaments and joint capsules, musculotendinous structures, and the skin, and

4. identify the four major components of the motor control system and describe the role of each in neuromuscular coordination, postural control, and balance.

An intact, properly functioning sensorimotor system is essential to safe and efficient performance of sports activities, as well as routine activities of daily living. The motor systems of the body rely on a continuous flow of sensory information from a variety of sources, which when integrated and interpreted, forms the basis for appropriate neuromuscular responses. In a broad sense, the sensorimotor functions of the body are dependent on intact neural mechanisms associated with somatosensory mechanoreceptors located in peripheral anatomical structures (e.g., ligaments and joint capsules, muscles), mechanoreceptors in the vestibular apparatus of the inner ear, and photoreceptors in the retina. Collectively, sensory input from these three primary sources provides the neural foundation for motor skill performance requiring neuromuscular coordination, postural control, and balance.

The term *sensation* has been defined as "a feeling or awareness of conditions within or without the body resulting from the stimulation of sensory receptors" (Thomas 1993). Taste, hearing, sight, smell, and touch are among the five familiar senses. Historically, the term *sixth sense* has been associated with a sensation involving a general awareness of normal body functions (Thomas 1993). During the early 1990s, awareness of joint position and movement, sensations referred to as *proprioception*, became more closely associated with existence of a sixth sense (Parkhurst and Burnett 1994). Contemporary thought, however, supports the view that proprioception is a variation of the basic sense of touch. Currently, proprioception is considered to include the awareness of static joint position, referred to as *joint position sense*, and the perception of joint movement, or *kinesthesia* (Lephart 1994). By definition, *proprioception* implies cognitive awareness, or perception, of these two components at cortical levels of the brain.

For discussion purposes, it is important to establish a distinction between proprioception and sensorimotor function. Current views restrict the definition of *proprioception* to the neural mechanisms associated with stimulation of mechanoreceptors, relay of afferent (sensory) information to the central nervous system, and processing by higher brain centers (Lephart, Rieman, and Fu 2000). This definition, however, does not include the neural processes through which motor signals are conveyed through efferent (motor) pathways. Sensorimotor function, on the other hand, is a more inclusive concept that incorporates and integrates processes associated with afferent (sensory) input, central processing of information, and efferent (motor) output. Thus, proprioception is a component, albeit a crucial component, of sensorimotor activity.

Rationale for discussion of proprioception and sensorimotor function in this book is based on the premise that proprioceptive deficits represent a pathological component of common sports injuries to the musculoskeletal system. Trauma to body tissues that house somatosensory receptors for proprioception (e.g., ligaments, joint capsules) may include disruption of the receptors as well as degeneration of their afferent (sensory) nerve fibers. Resulting proprioceptive deficits may include not only impairments in joint position sense and kinesthesia but also deficits in dynamic joint stabilization, postural control, and balance. To the extent that these impairments are associated with sports injuries, they represent increased risk factors for the sports participant that require therapeutic attention during the rehabilitation process.

As a basis for discussion of proprioceptive and sensorimotor training programs in chapter 9, the relevant neuroanatomy and neurophysiology associated with proprioception and sensorimotor function is reviewed in this chapter. For discussion purposes, neural pathways associated with sensory input from somatic mechanoreceptors (i.e., joint, musculotendinous, and skin receptors) are designated as the peripheral proprioceptive system, as distinguished from the vestibular system and the visual system. This distinction, however, is not intended to ignore the more inclusive concept that sensorimotor activities are an integrated function of all three systems. Hence, neural mechanisms associated with each of these systems and their relationship to proprioception and neuromuscular control are reviewed as a foundation for development of comprehensive sensorimotor training programs.

The Peripheral Proprioceptive System

As categorized for discussion purposes, the peripheral proprioceptive system includes somatosensory mechanoreceptors (i.e., joint, musculotendinous, and skin receptors) and their afferent (sensory) neurons, as well as ascending spinal cord pathways, the cerebral cortex and associated subcortical structures (i.e., basal ganglia, cerebellum), and descending (motor) spinal cord pathways. Although designated as the peripheral proprioceptive system, it is important to note that this taxonomy includes major components of the motor control system. Thus, discussion in this section includes a review of the neuroanatomy associated with stimulation of peripheral mechanoreceptors.

Peripheral Mechanoreceptors

Proprioception is dependent, in part, on afferent input to the central nervous system from somatosensory receptors located in joint capsules and ligaments, musculotendinous structures, and the skin (Lephart 1994). These sensory receptors, which represent the distal terminals of afferent (sensory) neurons, are referred to as *mechanoreceptors*, or *proprioceptors*, because of their sensitivity to mechanical stimuli involving tension, stretch, or pressure. Histological examination of articular soft tissues (i.e., ligaments, joint capsules, synovial membrane), musculotendinous tissues, and the skin has revealed several types of mechanoreceptors that play an integral role in the peripheral proprioceptive system (Rowinski 1997). The general morphology and function of mechanoreceptors in each of these tissue types is reviewed as a basis for appreciation of their contribution to proprioception. Clinically significant neural mechanisms associated with mechanoreceptor stimulation, generation of nerve impulses, and receptor adaptation are also discussed in subsequent sections of this chapter.

Joint Receptors

In the mid 1800s, John Hilton, a British surgeon, described the innervation of various joints and discovered that nerves supplying the muscles that cross a particular joint also send branches to articular structures and to the skin overlying the muscle insertions (Thomas 1993). This principle is referred to as *Hilton's law* (Barrack and Skinner 1990). Since the 1800s, several investigators have attempted to clarify the innervation of various joints of the body as well as the distribution of nerve branches to specific joint structures. Although studies commonly reveal a certain amount of variability in distribution of articular nerve branches, predominant patterns of innervation have been established for most major joints of the body. The specific pattern of innervation in the human knee, for example, has been summarized by Kennedy, Alexander, and Hayes (1982). Extension of nerve branches from periarticular muscles to articular structures with termination as mechanoreceptors in joint capsules and ligaments provides an anatomical basis for dynamic joint stability, particularly as related to the neural mechanisms of reflex muscle contraction.

Historically, most histological studies of joint receptors have used animal models. In recent years, however, an increasing number of investigations have confirmed the presence of several types of mechanoreceptors in various articular structures in humans. Articular mechanoreceptors have been identified in joint capsules, ligaments, and synovial tissues. Mechanoreceptors have also been found in the menisci and periarticular fat pads of the knee. Most histological studies have focused on the major joints of the lower extremities (i.e., the ankle and knee) and, to a lesser extent, the glenohumeral joint (Lephart 1994). A review of the literature indicates that joint receptors have been classified, morphologically and functionally, into four basic types: (1) pacinian corpuscles, (2) Ruffini's corpuscles, (3) Golgi ligament endings (Golgi tendon organlike endings), and (4) free nerve endings (Borsa et al. 1994; Freeman and Wyke 1965; Nyland et al. 1994). These receptors differ not only in their morphological characteristics but also in their specific neural functions.

Pacinian corpuscles

Named after the Italian anatomist Filippo Pacini, pacinian corpuscles (Pacini's corpuscles) are oval shaped, encapsulated (i.e., enclosed by connective tissue) single terminal endings typically located near small blood vessels at the junction of the joint capsule and adjacent synovial membrane (figure 8.1). Histological studies have demonstrated a higher density of pacinian corpuscles in distal joints compared to proximal joints (Nyland et al. 1994; Tortora and Grabowski 1993). As noted by Grigg (1994), compressive forces acting on capsular tissues during extremes of joint movement appear to provide the primary stimulus for activation of pacinian corpuscles. In contrast to other types of joint mechanoreceptors (i.e., Ruffini's corpuscles, Golgi ligament endings), pacinian corpuscles are categorized as rapidly adapting receptors with a very low threshold for mechanical stimulation. As such, they respond readily to rapid changes in joint position involving acceleration and deceleration of angular velocity (Rowinski 1997). The clinical significance of mechanoreceptor adaptation to sensory stimulation is discussed in a later section of this chapter.

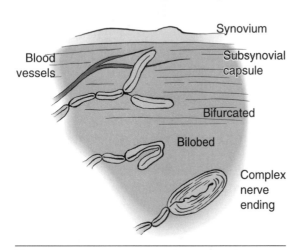

Figure 8.1 Neuroanatomy of pacinian corpuscles.

Reprinted, by permission, from M.J. Rowinski, 1997, Neurobiology for orthopedic and sport physical therapy. In *Orthopedic and sports physical therapy*, 3rd ed., edited by T.R. Malone, T.G. McPoil, and A.J. Nitz (St. Louis: Mosby-Yearbook), 50.

Ruffini's corpuscles

Angelo Ruffini, an Italian anatomist, was the first to identify the mechanoreceptors in joint capsules that bear his name. Morphologically, Ruffini's corpuscles are thinly encapsulated, spray-type sensory receptors embedded within the collagenous framework of the joint capsule (figure 8.2). Unlike pacinian corpuscles, Ruffini's corpuscles are comparatively dense in proximal joints. Anatomically, they are found predominately in areas of the joint capsule that are subjected to the greatest amount of stress. In hinge joints, for example, Ruffini's corpuscles are concentrated in areas of the capsule that are stretched during extension (e.g., the posterior joint capsule of the knee). Stimulation is proportional to the extent of articular tissue loading, or stretch. Because Ruffini's corpuscles are thought to be activated when a joint approaches its extended range, they have been referred to as "limit detectors" (Grigg 1994). Classified as slowly adapting receptors, these mechanoreceptors appear to play an important role in detection of static joint position and slow changes in joint position (Borsa et al. 1994). Ruffini's corpuscles are also thought to be sensitive to intracapsular pressure such as that associated with joint effusion and edema (Rowinski 1997). The effects of joint effusion and capsular distention on proprioception and neuromuscular function are discussed further in chapter 9.

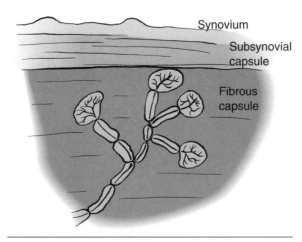

Figure 8.2 Neuroanatomy of a Ruffini's corpuscle.

Reprinted, by permission, from M.J. Rowinski, 1997, Neurobiology for orthopedic and sport physical therapy. In *Orthopedic and sports physical therapy*, 3rd ed., edited by T.R. Malone, T.G. McPoil, and A.J. Nitz (St. Louis: Mosby-Yearbook), 50.

Golgi ligament endings

Golgi ligament endings, named after Italian anatomist Camillo Golgi, resemble Golgi tendon organs. Thus, they are also referred to as *Golgi tendon organlike endings*. Structurally, Golgi ligament endings are encapsulated mechanoreceptors with numerous terminal branches, or spray endings. These receptors are located predominately in ligaments, primarily near ligamentous attachments to bone (figure 8.3). Golgi ligament endings are slowly adapting mechanoreceptors with a comparatively high threshold for mechanical stimuli. Correspondingly, they appear to be sensitive to sustained ligament stretch, or tension. As such, they are particularly responsive to mechanical deformation that occurs at the extremes of joint motion (Nyland et al. 1994). Along with Ruffini's corpuscles, the importance of Golgi ligament endings in detection of slow changes in joint position has been noted (Borsa et al. 1994).

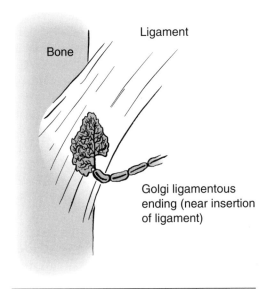

Figure 8.3   Neuroanatomy of a Golgi ligament ending.

Reprinted, by permission, from M.J. Rowinski, 1997, Neurobiology for orthopedic and sport physical therapy. In *Orthopedic and sports physical therapy*, 3rd ed., edited by T.R. Malone, T.G. McPoil, and A.J. Nitz (St. Louis: Mosby-Yearbook), 51.

Free nerve endings

Free nerve endings represent a fourth category in the morphological and functional classification of joint receptors. These receptors are thin, naked (i.e., not encapsulated by connective tissue) afferent nerve endings found in joint capsules, ligaments, and synovium, as well as fat pads and other periarticular tissues (see chapter 4, figure 4.5). Whereas pacinian corpuscles, Ruffini's corpuscles, and Golgi ligament endings are classified as mechanoreceptors, free nerve endings are generally considered nociceptors, which respond primarily to noxious stimuli. Some authorities have suggested, however, that some free nerve endings in articular tissues may be highly sensitive mechanoreceptors (Rowinski 1997). Whereas some free nerve endings are particularly responsive to noxious mechanical stimulation, others appear to be sensitive to nonnoxious mechanical stimuli (Grigg 1996). The nociceptive function of free nerve endings and their afferent (sensory) neurons was discussed in chapter 4.

Musculotendinous Receptors

Mechanoreceptors located in muscles and tendons function as a second categorical source of sensory information in the peripheral proprioceptive system. These receptors include (1) muscle spindles and (2) Golgi tendon organs. A brief review of the morphology and function of muscle spindles and Golgi tendon organs is presented in this section. In addition, the reflex arcs associated with stimulation of each of these sensory receptors are discussed, primarily as a basis for an understanding of dynamic joint stabilization and postural control.

Muscle spindles

Muscle spindles represent both sensory and motor units that lie, in a parallel orientation, within skeletal muscles. Their primary function is to monitor change, and the rate of change, in muscle length. Muscle spindles consist of specialized *intrafusal fibers* partially encased in a connective tissue capsule. This capsule, in turn, is surrounded by larger muscle fibers called *extrafusal fibers* (see chapter 4, figure 4.13). The central, noncontractile portion of the intrafusal fibers is innervated by afferent (sensory) nerve fibers that spiral around (i.e., Type Ia fibers) or are embedded within the intrafusal fibers (i.e., Type II fibers). The terminals of these fibers represent the sensory receptors (i.e., mechanoreceptors) of the muscle spindle that respond to mechanical deformation. When these mechanoreceptors are stimulated by sudden or sustained stretch of the central intrafusal fibers, sensory impulses are transmitted to the spinal cord via Type Ia and Type II afferent nerve fibers. Small efferent (motor) nerve fibers called *gamma motor neurons* also innervate the muscle spindle, terminating as *motor end plates* at the ends of the intrafusal fibers. Because the polar regions of intrafusal fibers contain actin and myosin filaments, they represent the contractile portion of intrafusal fibers (Kandel, Schwartz, and Jessell 1995). Larger efferent (motor) nerve fibers known as *alpha motor neurons* innervate the extrafusal muscle fibers (Tortora and Grabowski 1993). Compared to smaller intrafusal fibers that produce contractile forces of a lesser magnitude, extrafusal fibers produce greater contractile forces and, thus, represent the primary contractile unit.

The stretch reflex is a manifestation of the integrated sensory and motor functions of muscle spindles and, as such, is an important neural mechanism associated with reflex periarticular muscle contraction and dynamic joint stabilization. The reflex arc that occurs in the spinal cord as a result of muscle spindle stimulation is illustrated in figure 8.4. When the intrafusal fibers of the muscle spindle are subjected to a continuous or sudden mechanical stretch, a *monosynaptic reflex arc* is initiated (i.e., a reflex arc involving two neurons, a sensory neuron and a motor neuron, and a single synapse). Whereas muscle spindle response to continuous efferent impulses is referred to as a *static stretch reflex*, muscle spindle response to a rapid stretch is referred to as a *dynamic stretch reflex*, the type of reflex that provides rationale for dynamic joint control (Bierdert 2000). Mechanical stretch of the intrafusal fibers generates sensory impulses that are transmitted to the spinal cord via afferent (sensory) neurons (i.e., Type Ia and Type II fibers). These afferent neurons synapse with efferent (motor) neurons in the spinal cord, thus forming the neural framework for the monosynaptic reflex arc. Efferent (motor) nerve impulses are directed to the polar regions of the intrafusal fibers through the gamma motor neurons and to the extrafusal fibers by the alpha motor neurons (see chapter 4, figure 4.13). As a result, reflex muscle contraction occurs on the ipsilateral side, primarily as the result of extrafusal muscle fiber contraction. With simultaneous stimulation, or *coactivation*, of gamma motor neurons and alpha motor neurons, contraction of both the intrafusal and the extrafusal fibers of the muscle spindle occurs (Bierdert 2000). As discussed in chapter 9, muscle spindle excitation and the dynamic stretch reflex have clinically significant implications for a wide range of sensorimotor training techniques and functional rehabilitation protocols.

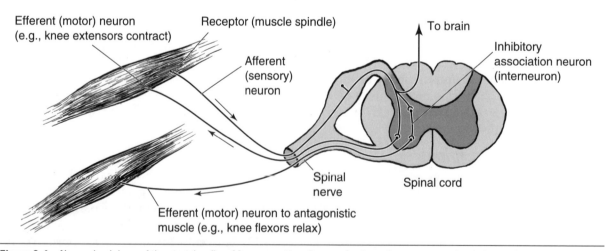

Figure 8.4 Neurophysiology of the stretch reflex. Monosynaptic reflex arc produces homonymous (same) muscle contraction (knee extensors). Polysynaptic reflex arc (inhibitory) causes antagonistic muscle relaxation (knee flexors).

Adapted from G.J. Tortora and S.R. Grobowski, 1993, *Principles of anatomy and physiology*, 7th ed. (New York: Harper Collin's College Publishers), 385. Copyright © 1993, John Wiley & Sons, Inc. This material is used by permission of John Wiley & Sons, Inc.

An additional neural mechanism associated with muscle spindle activity, referred to as *reciprocal inhibition*, is also a relevant consideration in functional rehabilitation of the injured sports participant, including sensorimotor training. As illustrated in figure 8.4, afferent (sensory) neurons originating in muscle spindles also synapse with *inhibitory association neurons* (i.e., interneurons) in the spinal cord. These interneurons, in turn, synapse with efferent (motor) neurons that innervate antagonistic muscles. Because three neurons (i.e., a sensory neuron, an association neuron, and a motor neuron) and two synapses are involved, stimulation of this mechanism produces a *polysynaptic reflex arc*. Inhibitory motor impulses cause the antagonistic muscles to relax while agonistic muscles are contracting. Thus, reciprocal inhibition allows for alternating contraction and relaxation of antagonistic muscle groups, which is essential for coordinated muscular activity and unrestricted movement (Nyland et al. 1994; Tortora and Grabowski 1993).

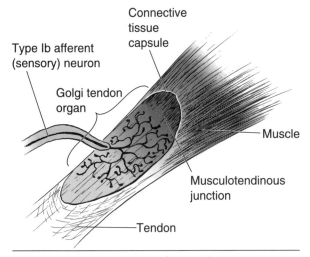

Figure 8.5 Neuroanatomy of a Golgi tendon organ.

Adapted from G.J. Tortora and S.R. Grobowski, 1993, *Principles of anatomy and physiology*, 7th ed. (New York: Harper Collin's College Publishers), 450. Copyright © 1993, John Wiley & Sons, Inc. This material is used by permission of John Wiley & Sons, Inc.

Golgi tendon organs

Golgi tendon organs are mechanoreceptors located in tendinous tissues near the musculotendinous junction. Whereas muscle spindles respond to mechanical stimuli involving stretch (i.e., elongation), Golgi tendon organs monitor changes in intramuscular tension, such as that created during muscle contraction (Tortora and Grabowski 1993). A primary function of Golgi tendon organs is protection of muscles from excessive tension. Structurally, Golgi tendon organs represent the terminals of Type Ib afferent nerve fibers that are embedded within an encapsulated unit of collagen fibers (figure 8.5). When Golgi tendon organs are mechanically stimulated by increased intramuscular tension, sensory impulses are transmitted to the spinal cord via Type Ib afferent nerve fibers and an inhibitory reflex arc is activated. As illustrated in figure 8.6, this reflex arc involves three neurons (i.e., a sensory neuron,

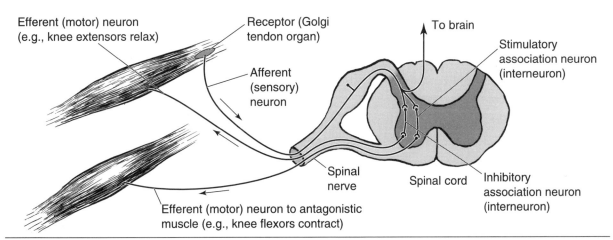

Figure 8.6 Neurophysiology of Golgi tendon organ function. Polysynaptic reflex arc (inhibitory) causes homonymous (same) muscle relaxation (knee extensors). Polysynaptic reflex arc (stimulatory) causes antagonistic muscle contraction (knee flexors).

Adapted from G.J. Tortora and S.R. Grobowski, 1993, *Principles of anatomy and physiology*, 7th ed. (New York: Harper Collin's College Publishers), 382. Copyright © 1993, John Wiley & Sons, Inc. This material is used by permission of John Wiley & Sons, Inc.

an interneuron, and a motor neuron) and two synapses. Thus, it represents a polysynaptic reflex arc. In the spinal cord, the afferent (sensory) neurons synapse with *inhibitory association neurons* (i.e., interneurons) which, in turn, synapse with efferent (motor) neurons leading to the homonymous muscle. As inhibitory efferent impulses are conducted to muscle tissues, relaxation occurs, thereby protecting the muscle from excessive tension and potential injury (Tortora and Grabowski 1993). Activation of reflex inhibitory mechanisms that result in homonymous muscle relaxation is referred to as *autogenic inhibition* (Ganong 1995). This neuromuscular response is illustrated during the use of proprioceptive neuromuscular facilitation (PNF) relaxation techniques designed to facilitate muscle stretching (e.g., contract-relax, hold-relax), as described in chapter 5.

Afferent (sensory) neurons originating from Golgi tendon organs also synapse with *stimulatory association neurons* (i.e., interneurons) in the spinal cord. These association neurons, in turn, synapse with efferent (motor) neurons leading to antagonistic muscles, rather than the muscles that gave rise to the original stimulus. Motor impulses arising from this polysynaptic reflex arc produce contraction of the antagonistic muscles. Thus, Golgi tendon organ stimulation and the resulting reflex arcs also illustrate the concept of reciprocal inhibition (Tortora and Grabowski 1993).

Cutaneous Receptors

Tactile sensations of the skin include touch, pressure, and vibration. These sensations are mediated by cutaneous and subcutaneous sensory receptors that are sensitive to mechanical deformation (figure 8.7). Several types of mechanoreceptors are located in the epidermis (e.g., Meissner's corpuscles, tactile discs), the underlying dermis (e.g., Type II cutaneous mechanoreceptors, or end organs of Ruffini), and subcutaneous tissues (e.g., pacinian corpuscles) (Tortora and Grabowski 1993). Although cutaneous sensory receptors are known to respond to mechanical stimuli involving touch, pressure, and vibration, their role in joint position sense and kinesthesia is less clear. Theoretically, joint motion that produces stretching and deformation of the skin can provide the mechanical stimuli necessary to activate cutaneous receptors. Although the potential role of skin receptors in detection of joint movement (i.e., kinesthesia) has been acknowledged, their contribution appears to be minor, perhaps only complimentary to the role of joint and musculotendinous receptors (Grigg 1994). Nevertheless, stimulation of cutaneous and subcutaneous mechanoreceptors through the use of external compression devices (e.g., knee braces, elastic wraps) may function to augment somatosensory proprioceptive input from joint and musculotendinous receptors. Clinical implications for the use of external compression devices and braces are discussed further in chapter 9.

Neurophysiology of Mechanoreceptors

The peripheral somatosensory receptors subserving the proprioceptive system have been identified for many years. Authorities generally agree that proprioception is dependent on cumulative and integrated sensory input from mechanoreceptors in joint capsules and ligaments, musculotendinous structures, and the skin. As such, proprioception differs from other senses (e.g., vision, hearing) because stimulation originates within body tissues, through mechanical deformation of tissues that house the receptors of afferent (sensory) neurons. Nevertheless, the neural mechanisms associated with other types of sensory receptors are also applicable to mechanoreceptor function. Relevant concepts include those related to *receptive field* stimulation, generation of afferent nerve impulses, and receptor adaptation.

Receptive Fields

Certain types of mechanoreceptors are stimulated when specific areas of a joint capsule are deformed. These areas are referred to as the *receptive field* of a particular mechano-

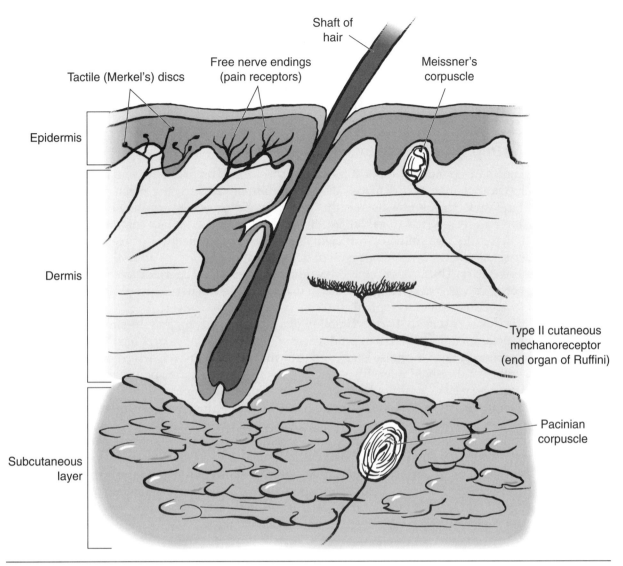

Figure 8.7   Neuroanatomy of the skin and cutaneous sensory receptors.

Adapted from G.J. Tortora and S.R. Grobowski, 1993, *Principles of anatomy and physiology*, 7th ed. (New York: Harper Collin's College Publishers), 447. Copyright © 1993, John Wiley & Sons, Inc. This material is used by permission of John Wiley & Sons, Inc.

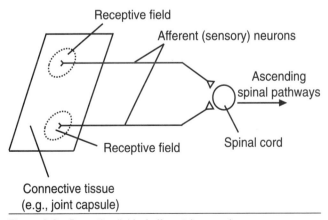

Figure 8.8   Receptive field of afferent (sensory) neurons.

Adapted from E.R. Kandel, J.H. Schwartz, and T.M. Jessell, eds., 1991, *Principles of neural science*, 3rd ed. (Norwalk, Connecticut: Appleton & Lange), 374. Reproduced with the permission of The McGraw-Hill Companies.

receptor. Rowinski (1997, p. 55) described a receptive field as an "area of the joint capsule, ligament, or other periarticular tissue whose mechanical distortion leads to excitation of a given joint afferent fiber." The concept of receptive field stimulation is illustrated in figure 8.8. Mechanical deformation of a particular receptive field, and thus stimulation of its sensory receptors, is related to joint position and movement. Most mechanoreceptors are maximally sensitive at the extremes of a joint range (Borsa et al. 1994; Grigg 1994). For example, Ruffini's corpuscles, which are located predominately in the posterior capsule of the knee, are activated as the joint approaches extension. Thus, the receptive field for these Ruffini's corpuscles is the posterior joint capsule, which is subject to mechanical deformation (i.e., stretch) during terminal extension. The likelihood of mechanoreceptor stimulation and afferent (sensory) nerve firing is optimal during this range (Rowinski 1997). In this regard, joint motions that produce receptive field deformation, and thus mechanoreceptor stimulation, during proprioceptive and sensorimotor training represent a significant clinical consideration. Generally, full range of joint motion is indicated unless precluded by existing pathology, incomplete tissue repair, or pain.

Electrophysiology of Mechanoreceptors

When a mechanoreceptor is stimulated by deformation of tissues in a receptive field, an electrical change occurs across its cell membrane. At rest, the mechanoreceptor membrane is electrically positive on the outside and electrically negative on the inside. This difference is referred to as the *resting membrane potential*. When the mechanoreceptor is subjected to a stimulus of sufficient intensity, a neutralization of electrical polarity, or *depolarization*, occurs. As the result of depolarization, an *action potential*, or nerve impulse, is produced. Thus, the mechanoreceptor functions as a generator to convert mechanical energy into electrical energy, resulting in conduction of a nerve impulse along the afferent (sensory) neuron to the spinal cord.

The relative sensitivity, or excitability, of a mechanoreceptor and the strength of the stimulus determine the potential to produce a nerve impulse. The degree of stimulation required to produce a nerve impulse is referred to as the *threshold*, or *firing level* (Ganong 1995). Once a sufficient threshold intensity is reached, a sensory receptor responds according to the *all-or-none principle*. Accordingly, a nerve impulse of optimal magnitude is generated or is not generated at all (Tortora and Grabowski 1993). Considering these principles, it becomes clear that mechanical stimuli applied for a therapeutic effect must be of sufficient intensity to produce depolarization of the mechanoreceptor cell membrane. Optimal stimulation of joint receptors occurs within their receptive field, usually toward the extremes of joint range where joint capsules are subjected to maximal deformation. In this example, joint motion that produces sufficient receptive field deformation, and thus threshold stimulation of joint receptors, suggests clinically important implications for proprioceptive and sensorimotor training in the management of sport-related musculoskeletal injuries.

Receptor Adaptation

Traditionally, mechanoreceptors have been classified as *rapidly adapting receptors* or *slowly adapting receptors*. Adaptation refers to the decline in an afferent nerve impulse rate (i.e., the number of impulses per second), and thus sensation, after receptor stimulation of constant intensity (Ganong 1995; Waxman and deGroot 1995). Stimulation of rapidly adapting receptors elicits a rapid increase in afferent impulses followed by a comparatively rapid decline in the impulse rate (figure 8.9). In some receptors, the generated nerve impulses decrease to extinction within milliseconds after stimulation. Thus, the response of rapidly adapting receptors is transient, occurring only at the onset and termination of the stimulus (Kandel, Schwartz, and Jessell 1995). These types of mechanoreceptors are particularly sensitive to sudden mechanical deformation of tissues and, as such, are associated with detection of rapid acceleration and deceleration of joint motion (Barrack and Skinner 1990). Pacinian corpuscles, for example, function as rapidly adapting mechanoreceptors. In contrast,

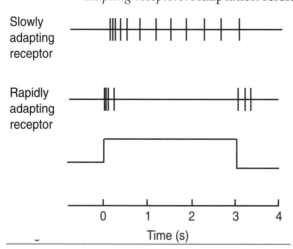

Figure 8.9 Sensory receptor adaptation.

Adapted from E.R. Kandel, J.H. Schwartz, T.M. Jessell, 1991, *Principles of neural science*, 3rd ed. (Norwalk, Connecticut: Appleton & Lange), 380. Reproduced with the permission of The McGraw-Hill Companies.

stimulation of slowly adapting receptors such as Ruffini's corpuscles and Golgi ligament endings elicits continued firing throughout the duration of a stimulus of consistent intensity with a slower rate of decline (see figure 8.9). Consequently, slowly adapting mechanoreceptors have been associated with detection of joint position and slow changes in joint position (Borsa et al. 1994; LaRiviere and Osternig 1994). Slow adaptation allows for perception of joint position or slow changes in joint position over a period of time, as opposed to perception only at the beginning and end of movement.

Traditionally, designation of mechanoreceptors as rapidly adapting or slowly adapting receptors has been directly related to their morphological characteristics and typological classification. The implication is, for example, that pacinian corpuscles function only as rapidly adapting receptors and that Ruffini's corpuscles and Golgi ligament endings act solely as slowly adapting receptors. Rowinski (1997), however, noted exceptions to these relationships and cautioned against unchallenged acceptance of a positive correlation between receptor morphology and receptor adaptation. Nevertheless, the presence of sensory receptors that adapt to mechanical stimuli at different rates presents relevant implications for proprioceptive training, particularly when the speed of movement and angular velocity of joint motion must be determined. The clinical significance of receptor adaptation as related to proprioceptive testing and sensorimotor training is discussed further in chapter 9.

Integration of Mechanoreceptor Functions

It is generally accepted that joint position sense and kinesthesia are dependent on sensory information arising from deformation of mechanoreceptors located in various soft tissues of the body. Historically, somatosensory receptors located in ligaments and joint capsules, musculotendinous tissues, and the skin have been considered to be three independent categories of mechanoreceptors that function in a parallel manner to provide proprioceptive information. In recent years, however, this strict compartmentalization of mechanoreceptor populations has been questioned in favor of more integrated mechanoreceptor functions (Grigg 1994). In this regard, it is significant to note that joint motion most likely causes simultaneous deformation and, thus, excitation of multiple mechanoreceptor populations. For example, active joint motion causes tissue deformation and activation of mechanoreceptors in periarticular musculotendinous tissues, ligaments and joint capsules, and the overlying skin. Thus, mechanoreceptors in these three tissue types represent potential sources of simultaneous somatosensory input. This observation has challenged investigators to determine the specific role of various mechanoreceptors in proprioception. It has been suggested that, while integrated sensory input from mechanoreceptors in all tissue types contributes to proprioception, the specific type and extent of proprioceptive information provided may differ among the various mechanoreceptor populations (Grigg 1994).

Historically, the comparative contribution of mechanoreceptors in articular structures and those located in musculotendinous tissues has been debated. Some authorities have placed a greater emphasis on the importance of joint receptors, whereas others have emphasized the significance of muscle receptors. During the 1960s, joint receptors were commonly thought to be the primary determinants of joint position sense and kinesthesia. More recent studies, however, led investigators to place less emphasis on the importance of joint receptors and greater emphasis on the role of muscle receptors (Clark et al. 1979; Clark, Burgess, and Chapin 1986). This view is supported by observations that total knee joint arthroplasty and anesthetization of articular structures results in little or no proprioceptive impairment (Grigg 1994; Skinner et al. 1984). Furthermore, the observation that mechanoreceptors located in joint capsules are activated by capsular deformation that occurs at the extremes of a joint range (e.g., excitation of Ruffini's corpuscles in the posterior capsule during knee extension) has led to the suggestion that joint mechanoreceptors play a minimal role in proprioception when a joint is in the midrange position. Consequently, joint position sense and perception of joint motion that occurs during midrange is attributed to sensory input from muscle receptors (Grigg 1996). Rowinski (1997) suggested that muscle spindles are the most crucial structures in detection of joint position and that they are supported in this function by joint and cutaneous receptors. Nevertheless, Lephart (1994) proposed that joint receptors and muscle receptors form an intricate afferent system and that their respective functions are complementary.

Despite evidence indicating the importance of muscle receptors in proprioception, the role of joint receptors, especially in detection of joint position and movement toward the limits of joint motion, is generally acknowledged. For example, Ruffini's corpuscles located in the posterior capsule of the knee are optimally stimulated during deformation of the capsule that occurs in the extended range. Thus, the designation of Ruffini's corpuscles as "limit detectors" (Grigg 1994). The role of joint receptors as limit detectors appears to be substantiated by studies demonstrating greater joint position sense and kinesthetic awareness toward the limits of joint motion compared to proprioceptive awareness in the midrange position (Lephart et al. 1992). In addition to their contribution to joint position sense and kinesthesia, the role of joint mechanoreceptors in reflex muscle contraction and dynamic joint stabilization has been examined. Several investigators have suggested a relationship between excitation of capsuloligamentous mechanoreceptors and reflex periarticular muscle contraction (Barrack, Lund, and Skinner 1994; Wilkerson and Nitz 1994). In contrast, Grigg (1996) questioned the validity of some studies suggesting that joint mechanoreceptors are a significant origin of afferent nerve impulses that mediate reflex muscle contraction and dynamic joint stabilization. Nevertheless, Grigg acknowledged the protective role of joint mechanoreceptors in detection of extreme joint positions in which taut joint structures are vulnerable to excessive tensile loading and capsuloligamentous injury.

Although not proprioceptive in nature, a protective mechanism involving excitation of nociceptive free nerve endings in the soft tissues of a joint has been proposed (Grigg 1996). These nociceptive nerve endings, or pain receptors, are sensitive to mechanical stimuli resulting from forceful movement into the limits of joint motion, especially when sensitized by soft tissue inflammation. Because these joint motions signal potential tissue injury, they have been referred to as *noxious rotations*. As proposed, noxious joint rotations initiate a nociceptive flexor reflex that produces flexion withdrawal and unloading of a joint, thereby protecting ligaments and joint capsules from injury (Grigg 1996). In the event of noxious rotations of the knee, for example, excitatory motor impulses to the hamstring muscles, in combination with inhibitory impulses to the quadriceps, produces reflex knee flexion and unloading of joint structures. An integrated protective function of joint mechanoreceptors (e.g., Ruffini's corpuscles) as sensors of joint motion limits and nociceptors as detectors of noxious joint rotations is suggested by the observation that an individual may adopt movement strategies that avoid excitation of both types of joint receptors, which would ordinarily signal a potentially damaging end-range position (Grigg 1996). Other investigators, however, have questioned nociceptor excitation as a significant protective mechanism compared to the role of mechanoreceptor stimulation (Barrack, Lund, and Skinner 1994). This comparison is based on the observation that proprioceptive impulses originating from capsuloligamentous mechanoreceptor stimulation are conducted to the central nervous system by large-diameter A fibers at a much faster rate than pain impulses that are conducted by small-diameter A-delta and C fibers. Consequently, the neural response associated with mechanoreceptor stimulation (i.e., reflex muscle contraction) would be expected to be significantly faster than the flexion withdrawal response associated with nociceptor activation, thereby representing the predominant protective mechanism (Barrack and Skinner 1990).

Aside from mechanoreceptors in articular and musculotendinous structures, cutaneous mechanoreceptors represent a potential source of proprioceptive information related to joint position sense and kinesthesia. Mechanoreceptors located in the skin and subcutaneous tissues include tactile discs, Meissner's corpuscles, end organs of Ruffini, and pacinian corpuscles (see figure 8.7). Like joint receptors and muscle receptors, these receptors respond to mechanical deformation of the tissues in which they are located. Thus, stretching of the overlying skin that occurs during joint movement represents a potential source of mechanical stimulation. Additionally, evidence exists that cutaneous mechanoreceptors are sensitive to pressure, such as that provided by elastic wraps, braces, and other external compression devices commonly used in the management of sports injures (Lephart et al. 1992). Several investigators have attempted to determine the contribution of cutaneous mechanoreceptors to joint position sense and kinesthesia in the absence of external pressure. Clark et al. (1979), for example, concluded that static knee position sense is not dependent on sensory input from cutaneous receptors. In a later study, Clark, Burgess, and Chapin (1986) reported that anesthesia of the skin adjacent to interphalangeal joints of the fingers did not affect proprioception. LaRiviere and Osternig (1994) studied the effect of ice immersion, which presumably produced partial anesthesia of periarticular muscles and the overlying skin, on proprioception in the ankle. These investigators reported that five- or 20-minute ice immersions had no effect on joint position sense. In general, the contribution of cutaneous receptors to joint position sense and perception of joint motion appears to be minor compared to proprioceptive input derived from joint and musculotendinous mechanoreceptor stimulation (Grigg 1994).

The Dorsal Column-Medial Lemniscal System

Stimulation of peripheral somatosensory receptors generates nerve impulses that are transmitted to the cerebral cortex through one of two primary ascending spinal cord pathways, the *anterolateral system* or the *dorsal column-medial lemniscal system* (Martin 1996). The anterolateral system, which conducts somatosensory impulses for pain and temperature, was discussed in chapter 4. The ascending pathway for proprioception, as well as touch and vibration, is the dorsal column-medial lemniscal system (figure 8.10). In both systems, nerve impulses are transmitted through three levels of sensory neurons referred to as *first order neurons*, *second order neurons*, and *third order neurons*. Transmission of nerve impulses from one level to the next occurs at a *synaptic junction*, or *synapse* (see chapter 4). Despite anatomical similarities between the two major ascending pathways, the neural structures in which the three levels of sensory neurons terminate, synapse, and decussate (i.e., cross) in the dorsal column-medial lemniscal system differ from those of the anterolateral system. In an attempt to foster an understanding of the ascending pathways for proprioception, the three levels of sensory neurons in the dorsal column-medial lemniscal system are compared and contrasted to those of the anterolateral system.

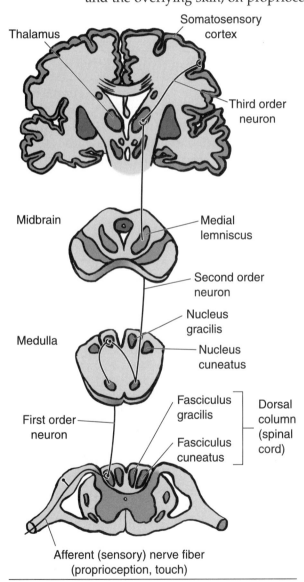

Figure 8.10   The dorsal column-medial lemniscal system.

Adapted from G.J. Tortora and S.R. Grobowski, 1993, *Principles of anatomy and physiology*, 7th ed. (New York: Harper Collin's College Publishers), 451. Copyright © 1993, John Wiley & Sons, Inc. This material is used by permission of John Wiley & Sons, Inc.

Afferent (Sensory) Neurons

Somatosensory afferent (sensory) neurons are typically classified as A or C according to whether they are myelinated (i.e., covered with a fat-like myelin sheath), their size (i.e., diameter), and their rate of conduction (see chapter 4, table 4.2). In contrast to pain impulses, which are transmitted to the spinal cord by small-diameter A-delta and C fibers, afferent nerve impulses associated with mechanical stimuli are conducted by large-diameter, myelinated A fibers (i.e., A-alpha and A-beta) at a comparatively rapid rate of conduction. Mechanoreceptors located in ligaments and joint capsules, musculotendinous tissues, and the skin represent the distal terminals of these afferent neurons.

Ascending Spinal Cord Pathways

As afferent (sensory) neurons in both the anterolateral system and the dorsal column-medial lemniscal system project to the spinal cord, they enter through the dorsal root on the ipsilateral side. Thereafter, most afferent pain fibers (i.e., first order neurons) of the anterolateral system (i.e., A-delta and C fibers) enter the dorsal horns, the dorsolateral extensions of the gray matter, where they synapse with second order neurons (i.e., ascending spinal cord pathways). Most second order neurons in the anterolateral system cross (i.e., decussate) to the contralateral side of the spinal cord before ascending through the lateral gray matter to the thalamus (see chapter 4). In contrast, afferent neurons in the dorsal column-medial lemniscal system enter the dorsal white matter of the spinal cord, rather than the dorsal horns of the gray matter, where they form ipsilateral ascending tracts (i.e., the fasciculus gracilis and fasciculus cuneatus) to the medulla without crossing. Thus, the first order neurons of the dorsal column-medial lemniscal system include afferent neurons (e.g., A fibers) as well as the ascending spinal cord pathways to the medulla (see figure 8.10). These first order neurons synapse with second order neurons in the medulla rather than the spinal cord, as is the case in the anterolateral system. Second order neurons in the dorsal column-medial lemniscal system cross to the contralateral side in the lower medulla before ascending through the *medial lemniscus* (see figure 8.10). The medial lemniscus represents an ascending neural pathway to the thalamus formed by relay nuclei in the medulla (i.e., the nucleus gracilis and nucleus cuneatus). As is the case in the anterolateral system, second order neurons in the dorsal column-medial lemniscal system synapse with third order neurons (i.e., thalamocortical projection neurons) in the thalamus. In both ascending pathways, third order neurons, in turn, project through the internal capsule of the cerebrum to the somatosensory area of the cerebral cortex (see figure 8.10).

Although anatomically distinct from the dorsal column-medial lemniscal system, two additional ascending spinal cord pathways, the spinocerebellar tracts, convey proprioceptive information from peripheral somatosensory receptors (e.g., muscle spindles, Golgi tendon organs) to the brain. In contrast to the dorsal column-medial lemniscal system, however, the *dorsal spinocerebellar tract* and the *ventral spinocerebellar tract* conduct proprioceptive information to the cerebellum, rather than the cerebral cortex (Waxman and deGroot 1995). These ascending spinal pathways project to the cerebellum to form the *spinocerebellum*, a functional division of the cerebellum that provides indirect subcortical regulation of voluntary motor activities (Martin 1996). The functional divisions of the cerebellum as related to motor control are discussed shortly.

The Thalamus

The primary neural components of the central nervous system are connected by groups of specialized nerve cells that relay and distribute sensory or motor information to various areas of the brain. These nerve cells, called *relay nuclei*, are the sites of excitatory or inhibitory synaptic connections through which neural information is transmitted and, in some cases, modified before distribution to other areas of the central nervous system (Kandel, Schwartz, and Jessell 1995). The thalamus, which is composed of several functionally specific relay nuclei, is the primary center for relay of somatosensory information from other areas of the central nervous system to the cerebral cortex (see chapter 4, figure 4.10). Nearly all sensory information that reaches the cerebral cortex passes through the thalamus, including the somatosensory information transmitted by both the dorsal column-medial lemniscal system and the anterolateral system.

Somatic proprioceptive information reaching the thalamus via the ascending dorsal column-medial lemniscal pathway is relayed to the primary somatosensory area of the cerebral cortex by the *ventral posterior nucleus* of the thalamus (Martin 1996). Sensory information from the ventral posterior nucleus is transmitted through the internal capsule of the cerebrum by third order neurons called *thalamocortical projection*, or *relay*, *neurons* (Kandel, Schwartz, and Jessell 1995). Because of the functional specificity of thalamic nuclei, which receive sensory input through specific ascending spinal cord pathways, preliminary identification of some types of sensation is thought to occur in the thalamus (Waxman and deGroot 1995). Thus, the *modality of sensation* (e.g., touch) is determined by stimulation of specific sensory receptors (e.g., mechanoreceptors), transmission of nerve impulses to functionally discrete thalamic nuclei (e.g., the ventral posterior nucleus), and projection to distinct sensory areas of the *cerebral cortex* where conscious awareness occurs (Waxman and deGroot 1995). In addition to determination of the sensory modality, the thalamus also functions to identify the general area of the body from which stimuli originate. Determination of the precise anatomical source of a sensory impulse, however, is a function of the cerebral cortex.

The Cerebral Cortex

The outermost portion of the cerebrum, the cerebral cortex, represents the highest functional level of the central nervous system. Whereas neural mechanisms operating at various subcortical levels of the brain are primarily associated with subconscious responses, conscious awareness of conditions associated with proprioception (e.g., joint position and kinesthesia) occurs when sensory input reaches the cerebral cortex. Receipt of proprioceptive input from various sources (e.g., somatosensory mechanoreceptors, vestibular receptors), interpretation and integration of sensory information, and mediation of voluntary motor responses are the primary functions of the cerebral cortex. Collectively, these processes are mediated by three general functional divisions of the cerebral cortex that provide a neural foundation for the *sensorimotor system* of the body (Lephart, Rieman, and Fu 2000). These divisions include the sensory area, association areas, and the motor area.

The *primary somatosensory area*, located in the postcentral gyrus of the parietal lobe, receives somatic sensory input from the ventral posterior nucleus in the thalamus via third order projection neurons. Orderly arrangement of thalamic relay projections to the primary somatosensory cortex is such that specific functional areas, referred to as *Brodmann's areas* (areas numbered 1, 2, and 3), receive input from different body parts (see chapter 4, figure 4.11). Thus, each body part is spatially represented, allowing for conscious localization of the anatomical origin of a sensory stimulus. Organization of sensory input is referred to as *somatotopy* (Martin 1996). Somatotopic organization of the primary somatosensory area of the cerebral cortex is commonly depicted as the *sensory homunculus* (see chapter 4, figure 4.12).

Association areas of the cerebral cortex represent a complex circuitry of cortical association neurons that connect various sensory and motor areas. Interpretation and integration of sensory input (e.g., the relationship of one body part to another) is a primary function of the *somatosensory association area*, which is identified as Brodmann's area 5 (see chapter 4, figure 4.11). The somatosensory association area also mediates higher level integrative functions associated with proprioception, including learning and memory. Thus, proprioceptive information can be stored and perceived in the future on the basis of previous movement experiences (Tortora and Grabowski 1993). It is commonly recognized, for example, that joint motion is most readily perceived during movement patterns that have been learned and practiced in the past. Another association area in the cerebral cortex, the *premotor area* (Brodmann's area 6), is a motor association area that mediates learned movement patterns of a complex, sequential nature (see chapter 4, figure 4.11). In addition, memory of skilled motor activities is stored in the premotor area. A *supplementary motor area*, located in the upper part of Brodmann's area 6, is involved in the planning and programming of body movements.

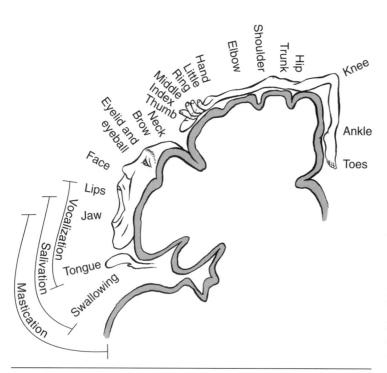

Figure 8.11   Motor homunculus.

Adapted from G.J. Tortora and S.R. Grobowski, 1993, *Principles of anatomy and physiology*, 7th ed. (New York: Harper Collin's College Publishers), 453. Copyright © 1993, John Wiley & Sons, Inc. This material is used by permission of John Wiley & Sons, Inc.

Located in the precentral gyrus of the frontal lobe, the *primary motor area* (Brodmann's area 4) receives input from premotor association areas and, in turn, projects to the spinal cord and the brain stem via descending (motor) pathways (see chapter 4, figure 4.11). These descending tracts synapse with somatic efferent neurons (i.e., lower motor neurons) in the spinal cord that innervate specific skeletal muscles, or muscle groups. Thus, the primary motor cortex represents the major control center for initiation of voluntary, goal-directed body movements (Martin 1996). As is the case in the primary somatosensory area, different body parts are spatially represented in the primary motor area. The cortical origins of direct descending motor tracts (i.e., corticospinal and corticobulbar tracts) in specific areas of the primary motor area are discussed shortly. This orderly arrangement allows for motor control of specific body parts by the primary motor cortex. Somatotopic organization of the primary motor cortex is depicted by the *motor homunculus* (figure 8.11). The cerebral cortex, along with the brain stem, represents one of the four major components of the central nervous system that mediate motor activities. The other three major components include the basal ganglia, the cerebellum, and descending (motor) pathways from the motor cortex and the brain stem. Collectively, these four components are referred to as the *motor control system* (Martin 1996).

Basal Ganglia and the Cerebellum

Whereas the primary motor cortex represents the major control center for voluntary body movements, two subcortical structures have significant regulatory influence on motor activities at the subconscious level. These two structures, the *basal ganglia* and the *cerebellum*, are considered the second and third major components of the motor control system (Martin 1996). Because neither the basal ganglia nor the cerebellum project motor neurons directly to the spinal cord, their influence on motor activity occurs indirectly, primarily through neural connections with the motor cortex (Kandel, Schwartz, and Jessell 1995).

Various interconnections between these subcortical structures and the cerebral cortex, as well as the brain stem and the thalamus, provide a neural framework for planning and coordination of voluntary movements, postural control, and balance (Martin 1996; Waxman and deGroot 1995).

Basal Ganglia

The basal ganglia represent five functionally related groups of gray matter, or *cerebral nuclei*, that lie deep within each cerebral hemisphere. As illustrated in figure 8.12, the basal ganglia include the caudate nucleus, putamen, globus pallidus, subthalamic nucleus, and the substantia nigra. In addition to their neural interconnections with each other, the basal ganglia combine with the thalamus and the cerebral cortex to form a functional feedback system that mediates motor activities (Kandel, Schwartz, and Jessell 1995). In this system, referred to as the *motor circuit*, the basal ganglia receive afferent input from the sensory, motor, and association areas of the cerebral cortex (figure 8.13). In turn, the basal ganglia project back to the motor cortex via the ventral anterior and ventral lateral nuclei of the thalamus (see chapter 4, figure 4.10). Through this circuitry, the basal ganglia influence efferent information projected from the motor cortex via descending motor pathways (i.e., the corticospinal and corticobulbar tracts). Thus, the basal ganglia function to monitor several motor activities, including planning and execution of voluntary movements, eye movements, postural control, and balance (Ganong 1995; Martin 1996). The important regulatory role of the basal ganglia in motor activity is dramatically illustrated by Parkinson's disease, a pathological deterioration of neurons in the basal ganglia that results in uncontrollable movements (i.e., tremor) and muscle rigidity (Tortora and Grabowski 1993).

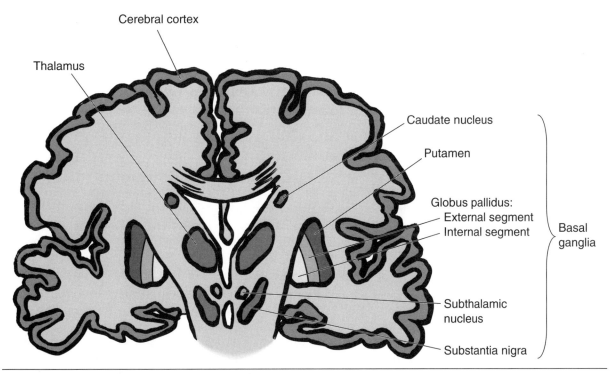

Figure 8.12   Basal ganglia.

Reprinted from E.R. Kandel, J.H. Schwartz, and T.M. Jessell, 1991, *Principles of neural science*, 3rd ed. (Norwalk, Connecticut: Appleton & Lange), 545. Reproduced with the permission of The McGraw-Hill Companies.

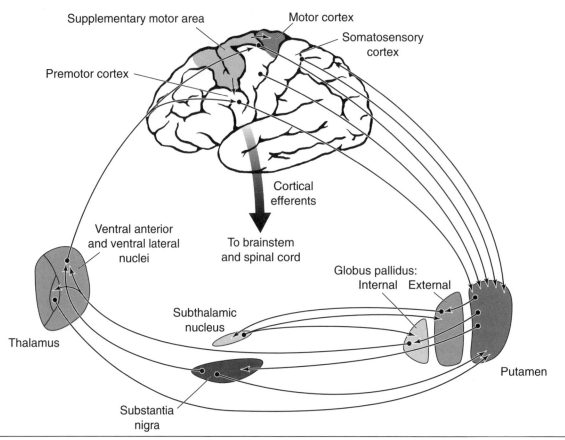

Figure 8.13   The motor circuit of the basal ganglia, thalamus, and cerebral cortex.

Adapted from E.R. Kandel, J.H. Schwartz, and T.M. Jessell, 1991, *Principles of neural science,* 3rd ed. (Norwalk, Connecticut: Appleton & Lange), 548. Reproduced with the permission of The McGraw-Hill Companies.

The Cerebellum

The cerebellum has several functional roles related to motor control and movement. These functions include planning and coordination of voluntary body movements, as well as postural control and balance (Waxman and deGroot 1995). Various afferent and efferent neural connections with the cerebral cortex, the spinal cord, and the vestibular labyrinth form three functional divisions of the cerebellum that provide indirect regulation of motor activity (Kandel, Schwartz, and Jessell 1995). These divisions are depicted in figure 8.14. Neural connections between the cerebellum and the cerebral cortex form the *cerebrocerebellum*, which plays a primary role in the planning of voluntary body movements. In this division, the cerebellum receives afferent input from the sensory, motor, and association areas of the cerebral cortex via the pontine nuclei in the pons. In turn, efferent output from the cerebellum is projected to the thalamus (ventral lateral nucleus), which relays information back to the premotor area and the primary motor area of the cerebral cortex (Martin 1996). In the *spinocerebellum* division, the cerebellum receives afferent somatosensory input from peripheral mechanoreceptors (i.e., joint and musculotendinous receptors) via the ascending *spinocerebellar tracts* and, through efferent projections to the motor cortex, functions to control posture and movements of the trunk and limbs (Martin 1996). Afferent and efferent neural connections between the cerebellum and the vestibular system in the inner ear form the *vestibulocerebellum*, the third functional division of the cerebellum. This division governs eye movements in response to movements of the head detected by mechanoreceptors in the vestibular labyrinth. The cerebellum receives afferent input directly through afferent neurons from the vestibular labyrinth and indirectly through the vestibular nucleus in the brain stem. In turn, the cerebellum projects back to the vestibular nucleus (Martin 1996). Thus, the

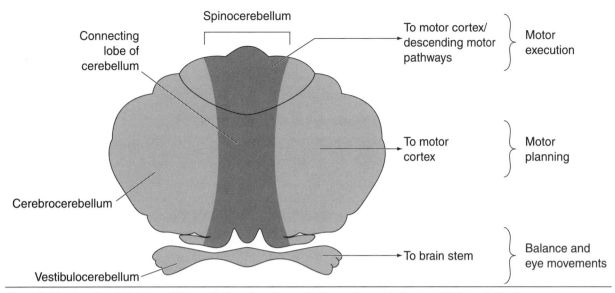

Figure 8.14 Functional divisions of the cerebellum (cerebrocerebellum, spinocerebellum, vestibulocerebellum).

Adapted from E.R. Kandel, J.H. Schwartz, and T.M. Jessell, 1991, *Principles of neural science*, 3rd ed. (Norwalk, Connecticut: Appleton & Lange), 539. Reproduced with the permission of The McGraw-Hill Companies.

vestibulocerebellum division functions to regulate eye movements and balance (Ganong 1995). These functions and the specific role of the vestibular system, as related to proprioception and motor control, are discussed further in a following section of this chapter. Although through different neural circuitry, each of the three functional divisions of the cerebellum function to regulate output from the motor cortex or the brain stem. The crucial role of the cerebellum in motor control is illustrated by cerebellar pathology that results in *ataxia*, an uncontrollable, staggering walking gait. Cerebellar dysfunction may also be manifested by uncontrolled oscillatory movements of the trunk or limbs (i.e., tremor) or involuntary oscillation of the eyes (nystagmus) (Martin 1996).

Descending (Motor) Pathways

The cerebral cortex and the brain stem, the basal ganglia, and the cerebellum represent three of the major components of the motor system. The descending (motor) pathways represent a fourth primary component (Martin 1996). Descending neural pathways that mediate motor activities originate from two primary areas in the central nervous system, the motor cortex and the brain stem. Motor pathways from the cerebral cortex are referred to as *direct (pyramidal) pathways*, whereas those that originate from various brain stem nuclei or the reticular formation are called *indirect (extrapyramidal) pathways*. Neurons that constitute motor pathways in the brain and spinal cord are referred to as *upper motor neurons*. As illustrated in figure 8.15, various upper motor neurons in both the direct and the indirect

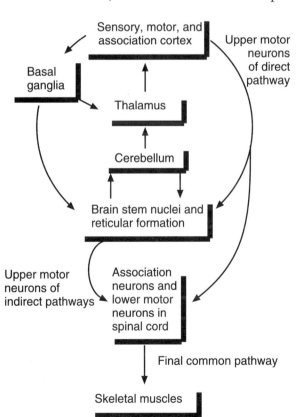

Figure 8.15 Descending direct (pyramidal) and indirect (extrapyramidal) motor pathways.

Reprinted from G.J. Tortora and S.R. Grobowski, 1993, *Principles of anatomy and physiology*, 7th ed. (New York: Harper Collin's College Publishers), 456. Copyright © 1993, John Wiley & Sons, Inc. This material is used by permission of John Wiley & Sons, Inc.

descending pathways synapse with somatic efferent neurons in the spinal cord to form a "final common pathway" to skeletal muscles (Tortora and Grabowski 1993). Motor neurons that exit the spinal cord and terminate in skeletal muscles are referred to as *lower motor neurons*. Ultimately, all motor impulses mediated by the motor cortex, the basal ganglia, and the cerebellum influence the lower motor neurons.

Direct (Pyramidal) Pathways

Cortical control of motor functions occurs through two primary descending pathways, the *corticospinal tracts* (lateral and anterior) that project to the spinal cord and the *corticobulbar tract* that descends to the brain stem (Kandel, Schwartz, and Jessell 1995). The specific cortical origin of these descending motor tracts, as related to the somatotopic organization of the primary motor cortex, is illustrated in figure 8.16.

Corticospinal tracts

Motor neurons of the corticospinal tracts, most of which originate in the primary motor cortex (Brodmann's area 4), descend through a brain stem pathway called the *medullary pyramid* to form the *pyramidal tract* (Waxman and deGroot 1995). The descending corticospinal tracts are illustrated in figure 8.17. Most neurons in the corticospinal tracts (approximately 80%) descend through the *lateral corticospinal tract*, which crosses to the contralateral side at the *pyramidal decussation* in the medulla (Ganong 1995; Waxman and deGroot 1995). Descending motor fibers of the lateral corticospinal tract synapse with somatic efferent neurons in the spinal cord. These lower motor neurons, in turn, project to

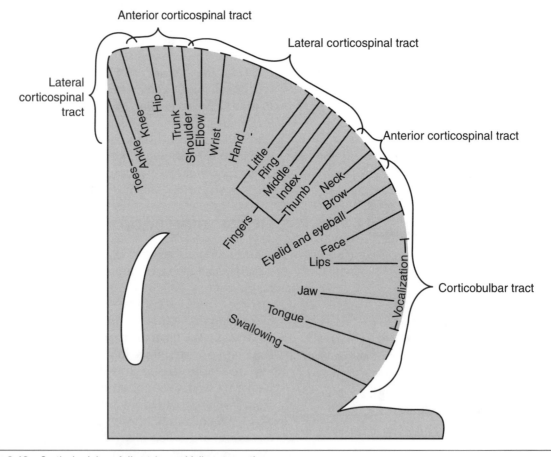

Figure 8.16 Cortical origins of direct (pyramidal) motor pathways.

Adapted from J.H. Martin, 1996, *Neuroanatomy*, 2nd ed. (Stamford, Connecticut: Appleton & Lange), 269. Reproduced with the permission of The McGraw-Hill Companies.

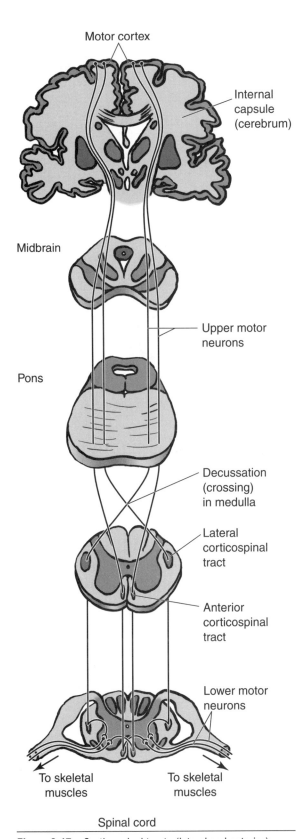

Figure 8.17 Corticospinal tracts (lateral and anterior).

Adapted from G.J. Tortora and S.R. Grobowski, 1993, *Principles of anatomy and physiology*, 7th ed. (New York: Harper Collin's College Publishers), 455. Copyright © 1993, John Wiley & Sons, Inc. This material is used by permission of John Wiley & Sons, Inc.

muscles of the distal extremities that mediate fine, skilled movements (Ganong 1995). Crossing, or decussation, of the lateral corticospinal tract in the medulla explains the control of movements on one side of the body by motor areas in the contralateral hemisphere of the cerebral cortex. Approximately 20% of the corticospinal fibers descend via the *anterior corticospinal tract* without crossing in the medulla (Ganong 1995). Instead, these neurons cross to the contralateral side in the spinal cord where they synapse with somatic efferent neurons that innervate muscles of the axial skeleton and proximal limbs (Tortora and Grabowski 1993). Consequently, the anterior corticospinal tract mediates motor responses associated with gross body movements and postural control (Ganong 1995).

The corticobulbar tract

As a counterpart to the corticospinal tracts, the corticobulbar tract also originates in the motor cortex. In contrast, however, this descending motor tract projects only to the brain stem level with termination in various cranial nerve nuclei. These nuclei, in turn, project efferent motor neurons to muscles of the head and face (see figure 8.16). As such, the corticobulbar tract does not have a significant role in postural control or movements of the trunk and limbs.

Indirect (Extrapyramidal) Pathways

In contrast to direct (pyramidal) pathways, which originate in the motor cortex, indirect (extrapyramidal) pathways project from various areas of the brain stem. The four primary indirect motor pathways are illustrated in figure 8.18. These upper motor neurons descend to various levels of the spinal cord and, like the corticospinal tracts, synapse with lower motor neurons that innervate various skeletal muscles. Medial descending pathways from the brain stem include the *vestibulospinal, reticulospinal,* and *tectospinal tracts* (figure 8.18a). The *rubrospinal tract* (figure 8.18b) forms a lateral descending pathway (Kandel, Schwartz, and Jessell 1995). The first medial pathway, the vestibulospinal tract, has two components. A *lateral vestibulospinal tract* descends from the vestibular nucleus in the medulla and projects motor impulses to antigravity muscles in response to head movements detected by the vestibular apparatus in the inner ear. Thus, this tract plays an important role in reflex postural control and balance. A *medial vestibulospinal tract*, which descends to the cervical and upper thoracic spinal cord, mediates control of head position. Postural control is also mediated by the reticulospinal tract, a second medial pathway, which

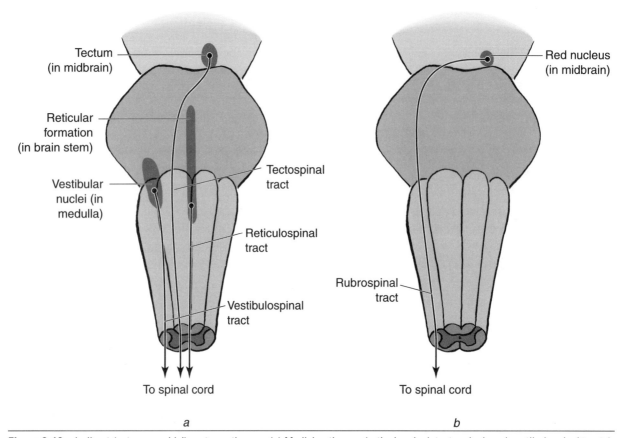

Figure 8.18   Indirect (extrapyramidal) motor pathways. (a) Medial pathways (reticulospinal, tectospinal, and vestibulospinal tracts). (b) Lateral pathway (rubrospinal tract).

Adapted from E.R. Kandel, J.H. Schwartz, and T.M. Jessell, 1991, *Principles of neural science*, 3rd ed. (Norwalk, Connecticut: Appleton & Lange), 497. Reproduced with the permission of The McGraw-Hill Companies.

originates from the reticular formation in the pons and medulla and descends throughout the spinal cord. The third medial pathway, the tectospinal tract, descends from the tectum (i.e., roof) of the midbrain to the cervical spinal cord and functions to coordinate head and eye movements. The fourth indirect motor pathway, the lateral descending rubrospinal tract, originates from the red nucleus in the midbrain. Collectively, the three medial descending tracts from the brain stem mediate postural control and balance through their connections with lower motor neurons that innervate muscles of the axial skeleton and proximal limbs. In contrast, the lateral descending pathway, the rubrospinal tract, is primarily associated with control of precise, voluntary movements of the distal extremities (Tortora and Grabowski 1993).

The Vestibular System

Motor control is dependent not only on sensory input from peripheral somatosensory mechanoreceptors but also on input from the vestibular system and the visual system. Discussion in this section is focused on the vestibular system and its contributions to proprioception and motor control. The relationship of the visual system is discussed in a subsequent section of this chapter. Major anatomical structures of the vestibular system that subserve proprioception and sensorimotor control include the vestibular receptors of the inner ear, afferent (sensory) pathways to the brain stem, the vestibular nucleus in the brain stem, and efferent (motor) projections from the vestibular nucleus to various areas of the central nervous system. An understanding of the neurophysiology associated with these structures is crucial to development of effective sensorimotor training programs involving postural control and balance. Thus, each component is reviewed as a basis for an understanding of the role of the vestibular system in proprioception and sensorimotor function.

Vestibular Receptors and Afferent (Sensory) Pathways

Postural control and maintenance of equilibrium, or balance, are primary functions of the vestibular apparatus in the inner ear. The inner ear, or *labyrinth*, contains sensory receptors for both static and dynamic equilibrium. In a general sense, balance involves the ability to maintain the center of body mass within the base of support (Irrgang, Whitney, and Cox 1994). Furthermore, balance is dependent on postural control, or the ability to maintain equilibrium despite the force of gravity. Orientation regarding the position of the head in space is referred to as *static equilibrium*, whereas maintenance of body position in response to sudden movements of the head is called *dynamic equilibrium* (Ganong 1995; Tortora and Grabowski 1993). Whereas some sports require static equilibrium (e.g., static body positions in gymnastics), most sports activities necessitate maintenance of dynamic equilibrium. Although input from the peripheral proprioceptive system (i.e., joint and musculotendinous mechanoreceptors) and the visual system contributes to postural control and balance, dynamic equilibrium is highly dependent on sensory input from the vestibular receptors in the labyrinth.

The labyrinth consists of two primary components, an outer *bony labyrinth* and an inner portion referred to as the *membranous labyrinth*. These structures are illustrated in figure 8.19. The bony labyrinth includes the three semicircular canals, the vestibule, and the

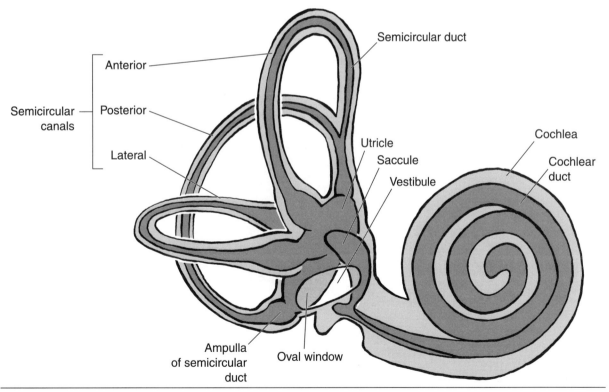

Figure 8.19 Major structures of the inner ear (labyrinth). Note the components of the vestibular labyrinth (semicircular ducts, saccule, utricle).

cochlea. Components of the membranous labyrinth that constitute the vestibular system are the semicircular ducts, the saccule, and the utricle. Each of these structures, collectively referred to as the *vestibular labyrinth*, contain specialized sensory receptors called *hair cells*. Because mechanical deformation, and thus stimulation, of these receptors occurs in response to movements of the head, hair cells function as mechanoreceptors (i.e., proprioceptors).

A sensory receptor organ called a *macula* is located within both the saccule and the utricle (figure 8.20). The macula contains the hair cells that provide sensory input about the position of the head in space. As such, these receptors are associated with detection of linear acceleration, both horizontal and vertical, and static equilibrium (Waxman and deGroot 1995). The enlarged end of each semicircular duct, referred to as an *ampulla* (see figure 8.19), contains a receptor organ called the *crista ampullaris* (figure 8.21a). The crista contains hair cells that respond to head movements involving angular rotation. Thus, vestibular receptors located in the semicircular ducts are associated with dynamic equilibrium. Angular rotation of the head detected by hair cells in the crista (see figure 8.21a) provides the stimulus for body righting reflexes, as well as the stimulus for reflex adjustment of gaze that contributes to dynamic equilibrium (Ganong 1995). Stimulation of receptors in the three components of the vestibular labyrinth (i.e., semicircular ducts, saccule, utricle) generates afferent sensory impulses that are transmitted to the brain stem via the vestibular branch of the vestibulocochlear nerve (i.e., cranial nerve VIII) (see figure 8.20). In comparison, the cochlear division of the vestibulocochlear nerve conducts sound waves from the cochlea to the brain stem and, thus, represents a component of the auditory system.

Vestibular Nuclei and Efferent (Motor) Projections

Afferent (sensory) neurons from the vestibular labyrinth terminate in specific nuclei of the medulla oblongata in the brain stem. One of these nuclei, the *vestibular nucleus*, projects motor impulses that control eye movements, movements of the head, and movement of the axial skeleton. Postural control and balance are maintained, in part, through complex

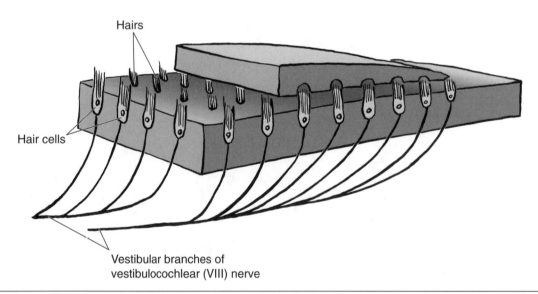

Figure 8.20 Cross section of a macula with hair cells (sensory receptors). Also, note the vestibular branches of the vestibulocochlear nerve.

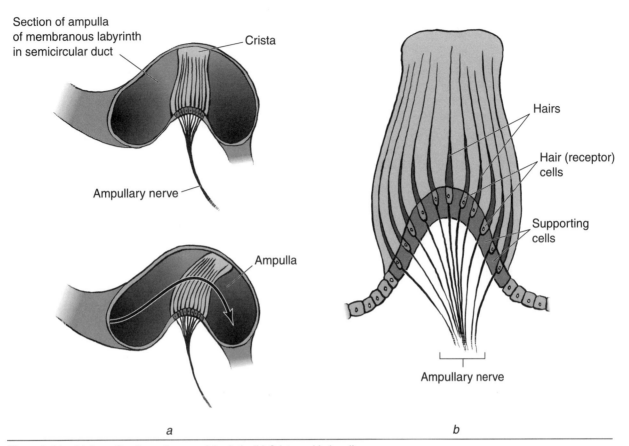

Section of ampulla
of membranous labyrinth
in semicircular duct

Crista

Ampullary nerve

Ampulla

Hairs

Hair (receptor)
cells

Supporting
cells

Ampullary nerve

a   *b*

Figure 8.21   (a) Ampulla of membranous labyrinth. (b) Crista and hair cells.

Adapted from G.J. Tortora and S.R. Grobowski, 1993, *Principles of anatomy and physiology*, 7th ed. (New York: Harper Collin's College Publishers), 496. Copyright © 1993, John Wiley & Sons, Inc. This material is used by permission of John Wiley & Sons, Inc.

integrated functions of these sensorimotor structures. Three neural pathways that project from the vestibular nucleus are noteworthy. These include (1) the medial longitudinal fasciculus that projects to specific ocular muscles, (2) the descending vestibulospinal tract to the spinal cord, and (3) vestibular projections to the cerebellum.

The medial longitudinal fasciculus represents an ascending neural pathway to the motor nuclei of the three pairs of cranial nerves that control movements of the eyes (figure 8.22). These cranial nerves include the *oculomotor nerve (III)*, the *trochlear nerve (IV)*, and the *abducens nerve (VI)*, which project to the ocular muscles (e.g., medial rectus, lateral rectus). Movement of the eyes is directly integrated with rotation of the head through a compensatory reflex adjustment of gaze referred to as the *vestibuloocular reflex*. For example, sudden rotation of the head in one direction is counteracted by reflex movement of the eyes in the opposite direction, thereby allowing for retention of fixation on a visual target during dynamic body movements. Simultaneous movement of both eyes in the same direction is referred to as *conjugate gaze movement* (see figure 8.22), whereas visual fixation on an object in the visual field is called *vergence* (Waxman and deGroot 1995). The vestibuloocular reflex is mediated by sensory input from the vestibular receptors (i.e., hair cells) in the inner ear, which is projected to the vestibular nucleus in the brain stem. The vestibular nucleus, in turn, projects to *lateral gaze centers* and a *vergence center* in the brain stem that control eye movements (Waxman and deGroot 1995).

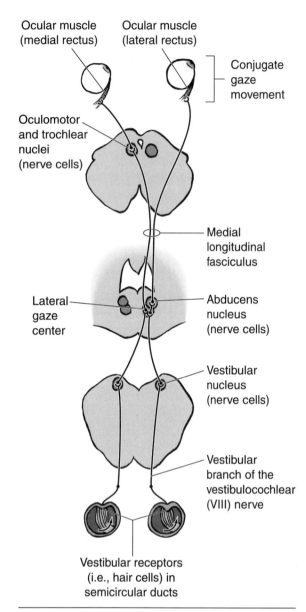

Ocular muscle (medial rectus)

Ocular muscle (lateral rectus)

Conjugate gaze movement

Oculomotor and trochlear nuclei (nerve cells)

Medial longitudinal fasciculus

Lateral gaze center

Abducens nucleus (nerve cells)

Vestibular nucleus (nerve cells)

Vestibular branch of the vestibulocochlear (VIII) nerve

Vestibular receptors (i.e., hair cells) in semicircular ducts

Figure 8.22 Neurophysiology of the vestibuloocular reflex. Note the conjugate gaze movement of the eyes.

Adapted from S.G. Waxman and J. de Groot, 1995, *Correlative neuroanatomy*, 22nd ed. (Norwalk, Connecticut: Appleton & Lange), 114. Reproduced with the permission of The McGraw-Hill Companies.

The *vestibulospinal tract* represents a second motor projection that arises from the vestibular nucleus. As illustrated in figure 8.18, the vestibulospinal tract is one of four major indirect (extrapyramidal) motor pathways from the brain stem to the spinal cord. A primary function of the vestibulospinal motor system is mediation of *body righting reflexes*, compensatory reflex actions that occur in response to sudden changes in body position (e.g., a fall). In response to changes in head position detected by the vestibular labyrinth (see figure 8.21), efferent nerve impulses are conducted via the descending vestibulospinal tract to muscles of the axial skeleton that act to adjust the position of the head and restore the body to the normal, upright position (Waxman and deGroot 1995). In addition to mediation of righting reflexes, the vestibulospinal tract contributes to postural control via efferent projections to antigravity muscles (Waxman and deGroot 1995).

A third important vestibular connection is represented by the *vestibulocerebellum*, one of the three functional divisions of the cerebellum that mediate motor activities (see figure 8.14). In addition to motor projections to the ocular muscles and the spinal cord, the vestibular nucleus projects to the cerebellum. The cerebellum also receives sensory input directly via afferent neurons from the vestibular labyrinth. In turn, the cerebellum projects back to the vestibular nucleus that, as previously discussed, is the origin of efferent (motor) neurons to the ocular muscles (i.e., the medial longitudinal fasciculus) and to muscles of the axial skeleton (i.e., the vestibulospinal tract). Collectively, these afferent and efferent connections provide a complex neural circuitry through which the cerebellum monitors eye movements and balance (Martin 1996).

The Visual System

Whereas the peripheral proprioception system and the vestibular system rely on stimuli arising from body tissues (i.e., deformation of mechanoreceptors), sensory input in the visual system is dependent on stimuli from the external environment. As such, the visual system is indirectly related to the proprioceptive mechanisms that mediate postural control and balance. Nevertheless, the visual system is directly related to motor systems that coordinate eye movements with movements of the head. Thus, a comprehensive discussion of postural control and balance necessitates consideration of the role of visual input. As in other sensorimotor systems, components of the visual system that contribute to postural control and balance include sensory receptors and afferent (sensory) pathways, cortical processing centers, and efferent (motor) projections.

Visual Receptors and Afferent (Sensory) Pathways

The sensory receptors for vision, *rods* and *cones*, are contained within the *retina*, the innermost layer of the eye. These receptors are classified as *photoreceptors* because of their selective sensitivity to light rays that provide the stimuli for activation. As in other sensory systems, visual receptors generate action potentials, or nerve impulses, which are conducted by afferent (sensory) neurons to central processing centers. In the visual system, the *optic nerve* (cranial nerve II) functions as the sensory nerve fiber that transmits visual impulses to the brain (Waxman and deGroot 1995). As illustrated in figure 8.23, fibers of the optic nerve form *optic tracts* that project to the thalamus (i.e., the lateral geniculate nucleus). The thalamus, in turn, relays visual information to the primary visual cortex where the form, color, and movement of objects in the visual field are perceived (Kandel, Schwartz, and Jessell 1995). A second optic nerve projection, to the *superior colliculus* in the midbrain, establishes a more direct sensory pathway through which visual input contributes to postural control and balance.

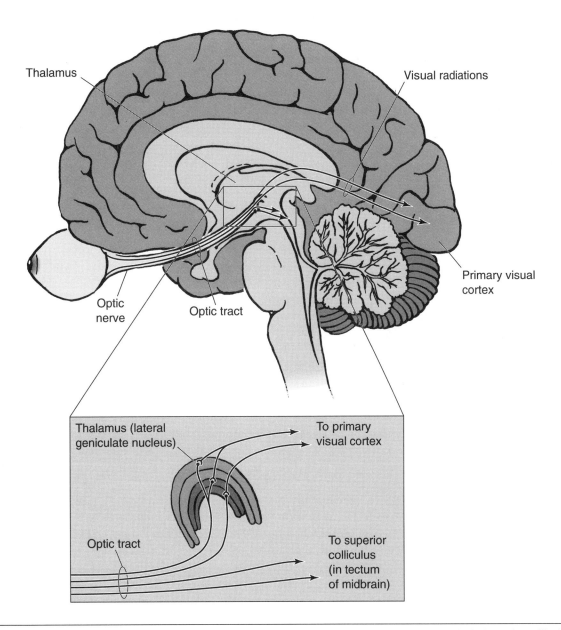

Figure 8.23   Afferent (sensory) projections from retina to the thalamus, primary visual cortex, and midbrain (superior colliculus).

Adapted from E.R. Kandel, J.H. Schwartz, and T.M. Jessell, 1991, *Principles of neural science*, 3rd ed. (Norwalk, Connecticut: Appleton & Lange), 429. Reproduced with the permission of The McGraw-Hill Companies.

The Superior Colliculus and Efferent (Motor) Projections

In addition to conduction of visual impulses to the thalamus, the optic nerve also projects to the superior colliculus (i.e., a small eminence) located in an area of the midbrain called the *tectum* (see figure 8.23). As illustrated in figure 8.18, the tectum is the anatomical origin of the tectospinal tract, one of the four major indirect (extrapyramidal) motor pathways from the brain stem to the spinal cord. The tectospinal tract descends to the level of the cervical spinal cord and projects, through efferent (motor) neurons, to muscles of the axial skeleton and proximal limbs, the muscle groups that control reflex movements of the head (Martin 1996; Waxman and deGroot 1995).

Because the optic nerve not only relays visual images from the retina, through the thalamus, to the primary visual cortex but also projects to the tectum, this integrated sensorimotor system is thought to play an important role in coordination of eye movements with movements of the head in response to visual stimuli (Martin 1996). As discussed in a previous section, eye movements and movements of the head are also mediated by the vestibular labyrinth through afferent (sensory) pathways to the vestibular nucleus in the brain stem and, in turn, through efferent (motor) projections from the vestibular nucleus to the ocular muscles (i.e., the medial longitudinal fasciculus) and the spinal cord (i.e., the vestibulospinal tract). These motor responses, however, occur as the result of mechanical stimuli (i.e., deformation of hair cells) rather than visual stimuli. Thus, both the visual system and the vestibular system contribute to postural control and balance, although through distinct neural pathways. Integration of these two systems is illustrated, for example, by dynamic balance training during which an athlete is asked to perform cutting maneuvers while catching a ball.

Summary

Proprioception is considered a variation of the sense of touch that includes an awareness of static joint position, or joint position sense, as well as the perception of joint motion, or kinesthesia. In a broad sense, the sensorimotor system of the body relies on afferent input from peripheral somatosensory mechanoreceptors, mechanoreceptors in the vestibular apparatus of the inner ear, and photoreceptors in the retina. Integration of sensory information from these three primary sources provides the basis for motor activity requiring neuromuscular control, postural control, and balance. These sensorimotor functions are dependent on intact neural mechanisms at various levels of the central nervous system, including the spinal cord, the brain stem, and the brain.

Sensory information in the peripheral proprioceptive system is derived from mechanical stimulation of receptors located in joint capsules and ligaments, musculotendinous structures, and the skin. Peripheral nerve branches that innervate periarticular muscles and the overlying skin terminate in joint receptors that have traditionally been classified as pacinian corpuscles, Ruffini's corpuscles, Golgi ligament endings, and free nerve endings. Whereas pacinian corpuscles, Ruffini's corpuscles, and Golgi ligament endings are considered mechanoreceptors, free nerve endings function primarily as nociceptors. Mechanoreceptors located in musculotendinous structures include muscle spindles, which are sensitive to a change in muscle length, and Golgi tendon organs that respond to increased intramuscular tension. Several types of mechanoreceptors are located in the epidermis, the dermis, and deeper subcutaneous tissues. Contemporary views generally consider proprioception an integrated function of all three types of somatosensory mechanoreceptors, although the comparative contribution of each mechanoreceptor population has been a subject of debate for many years. Somatosensory proprioceptive information reaching the cerebral cortex is transmitted through the ascending dorsal column-medial lemniscal system to the primary somatosensory cortex where integration and interpretation of sensory input occurs. In response, the primary motor cortex mediates voluntary motor responses that are regulated by two primary subcortical structures: the basal ganglia and the cerebellum. Direct and indirect descending motor pathways originating from the motor cortex and the brain stem, respectively, conduct efferent information to the skeletal muscles responsible for coordinated body movements, postural control, and balance.

Postural control and balance are primary functions of the vestibular system, which mediates both static and dynamic equilibrium. The vestibular labyrinth of the inner ear is composed of the semicircular ducts, the saccule, and the utricle, each of which contains hair cells that respond to mechanical deformation. Afferent sensory information from these mechanoreceptors reaches the vestibular nucleus in the brain stem via the vestibular branch of the vestibulocochlear nerve, which in turn projects efferent motor information to the ocular muscles, the spinal cord, and the cerebellum. Thus, the vestibular system provides the neural circuitry for control and coordination of eye movements, movements of the head, and movements of the axial skeleton. The vestibuloocular reflex and body righting reflexes are manifestations of this integrated sensorimotor system.

The third primary source of sensory input that mediates the sensorimotor functions of the body is provided by the visual system. Sensory information from photoreceptors located in the retina, the innermost lining of the eye, is transmitted by an optic nerve projection to the superior colliculus in the tectum of the midbrain, which, in turn, projects to the spinal cord through the descending tectospinal tract. Thus, this integrated network provides the neural framework for coordination of eye movements with movements of the head in response to visual stimuli. Optimal dynamic equilibrium is dependent on an operative vestibuloocular system.

References

Barrack, R.L., and H.B. Skinner. 1990. The sensory function of knee ligaments. In *Knee ligaments: Structure, function, injury, and repair*, edited by D. Daniel et al. New York: Raven Press.

Barrack, R.L., P.J. Lund, and H.B. Skinner. 1994. Knee joint proprioception revisited. *Journal of Sport Rehabilitation* 3:18-42.

Bierdert, R.M. 2000. Contribution of the three levels of nervous system motor control: Spinal cord, lower brain, cerebral cortex. In *Proprioception and neuromuscular control in joint stability*, edited by S.M. Lephart and F.H. Fu. Champaign, Ill.: Human Kinetics.

Borsa, P.A., S.M. Lephart, M.S. Kocher, and S.P. Lephart. 1994. Functional assessment and rehabilitation of shoulder proprioception for glenohumeral instability. *Journal of Sport Rehabilitation* 3:84-104.

Clark, F.J., R.C. Burgess, and J.W. Chapin. 1986. Proprioception with the proximal interphalangeal joint of the index finger: Evidence for a movement sense without a static position sense. *Brain* 109:1195-208.

Clark, F.J., K.W. Horch, S.M. Bach, and G.F. Larson. 1979. Contributions of cutaneous and joint receptors to static knee position sense in man. *Journal of Neurophysiology* 42:877-88.

Freeman, M., and B. Wyke. 1965. The innervation of the cat's knee joint. *Journal of Anatomy* 98:299-300.

Ganong, W.F. 1995. *Review of medical physiology*, 17th ed. Norwalk, Conn.: Appleton and Lange.

Grigg, P. 1994. Peripheral neural mechanisms in proprioception. *Journal of Sport Rehabilitation* 3:2-7.

Grigg, P. 1996. Articular neurophysiology. In *Athletic injuries and rehabilitation*, edited by J.E. Zachazewski, D.J. Magee, and W.S. Quillen. Philadelphia: W.B. Saunders.

Irrgang, J.J., S.L. Whitney, and E.D. Cox. 1994. Balance and proprioceptive training for rehabilitation of the lower extremity. *Journal of Sport Rehabilitation* 3:68-83.

Kandel, E.R., J.H. Schwartz, and T.M. Jessell, eds. 1995. *Essentials of neural science and behavior*. Norwalk, Conn.: Appleton and Lange.

Kennedy, J.C., I.J. Alexander, and K.C. Hayes. 1982. Nerve supply of the human knee and its functional importance. *American Journal of Sports Medicine* 10:329-35.

LaRiviere, J., and L.R. Osternig. 1994. The effect of ice immersion on joint position sense. *Journal of Sport Rehabilitation* 3:58-67.

Lephart, S.M., M.S. Kocher, F.H. Fu, P.A. Borsa, and C.D. Harner. 1992. Proprioception following anterior cruciate ligament reconstruction. *Journal of Sport Rehabilitation* 1:188-96.

Lephart, S.M. 1994. Reestablishing proprioception, kinesthesia, joint position sense, and neuromuscular control in rehabilitation. In *Rehabilitation techniques in sports medicine*, 2nd ed., edited by W.E. Prentice. St. Louis: Mosby-Year Book.

Lephart, S.M., B.L. Rieman, and F.H. Fu. 2000. Introduction to the sensorimotor system. In *Proprioception and neuromuscular control in joint stability*, edited by S.M. Lephart and F.H. Fu. Champaign, Ill.: Human Kinetics.

Martin, J.H. 1996. *Neuroanatomy*, 2nd ed. Stamford, Conn.: Appleton and Lange.

Nyland, J., T. Brosky, D. Currier, A. Nitz, and D. Caborn. 1994. Review of the afferent neural system of the knee and its contribution to motor learning. *Journal of Sports Physical Therapy* 19:2-11.

Parkhurst, T.M., and C.N. Burnett. 1994. Injury and proprioception in the lower back. *Journal of Sports Physical Therapy* 19:282-95.

Rowinski, M.J. 1997. Neurobiology for orthopedic and sports physical therapy. In *Orthopedic and sports physical therapy*, 3rd ed., edited by T.R. Malone, T.G. McPoil, and A.J. Nitz. St. Louis: Mosby-Year Book.

Skinner, H.B., R.L. Barrack, S.D. Cook, and R.J. Haddad Jr. 1984. Joint position sense in total knee arthroplasty. *Journal of Orthopaedic Research* 1:276-83.

Thomas, C.L., ed. 1993. *Taber's cyclopedic medical dictionary*, 17th ed. Philadelphia: Davis.

Tortora, G.J., and S.R. Grabowski. 1993. *Principles of anatomy and physiology*, 7th ed. New York: Harper Collins College Publishers.

Waxman, S.G., and J. deGroot. 1995. *Correlative neuroanatomy*, 22nd ed. Norwalk, Conn.: Appleton and Lange.

Wilkerson, G.B., and A.J. Nitz. 1994. Dynamic ankle stability: Mechanical and neuromuscular interrelationships. *Journal of Sport Rehabilitation* 3:43-57.

Therapeutic Implications: Proprioceptive and Sensorimotor Deficits

CHAPTER

9

Pathology of Proprioceptive Deficits
  Impairment of Joint Position Sense and Kinesthesia
    Proprioception Testing
    Proprioception Research
  Diminished Dynamic Joint Stabilization
    Functional Joint Stability
    Reflex Muscle Splinting
    Cocontraction of Periarticular Muscles
    Research and Clinical Observations
  Deficits in Postural Control and Balance
    Static Balance
    Semi-Dynamic and Dynamic Balance
    Functional Balance
Therapeutic Implications
  Acute Injury Management
    Control of Effusion and Edema
    Early Tissue Mobilization

Surgical Considerations in Proprioception
    Postoperative Mechanoreceptor Repopulation
    Proprioceptive Effects of Surgery
  Proprioceptive and Sensorimotor Training
    Muscle Strength and Neuromuscular Control
    Sensorimotor Training: A Conceptual Model
    Sensorimotor Manipulation and Therapeutic Progression
    Proprioceptive Effects of External Support Devices
    Effects of Sensorimotor Training
Summary

Learning Objectives

After completion of this chapter, the reader should be able to

❶ describe the pathological basis for proprioceptive and sensorimotor deficits associated with musculoskeletal injuries,

❷ identify the clinical manifestations of sensorimotor deficits related to impairment of joint position sense and kinesthesia, dynamic joint stabilization, and postural control and balance,

❸ describe contemporary methods and techniques in proprioceptive testing, assessment of dynamic joint control, and balance testing,

❹ describe the relevant surgical considerations in preservation and restoration of proprioceptive and sensorimotor function, and

❺ identify appropriate sensorimotor training strategies for restoration of proprioception and neuromuscular control.

As discussed in previous chapters, the physiological responses to trauma and the processes of connective tissue repair present implications for therapeutic intervention in five primary areas: (1) control of hemorrhage and edema, (2) alleviation of pain and muscle spasm, (3) enhancement of connective tissue repair mechanisms, (4) prevention of contractures and adhesions, and (5) enhancement of the structural and functional properties of scar tissue. Discussion in this chapter is based on the premise that proprioceptive and sensorimotor deficits result from musculoskeletal injuries commonly affecting the sports participant or from factors associated with connective tissue repair. Preservation or restoration of proprioceptive and sensorimotor function represents therapeutic objectives that parallel and complement other areas of intervention in connective tissue repair and recovery from musculoskeletal injuries. Hence, proprioceptive and sensorimotor training is addressed as a sixth major category of therapeutic intervention in sports injury management. Prior to a discussion of therapeutic implications in this chapter, the pathology and clinical manifestations of proprioceptive deficits associated with sports injuries are reviewed as a basis for development of proprioceptive and sensorimotor training programs.

Pathology of Proprioceptive Deficits

In the absence of direct intracranial trauma and cerebral, vestibular, or visual dysfunction, sensorimotor deficits resulting from sports injuries are commonly attributed to disruption of joint structures that contain the somatosensory receptors for proprioception. The relationship of proprioceptive deficits to traumatic disruption of ligaments and joint capsules has been studied for many years. Research has consistently indicated that joint mechanoreceptors respond to the mechanical deformation of intact ligaments and joint capsules that occurs during joint motion. Acute disruption or residual attenuation of these static restraints, however, reduces the potential for development of tension that otherwise would occur in intact articular structures. Thus, the potential for mechanical stimulation of joint receptors is correspondingly reduced. Evidence also exists that joint trauma results in direct mechanoreceptor destruction and degeneration of afferent (sensory) neurons. A histological assessment of ruptured, nonsurgical anterior cruciate ligaments by Denti et al. (1994), for example, provided evidence of mechanoreceptor degeneration after acute knee injuries. After arthroscopic removal of ruptured anterior cruciate ligament (ACL) specimens from human knees, these investigators found normal mechanoreceptors in patients with injuries of three months' duration or less. However, examination of specimens from patients with ACL deficiencies of nine months' duration revealed a significant decrease in the number of mechanoreceptors. A total absence of ACL mechanoreceptors was found in patients with lesions of a one-year duration.

The neuropathology involving destruction of joint mechanoreceptors and degeneration of their afferent neurons has been referred to as *articular deafferentation* (Freeman, Dean, and Hanham 1965). Although the exact mechanisms are unclear, deafferentation implies interference with transmission of somatosensory impulses by afferent neurons that alter proprioceptive information reaching the central nervous system (Wilkerson and Nitz 1994). In addition to acute ligament and joint capsule disruption and direct destruction of joint mechanoreceptors, articular deafferentation has been attributed to a number of other factors inherent in the pathology of joint injuries. These pathological manifestations include (1) acute hemarthrosis with associated capsular distension, (2) fibrous scar formation in ligaments and joint capsules, (3) permanent joint capsule distension, (4) synovial hypertrophy, and (5) chronic ligament or joint capsule laxity (Rowinski 1997; Safran, Caldwell, and Fu 1994). These conditions represent consequences of acute tissue disruption or connective tissue repair that alter the normal structural and biomechanical properties of articular structures, thereby affecting their neural components (i.e., mechanoreceptors). In addition to proprioceptive dysfunction that results from acute ligament and joint capsule trauma, proprioceptive deficits have also been attributed to surgical disruption or resection of articular or periarticular structures (Safran, Caldwell, and Fu 1994), as well as postoperative immobilization and activity restrictions (Wilkerson and Nitz 1994).

It is significant to note that motor denervation, (i.e., de-efferentation of motor nerves), in addition to deafferentation, has been identified as a pathological component of joint injuries (Wilkerson and Nitz 1994). On the basis of needle electromyography studies, Nitz, Dobner, and Kersey (1985) reported that, at two weeks after injury, a majority of 31 subjects who had sustained severe inversion ankle sprains demonstrated motor denervation of the leg muscles innervated by the peroneal and tibial nerves. Although direct peripheral nerve trauma may be a cause, motor denervation may also result from neurogenic inflammation, an inflammatory reaction associated with inflammation of the joint. Thus, in the case of inversion ankle sprains, both deafferentation of afferent (sensory) nerves and de-efferentation of efferent (motor) nerves have been cited as etiological factors in impairment of reflex periarticular muscle splinting and a reduction in the potential for dynamic joint stabilization. With specific reference to ankle sprains, Wilkerson and Nitz (1994) presented a comprehensive schematic illustration of the theoretical relationships among acute joint injuries, chronic joint instability, and sensorimotor dysfunction (figure 9.1).

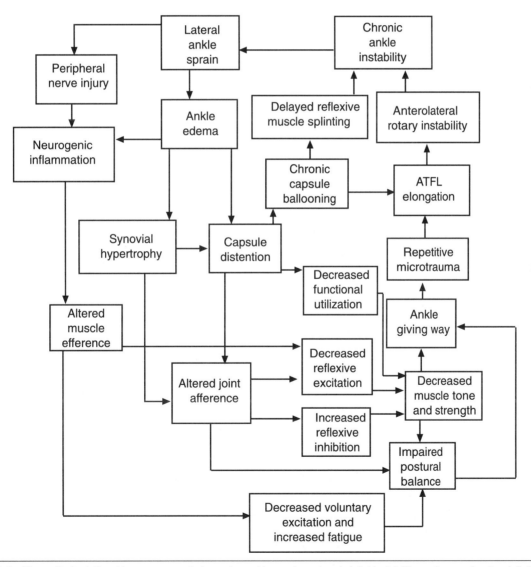

Figure 9.1   Theoretical relationships among acute inversion ankle sprains, chronic joint instability, and sensorimotor deficits.

Reprinted, by permission, from G.M. Wilkerson and A.J. Nitz, 1994, Dynamic ankle stability: Mechanical and neuromuscular interrelationships, *Journal of Sport Rehabilitation* 3 (1): 53.

During the past decade, evidence of mechanoreceptor degeneration and articular deafferentation has led to the numerous investigations regarding the effect of joint pathology on proprioception and sensorimotor function. Articular deafferentation with diminished somatosensory input may be manifested as sensorimotor deficits in three primary areas: (1) impaired joint position sense and kinesthesia, (2) diminished dynamic joint control with decreased functional joint stability, and (3) deficits in postural control and balance. The neuropathological basis of these sensorimotor deficits, an overview of proprioception testing protocols, and a review of research and clinical observations regarding sensorimotor dysfunction are presented in the following sections before a discussion of therapeutic implications.

Impairment of Joint Position Sense and Kinesthesia

Joint position sense, or identification of the static position of a joint within its available range, and kinesthesia, the awareness of joint movement, both imply conscious perception at the highest level of the central nervous system, the somatosensory area of the cerebral cortex. Thus, these proprioceptive functions are dependent on intact neural pathways at all levels of the dorsal column-medial lemniscal system (see chapter 8). Because peripheral somatosensory receptors are the primary source of sensory input, deficits in joint position sense and kinesthesia have been directly attributed to disruption of afferent neural impulses from mechanoreceptors located in articular structures (i.e., pacinian corpuscles, Ruffini's corpuscles, Golgi ligament endings) or musculotendinous tissues (i.e., muscle spindles, Golgi tendon organs).

Proprioception Testing

Traditionally, joint position sense and kinesthesia have been assessed by the use of three primary testing protocols (Borsa et al. 1994). Joint position sense is measured by reproduction of passive positioning (RPP) or reproduction of active positioning (RAP), whereas kinesthesia, or awareness of joint motion, is assessed by determining the threshold to detection of passive motion (TTDPM). Although specialized proprioceptive testing devices (PTDs) have been developed to implement these protocols, proprioception testing has also been assessed through the use of isokinetic dynamometers, electrogoniometers, and flexometers (Perrin and Shultz 2000). Collectively, these devices are used to assess joint position sense and kinesthesia associated with somatosensory cortex activity. During RPP and RAP assessment of joint position sense, the subject's ability to reproduce a particular static joint position by passive movement (RPP) or active movement (RAP) is determined. By comparison, TTDPM is used to assess the subject's ability to detect movement during slow, passive joint motion (Lephart 1994). It is significant to note that selective stimulation of articular or musculotendinous mechanoreceptors may occur during the use of PTDs, depending on the type of movement (i.e., passive or active) as well as the angular velocity of joint motion during the testing procedure. In general, the active reproduction movements performed during RAP testing stimulate musculotendinous receptors as well as joint receptors. Because RAP incorporates stimulation of mechanoreceptors in both articular tissues and musculotendinous tissues, it is considered a more functional assessment of afferent (sensory) nerve integrity compared to RPP and TTDPM test protocols that use passive joint motion (Lephart 1994).

Mechanoreceptor stimulation is also related to the angular velocity of joint motion and, thus, selective stimulation of slowly adapting joint receptors (i.e., Ruffini's corpuscles, Golgi ligament endings) or rapidly adapting receptors (i.e., pacinian corpuscles). As discussed in chapter 8, slowly adapting receptors have been associated with perception of slow changes in joint position. Because the slow, passive movements used during TTDPM are thought to selectively stimulate slowly adapting Ruffini's corpuscles and Golgi ligament endings with minimal stimulation of musculotendinous receptors, this technique is commonly used to assess proprioceptive deficits after capsular and ligamentous injuries (Lephart 1994). Selective mechanoreceptor stimulation is relevant not only to clinical assessment of joint position sense and kinesthesia but also to proprioceptive training, particularly when the use of active or passive therapeutic exercise and the most appropriate velocity of joint motion become therapeutic considerations. As an alternative to traditional proprioceptive testing (i.e., RPP, RAP, TTDPM), Myers and Lephart (2000) reported the use of an electromagnetic motion analysis system that permits subject reproduction of more functional sport-specific movement patterns.

Proprioception Research

Joint position sense and kinesthesia in subjects with diagnosed joint injuries have been studied for several years. Barrack, Skinner, and Buckley (1989) assessed threshold to detection of slow passive movement in 11 patients with midsubstance tears of the anterior cruciate ligament (ACL). Subjects determined to have acute knee joint instability (i.e., from three to six months post injury) and chronic instability (i.e., from 12 to 60 months post injury) were examined. Whereas the healthy reference group in this study demonstrated no significant difference in the ability to perceive changes in joint position between left and right knees, a statistically significant loss of joint position sense was found in the involved knee when compared to the contralateral uninvolved knee in ACL-deficient subjects. Similar deficits in joint proprioception after unilateral ankle sprains were demonstrated by Glencross and Thornton (1981), who reported decreased ability to replicate passive joint positioning in involved ankles. Garn and Newton (1988) found a decreased ability to sense passive dorsiflexion and plantar flexion movements in injured ankles. Other investigators found both TTDPM and RPP deficits in subjects with traumatic recurrent anterior glenohumeral instability when compared with contralateral stable joints (Lephart 1994; Smith and Brunolli 1989).

Using TTDPM and RAP techniques, Parkhurst and Burnett (1994) examined patients with a history of low back pathology. These investigators concluded that low back injury is an influential factor in proprioceptive asymmetry, although the relationship is weak. In contrast to other studies that cite joint receptors as a primary origin of proprioceptive deficits, Parkhurst and Burnett theorized that disruption of muscle receptors (i.e., muscle spindles and Golgi tendon organs) resulting from muscle strains is a source of proprioceptive dysfunction. They suggested that muscle spindles are particularly susceptible to the intramuscular hemorrhage, pressure, and ischemia associated with low back strains. Furthermore, these investigators suggested that Golgi tendon organs are vulnerable because of their anatomical concentration at the comparatively weak musculotendinous junction where tissue disruption is most likely to occur.

Diminished Dynamic Joint Stabilization

To the extent that connective tissue repair and remodeling of damaged ligaments and joint capsules are maximized, the structural integrity of the affected joint is restored. Healing of disrupted ligaments and joint capsules with optimal tensile strength and minimal joint laxity results in mechanical stability. In contrast, residual capsular or ligamentous laxity permits abnormal pathological joint motions that exceed normal physiological limits. Freeman, Dean, and Hanham (1965) referred to joint instability resulting from capsuloligamentous laxity as *mechanical instability*. Traditionally, surgical management of capsuloligamentous injuries has focused on restoration of the structural integrity of traumatized tissues to restore mechanical stability. In recent years, however, increased emphasis has been placed on preservation or restoration of the neural mechanisms that provide dynamic joint stabilization, or *functional stability*, through reflex periarticular muscle contraction and preactivated muscle stiffness (Myers and Lephart 2000).

Functional Joint Stability

Although the structural integrity of ligaments and joint capsules is generally considered an important prerequisite to safe, unencumbered sports participation, it is well known that athletes may exhibit functional deficits despite seemingly intact articular structures. The athlete who reports that a weight-bearing joint (e.g., a knee or ankle) "gives way" despite negative clinical laxity stress tests and apparent mechanical stability is familiar to the experienced sports health care clinician. In contrast, successful sports participation by athletes with demonstrable joint laxity and mechanical instability has been observed. Despite the association of proprioceptive deficits with joint pathology, several investigators have concluded that the degree of mechanical joint stability provided by capsuloligamentous structures correlates poorly with positive functional outcomes and patient satisfaction (Barrett 1991; Walla et al. 1985). These observations suggest that factors other than the structural integrity of ligamentous and joint capsules contribute to joint stability, particularly the functional stabilization necessary for safe and successful sports participation. As observed by Barrett (1991), successful return to sports activity after a joint injury may be more dependent on proprioception and neuromuscular control than on capsuloligamentous integrity.

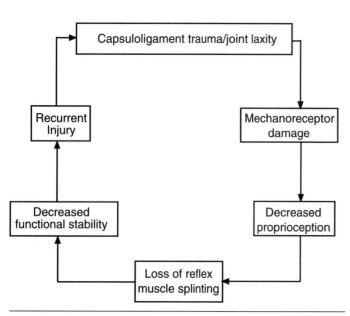

Figure 9.2   Cycle of capsuloligamentous trauma, proprioceptive deficit, and recurrent joint injury.

Several authors have attributed functional joint instability to impaired mechanoreceptor function and disruption of afferent neural impulses to the spinal cord (Borsa et al. 1994; Grigg 1994; Nyland et al. 1994; Wilk et al. 1994). These observations suggest that deficits in functional joint stability are directly associated with joint injuries commonly seen in the sports population. Although the cause and effect of this relationship has been debated, some investigators have suggested that deficits in mechanoreceptor function are both a cause and a consequence of joint pathology (Barrack, Lund, and Skinner 1994; Borsa et al. 1994). The purported cyclic relationship that exists among joint trauma, mechanoreceptor disruption, and recurrent injury is illustrated in figure 9.2. In this cycle, capsuloligamentous trauma and mechanoreceptor disruption lead to impaired proprioceptive feedback, loss of protective reflex muscle splinting, and decreased dynamic joint control. These consequences, in turn, become contributing factors to recurrent injury and degenerative joint disease (Borsa et al. 1994; Lephart 1994). As described in the following sections, dynamic joint stability is attributed to two related but distinct mechanisms of neuromuscular control: (1) reflex contraction of agonistic muscle groups and (2) cocontraction of antagonistic muscles. Respectively, these neuromuscular responses represent integrated feedback and feed-forward mechanisms that contribute to dynamic joint control (Myers and Lephart 2000). Regardless of the particular neuromuscular response, the synergy and synchrony of muscle firing patterns necessary for dynamic joint stabilization is dependent on intact proprioceptive mechanisms.

Reflex Muscle Splinting

Reflex contraction of periarticular muscles has traditionally been cited as the primary feedback mechanism of neuromuscular control associated with functional joint stability. Dynamic joint stabilization occurs, in part, as the result of mechanoreceptor stimulation, initiation of a monosynaptic reflex arc in the spinal cord, and reflex muscle contraction. These neural mechanisms were discussed in chapter 8 (see figure 8.4). The functional relevance of muscle spindle excitation is reflex contraction, or splinting, of periarticular muscles that occurs under conditions of joint stress (Rowinski 1997). Wilk et al. (1994) used the term *reactive neuromuscular control* to describe recognition of a vulnerable joint position and the reflex neuromuscular response to stabilize or reposition the joint. Most likely, these dynamic stabilizing mechanisms are mediated by the integrated functions of joint receptors and muscle receptors. The specific role and comparative contribution of these two mechanoreceptor types have been topics of debate over the years, however.

Research has indicated that reflex muscle splinting results from excitation of pacinian corpuscles, Ruffini's corpuscles, and Golgi ligament endings (Barrack, Lund, and Skinner 1994). Excitation of these joint receptors is thought to provide sensory input that directly mediates reflex muscle splinting and dynamic joint stabilization (Kennedy, Alexander, and Hayes 1982). As noted by Allen (2000), the rapidly adapting pacinian corpuscles, which respond readily to rapid acceleration and deceleration, are probably the primary joint receptors responsible for reflex periarticular muscle contraction. The neural link between joint mechanoreceptor function and reflex muscle splinting appears to be facilitated by periarticular muscle insertions into joint capsules (Rowinski 1997). When muscular contraction occurs, the tension placed on capsular structures produces mechanical deformation of the tissues in which mechanoreceptors are located. Although the exact mechanisms are somewhat unclear, the consequential stimulation of joint receptors activates motor impulses to the muscle spindles. Hence, reflex muscle contraction may result from transmission of efferent impulses to the intrafusal fibers of the muscle spindle by gamma motor neurons, by alpha motor neurons to surrounding extrafusal muscle fibers, or both (Barrack, Lund, and Skinner 1994; Wilkerson and Nitz 1994). As noted in chapter 8, simultaneous firing of gamma and alpha motor neurons is referred to as *coactivation* (Bierdert 2000).

Theoretically, reflex muscle splinting provides dynamic joint stabilization that serves to reduce injury risk during sports participation. Under conditions of moderate joint stress (e.g., vulnerable positions of the knee during running), mechanoreceptor stimulation initiates transmission of sensory impulses to the spinal cord by large-diameter afferent nerve fibers with a comparatively rapid conduction rate (i.e., A fibers), thereby initiating reflex periarticular muscle contraction. Despite the rapid conduction rate of large-diameter A fibers, however, the rate and magnitude of capsuloligamentous loading that sometimes occurs in contact sports, for example, may exceed the ability of reflex muscle splinting mechanisms to respond in a timely, protective manner (Barrack, Lund, and Skinner 1994). Nevertheless, reflex muscle splinting may be adequate to provide protective dynamic stabilization during moderate articular tissue loading, such as that associated with noncontact running, jumping, and throwing activities. These observations suggest that, in the absence of reflex muscle splinting, the incidence of noncontact joint injuries associated with sports participation may be higher, but that the incidence or severity of joint injuries resulting from rapidly applied external contact forces (e.g., blocking and tackling in football) may not be significantly reduced by reflex muscle contraction. In the event of excessive rapid loading, especially in the presence of capsuloligamentous laxity, the increased demand on dynamic stabilizers may render reflex muscle splinting ineffective in compensating for mechanical instability of the joint. In certain instances, dynamic joint stabilization may be more dependent on a feed-forward system of neuromuscular control involving anticipation of joint perturbation, cocontraction of antagonistic muscle groups, and preactivated muscle stiffness prior to joint loading (DeMont and Lephart 1998).

Cocontraction of Periarticular Muscles

Whereas reflex contraction of agonist muscle groups (i.e., the stretch reflex) with accompanying inhibition and relaxation of antagonistic muscles provides dynamic joint stabilization under certain conditions, functional joint stabilization during some types of motor activity is highly dependent on simultaneous contraction, or cocontraction, of antagonistic periarticular muscle groups, depending on the joint involved and the characteristic mechanism of joint stress (Osternig 2000). Although simultaneous contraction of antagonistic muscles would seemingly impair the function of agonists in development of the torque necessary to produce forceful movements, antagonist cocontraction that provides joint stiffness is an inherent component of many motor activities, thereby assisting joint capsules and ligaments in joint stabilization (Kandel, Schwartz, and Jessell 1995; Sale 1992). As related to functional joint stability, *muscle stiffness* refers to the ability of a muscle to absorb tension, thus alleviating potential traumatic forces that otherwise would be directed to articular structures (DeMont and Lephart 1998). For example, cocontraction of antagonistic muscles in a weight-bearing lower extremity during preparation for a cutting maneuver, or a rapid change of direction, contributes to knee joint stiffness at a time of increased ligament and capsular vulnerability.

As described by Johannson et al. (2000), functional joint stability, in a broad sense, is determined by the interactions of passive mechanical restraints (i.e., ligaments and joint capsules), joint geometry, intraarticular friction, and compression forces on the joint surfaces due to gravity and periarticular muscle contraction. The compression forces that contribute to joint stiffness and stability are increased significantly by simultaneous contraction of antagonistic periarticular muscle groups. In a comprehensive review of the role of quadriceps and hamstrings cocontraction in subjects with anterior cruciate ligament-deficient knees, Osternig (2000) noted the importance of eccentric hamstring contraction as a restraint to anterior tibial subluxation during active knee extension. In this example, optimal stiffness of the knee joint is dependent on cocontraction of the quadriceps and hamstring muscles, which significantly increases the articular compression forces.

In contrast to the monosynaptic reflex arc that governs muscle spindle excitation and reflex contraction of agonist muscles at the spinal cord level, cocontraction of antagonistic muscle groups is dependent on mechanisms of neuromuscular control and coordination at higher levels of the central nervous system. As described by Kandel, Schwartz, and Jessell (1995), cocontraction is mediated by descending corticospinal pathways from the motor cortex, which project to excitatory and inhibitory interneurons in the spinal cord. In turn, these interneurons connect with lower motor neurons leading to skeletal muscles. Hence, cocontraction of antagonistic muscle groups and the degree of joint stiffness are mediated by cortical structures that influence the balance of excitatory and inhibitory signals to interneurons in the spinal cord. With specific regard to dynamic joint stabilization, cocontraction of antagonistic muscles is a product of central programming and feed-forward neural mechanisms that transmit efferent impulses to periarticular muscles in anticipation of sudden joint perturbation (DeMont and Lephart 1998). As explained by Lephart, Riemann, and Fu (2000), feed-forward mechanisms of neuromuscular control are based on previous sensorimotor experiences that heighten awareness of joint position and movement. Feed-forward neural mechanisms involve alpha-gamma motor neuron coactivation that increases muscle spindle sensitivity, leading to more vigorous neuromuscular responses. When reflex muscle spindle activity is integrated with descending motor signals from higher brain centers, periarticular muscles become preactivated, stiffer, and more quickly responsive to sudden joint perturbation and loading.

Cortical control of simultaneous agonist and antagonist muscle contraction suggests that the neuromuscular coordination necessary for cocontraction is a learned motor activity and, therefore, subject to enhancement through proprioceptive and sensorimotor training (DeMont and Lephart 1998). Therapeutic attempts to facilitate the neural mechanisms of cocontraction are illustrated by the use of the proprioceptive neuromuscular facilitation (PNF) technique referred to as *rhythmic stabilization*. In this technique, the patient is asked to contract antagonistic muscle groups simultaneously, thereby producing cocontraction, joint stiffness, and resistance to manual movement by the clinician (Voss, Ionta, and Myers 1985). Rhythmic stabilization exercises incorporate preactivated joint stiffness and resistance to movement as well as neuromuscular responses to sudden multidirectional perturbations by the clinician. Consequently, they are thought to be effective in promotion of dynamic joint control (Myers and Lephart 2000).

Evidence exists that muscle firing patterns that provide dynamic stabilization in healthy joints are not necessarily the same as those required for protective stabilization of injured joints. Whereas cocontraction firing patterns in antagonistic muscles may be indicated for dynamic joint stabilization in some pathological conditions (e.g., multidirectional glenohumeral instability), other conditions may indicate the need for a comparative increase in firing of agonistic muscles. In these cases, the sports health care clinician may be challenged to identify particular dynamic stabilizers that provide restraint to specific pathological joint motions. For example, increased firing of the hamstring muscles has been recognized as a neural mechanism contributing to restraint of anterior tibial translation in an ACL-deficient knee (Solomonow et al. 1987). In another example, increased firing of the ankle evertors (i.e., peroneal muscles), as opposed to cocontraction of the invertors and evertors, may be a particularly protective neuromuscular response to sudden, excessive inversion/plantar flexion of a mechanically unstable ankle (Rivera 1994; Wilkerson and Nitz 1994). Although it is generally recognized that neural adaptation with enhanced muscle firing patterns is an early response to introduction of active and resistive exercise, further research is indicated to clarify the effect of sensorimotor training on alteration of cocontraction patterns in periarticular muscle groups (Sale 1992), as well as the effect of training programs on muscle firing patterns associated with specific sports injuries.

Research and Clinical Observations

Whereas joint position sense and kinesthesia are assessed by measuring RAP and RPP or TTDPM, respectively, reflex muscle contraction is commonly determined through the use of electromyography (EMG), which demonstrates neural firing patterns in periarticular muscle groups. Most EMG studies demonstrating the effect of joint capsule and ligament disruption on reflex muscle splinting have involved the knee, particularly the ACL-deficient knee. For the most part, these studies are based on a presumed relationship between joint mechanoreceptor disruption and diminished reflex periarticular muscle contraction. As previously indicated, reflex activation of the hamstring muscle group with corresponding inhibition of the quadriceps muscles is characteristically associated with tensile loading of the ACL (Branch, Hunter, and Donath 1989; Limbird et al. 1988). Based on a review of the literature, Barrack, Lund, and Skinner (1994) concluded that hamstring muscle contraction and quadriceps inhibition is the neural firing pattern consistently associated with stimulation of knee joint receptors. Considering the anatomical orientation of the hamstring muscles and the insertion of the medial hamstrings on the tibia, increased hamstring activity may function to control anterior translation of the tibia in an ACL-deficient knee, thus providing dynamic joint stabilization. A corresponding inhibition of quadriceps firing may facilitate this mechanism (Branch, Hunter, and Donath 1989). Solomonow et al. (1987) reported a significantly slower excitation of reflex hamstring activity in subjects with ACL-deficient knees compared to healthy subjects in a reference group. Although slower, retention of the hamstring reflex in an ACL-deficient knee suggests activation by secondary ligamentous or capsular restraints to anterior tibial translation. In the presence of ACL deficiency, stimulation of articular mechanoreceptors in secondary static restraints appears to be an important factor in activation of reflex hamstring muscle contraction and, thus, functional joint stability.

A clinical complication associated with altered muscle firing patterns in some ACL-deficient patients is an abnormal gait pattern referred to as a *quadriceps avoidance gait* (Berchuck et al. 1990). This gait pattern is characterized by decreased quadriceps muscle activity in conjunction with higher than normal hamstring muscle firing during walking and jogging (Andriacchi and Birac 1993; Berchuck et al. 1990). As demonstrated by Spencer, Hayes, and Alexander (1984) and Fahrer et al. (1988), reflex quadriceps inhibition, and thus a quadriceps avoidance gait, is associated with joint effusion (e.g., hemarthrosis). In the event of acute hemarthrosis, reflex inhibition is thought to result from the presence of fluid in the joint, rather than from ligamentous disruption. To the extent that fluid increases in the knee joint, intracapsular pressure increases and the capsule becomes progressively distended, thereby affecting joint mechanoreceptor function and, consequently, quadriceps muscle contraction. With regard to acute inversion ankle sprains, Wilkerson and Nitz (1994) also suggested a relationship between joint capsule distention and inhibited reflex muscle contraction. These authors noted that increased intraarticular fluid may result in a decrease in afferent (sensory) input to the central nervous system, resulting in inhibition of reflex peroneal muscle response.

Several investigators have found a positive relationship between functional joint instability in subjects with ACL-deficient knees and impaired performance on a variety of functional performance tests. Tegner et al. (1986), for example, determined the performance levels of a group of 26 active male subjects with ACL insufficiency to be generally inferior to those of a reference group of 66 healthy male soccer players on a battery of functional performance tests. Whereas most subjects with ACL insufficiencies achieved normal values on tests of straight running, fewer ACL-deficient subjects achieved normalcy on tests involving slope running, staircase running, and figure eight running. In a similar study, Barber et al. (1990) reported significantly lower scores on a single-leg hop test for distance in nonoperative ACL-deficient subjects compared to scores for subjects without a history of lower extremity injuries. Wilk et al. (1994) observed impaired performance on three types of single-leg hop tests among patients who had undergone arthroscopic ACL reconstruction within the previous 21 to 30 weeks.

During the past several years, research and clinical observations have indicated that physical characteristics such as mechanical joint stability, muscle strength, and limb girth are not necessarily valid indicators of functional ability and successful sports performance (Harter et al. 1988; Lephart, Perrin et al. 1992). These observations led to development of an increased number of performance tests that permit objective measurement of sport-related functional ability. For example, a battery of three tests (cocontraction test, a carioca crossover maneuver, shuttle run) was described by Lephart et al. (1991) as a tool for objective assessment of function in athletes with anterior cruciate ligament (ACL) insufficiency. Designed to elicit the pathological joint motions commonly associated with ACL insufficiency (e.g., the pivot shift phenomenon, anterior tibial subluxation), these tests require dynamic joint stabilization for optimal performance. Normative performance values on these three tests that have been developed for healthy male and female athletes in a variety of sports provide the sports health care clinician with a baseline for comparison when used for assessment of athletes with ACL deficiencies (Lephart et al. 1991). In another example of functional testing, Goldbeck and Davies (2000) reported the reliability of a closed kinetic chain stability test as a method for assessment of upper extremity function, particularly as related to the dynamic shoulder complex stabilization required for optimal performance of closed kinetic chain activities.

Deficits in Postural Control and Balance

Because disturbances in postural control and balance following musculoskeletal injuries of the lower extremities cannot be related to direct trauma of the vestibular system or the visual system, these deficits have been attributed to impairment of mechanoreceptor function associated with disruption of joint capsules and ligaments. Several studies have established a positive relationship between postural control and balance, and injuries to the ankle and knee. As noted by Wilkerson and Nitz (1994), an inability to maintain standing postural balance has been found to correlate highly with lower extremity functional joint instability. Unencumbered sensory input from somatosensory mechanoreceptors of the lower extremities appears to be an important factor in central control of balance and equilibrium (Irrgang, Whitney, and Cox 1994; Rivera 1994). During the past several years, a heightened awareness of balance deficits associated with sport-related lower extremity injuries has been accompanied by an increased array of balance-testing devices and protocols. In an effort to clarify conflicting terminology, Guskiewicz (1999) offered a useful classification of balance parameters for which assessment protocols have been developed. This classification includes tests for static balance, semi-dynamic balance, dynamic balance, and functional balance. These categories also provide a practical framework for discussion of balance training exercises. It is important to note that many balance-testing protocols also represent effective sensorimotor training exercises. As such, they are commonly incorporated into progressive functional rehabilitation programs designed to restore proprioception and dynamic joint control, as well as postural control and balance.

Static Balance

As commonly defined, static balance involves maintenance of the center of gravity (COG) of the body over a fixed base of support (i.e., the feet) while standing on a stable surface (e.g., the floor). Commonly, tests of static balance represent variations of Romberg's test, a subjective test traditionally used for assessment of postural sway associated with intracranial trauma. Variations of this test include single-leg standing, double-leg standing, and tandem standing during which one foot is placed behind the other. A review of the sports medicine literature reveals that single-leg stance tests are commonly used. During the past decade, objective assessment of standing balance has been enhanced by advances in forceplate technology, which permits quantitative measurement of postural sway by force sensors in a flat, rigid platform (Guskiewicz 1999; Irrgang, Whitney, and Cox 1994).

Several investigators have reported impaired standing balance in patients with ankle injuries and ACL insufficiency during single-leg balance testing. Zatterstrom et al. (1994) assessed single-leg standing balance in 26 patients with chronic ACL insufficiency. When compared with a group of subjects without a history of knee injuries, the ACL-deficient subjects demonstrated a significantly greater number of excessive sway movements and a greater speed of sway in the frontal plane. Studies involving subjects with unstable ankles have demonstrated single-leg stance deficits similar to those found in subjects with ACL-deficient knees. In an early study, Freeman, Dean, and Hanham (1965) used a modified Romberg's test to demonstrate impaired postural control in subjects with recent ankle sprains. Subsequent studies by Tropp, Odenrick, and Gillquest (1985) and Tropp and Odenrick (1988) revealed similar deficiencies in individuals with functional ankle instability. Using a modified Romberg's test, Lentell, Katzman, and Walters (1990) found significant single-leg balance asymmetry between the involved and uninvolved extremity in subjects with functional ankle stability. Of the 18 test subjects, 95% demonstrated standing balance deficits in the involved limb when compared with the contralateral uninvolved limb. In contrast, however, Bernier, Perrin, and Rijke (1997) found no significant difference in single-limb postural sway measurements between the involved and uninvolved limb in nine subjects with a 2- to 15-year history of unilateral functional instability of the ankle.

A concomitant finding in studies of standing balance by Lentell, Katzman, and Walters (1990) and Bernier, Perrin, and Rijke (1997) indicated that balance deficits in subjects with unilateral ankle instability are not necessarily related to muscular strength in the invertors and evertors of the ankle. These observations appear to be consistent with the conclusions of other investigators who suggested that intact proprioceptive mechanisms may be more important than periarticular muscle strength in functional joint stability (Ihara and Nakayama 1986; Wilk et al. 1994). A study by Hoffman et al. (1998) indicated that single-leg standing balance is also unrelated to lower limb dominance. These investigators found no significant difference in forceplate measurements between dominant and nondominant lower limbs in a group of 10 healthy young adults. As noted by the investigators, this finding may be particularly useful to the clinician who uses single-leg balance testing to monitor rehabilitation progress. With further confirmation of symmetry between dominant and nondominant limbs in healthy athletes, the sports health care clinician can more reasonably conclude that asymmetry in single-leg standing balance is a manifestation of sensorimotor dysfunction rather than lower limb dominance.

Semi-Dynamic and Dynamic Balance

In view of the integrated sensorimotor mechanisms involved, it seems plausible that an individual who demonstrates deficits in static balance as the result of lower extremity joint trauma will also exhibit deficiencies in dynamic balance. However, because tests of static balance (e.g., single-leg stance) involve continuous contact of the feet with a stable surface, they may not be valid measures of dynamic balance, which incorporate unstable surfaces, changes in the base of support, or both. According to the balance classification system presented by Guskiewicz (1999), semi-dynamic balance, in contrast to static balance, involves maintenance of the center of gravity (COG) over a fixed base of support while standing on a moving or unstable surface (e.g., foam mat, minitrampoline) rather than a stable surface. Alternately, subject movement of their COG over a fixed base of support while standing on a stable surface is also classified as semi-dynamic balance (e.g., minisquats, full squats). In comparison to static balance tests, commercial devices such as the Biodex Stability System (Biodex Medical Systems, Shirley, New York) incorporate mechanisms that permit measurable degrees of platform tilt, thereby allowing for varying surface stability during tests of standing balance (Arnold and Schmitz 1998). In another example of semi-dynamic balance testing with an unstable platform, Mattacola and Lloyd (1997) used a single-plane balance board that permitted platform tilting around an axis of rotation to demonstrate the effect of a strength and proprioceptive training program on subjects with a history of lateral ankle sprains.

In contrast to both static and semi-dynamic balance testing, during which the base of support is fixed (i.e., the feet), dynamic balance requires maintenance of the COG within maximum limits of stability (LOS) over a changing base of support (Guskiewicz 1999). Examples of dynamic balancing activities include step-ups, jumping exercises (e.g., hop test for distance, vertical jump test), figure eight running, shuttle runs, and the carioca maneuver, each of which requires changes of foot position in relation to the support surface (Irrgang, Whitney, and Cox 1994). It is significant to note that performance of these motor tasks begins to incorporate sport-specific functional balancing activities.

Functional Balance

In a general sense, the dynamic balancing tasks previously described are functional in nature because they simulate motor skills inherent in several sports activities. Nevertheless, in accordance with the classification system adopted for discussion, dynamic balance tests become functional balance activities when individualized sport-specific motor skills are incorporated (Guskiewicz 1999). For example, a basketball player may include dribbling during figure eight running and rebounding or basket shooting in jumping activities. In football, various crossover or cutting maneuvers can include catching a ball or defending a receiver (Lephart 1994). In these types of functional balance activities, subconscious dynamic balance control during concentration on a specific motor task is the primary criterion for successful performance.

Therapeutic Implications

With regard to management of proprioceptive deficits in surgical patients, Safran, Caldwell, and Fu (1994) identified the primary objectives as preservation of mechanoreceptors and their afferent nerve fibers, promotion of mechanoreceptor regeneration, and modification of protective reflex arcs. A review of the sports medicine literature, however, suggests that therapeutic intervention to preserve mechanoreceptor function actually begins with initial attempts to control hemorrhage and edema in an acute injury (Barrack, Lund, and Skinner 1994; Wilkerson and Nitz 1994). Furthermore, contemporary approaches to sports injury rehabilitation place an emphasis on preservation of proprioceptive input during the early stages of rehabilitation and incorporation of sensorimotor training into functional rehabilitation programs. With these observations in mind, the remainder of this chapter is devoted to a review of therapeutic intervention in three primary areas: (1) acute injury management, (2) surgery, and (3) proprioceptive and sensorimotor training.

Acute Injury Management

Although therapeutic management of proprioceptive deficits and impairment of motor function is typically addressed as a component of the intermediate and late stage of sports injury rehabilitation, intervention in the acute stage of sports injuries may be effective in preservation of mechanoreceptor function and retention of the somatosensory input necessary for neuromuscular control. Clinical observation suggests that proprioceptive deficits may be minimized through early therapeutic intervention that is directed to (1) control of effusion and edema and (2) early mobilization of the affected tissues.

Control of Effusion and Edema

Rationale for the use of pressure, ice, and elevation in the management of acute sports injuries was discussed in chapter 4. For the most part, use of these modalities to control hemorrhage and edema is directed to prevention of secondary hypoxic tissue damage and creation of a favorable physiological environment for tissue repair. In addition, however, control of joint effusion and edema may have a therapeutic value in preservation of mechanoreceptor function (Wilkerson 1991). As discussed in a previous section of this chapter, inhibition of protective reflex muscle contraction has been attributed to mechanoreceptor dysfunction, which results from joint effusion, increased intraarticular pressure, and distention of the joint capsule. Noting that a relatively small effusion of 20 ml in the knee produces reflex quadriceps inhibition, Spencer, Hayes, and Alexander (1984) stressed the importance of controlling hemarthrosis. For example, a positive effect of minimizing joint effusion may be prevention or alleviation of the quadriceps avoidance gait associated with quadriceps inhibition in acute knee injuries (Barrack, Lund, and Skinner 1994). With regard to control of joint effusion in acute inversion ankle sprains, Wilkerson (1991) suggested that capsular distention can be minimized by application of a U-shaped rubber "horseshoe" that provides focal joint compression. Theoretically, this procedure helps to restore normal intraarticular pressure, thereby creating a favorable environment for optimal proprioceptor stimulation and protective neuromuscular responses.

Control of joint effusion in acute injuries may contribute to preservation of mechanoreceptor function through additional avenues. Spencer, Hayes, and Alexander (1984) reported persistent neural inhibition despite a reduction in effusion and intraarticular pressure after knee injuries. These investigators suggested that residual distention of the joint capsule may be a more significant factor than acute joint effusion in inhibition of reflex muscle contraction. Noting that prolonged hemarthrosis may result in chronic capsular distention with fibrosis and hypertrophy of synovial tissues, Wilkerson and Nitz (1994) suggested that focal compression may reduce the potential for residual capsular distention and synovial hypertrophy. In addition, these authors theorized that reflex neuromuscular mechanisms may be adversely affected by increased intraarticular pressure that causes mechanical stimulation of joint nociceptors. As proposed, the resulting afferent pain impulses override sensory impulses from mechanoreceptors, thereby altering the proprioceptive input necessary for protective neuromuscular responses. Preservation of proprioception may therefore result from early efforts to control the pain responses associated with acute inflammation in the affected tissues.

Early Tissue Mobilization

Notwithstanding contraindications to premature mobilization of traumatized tissues, especially in view of hemorrhage and acute inflammation, early mobilization may minimize loss of proprioception. Contemporary approaches to preservation of mechanoreceptor function commonly include recommendations for initiation of low-risk proprioceptive training exercises during the early stages of rehabilitation (Lephart 1994; Myers and Lephart 2000). Early proprioceptive training may include simple passive or active joint repositioning with progression to closed kinetic chain weight-bearing activities. With regard to therapeutic management of acute ankle sprains, Wilkerson (1991) noted the rapid deterioration of neural connections between static and dynamic joint stabilizers that occurs with inactivity. Contending that joint proprioception is easier to maintain than to restore, Wilkerson suggested that early initiation of weight-bearing activities (e.g., partial weight-bearing crutch gaits) promotes mechanoreceptor stimulation and preservation of the neural mechanisms necessary for protective reflex muscle contraction. Effective control of joint effusion facilitates joint motion, which in turn permits earlier functional weight bearing. As edema control and tissue repair permit, early progressive resumption of weight bearing is encouraged, provided that damaged tissues can be protected from undue stress. For example, progression from non-weight-bearing crutch gaits (e.g., swing-through) to partial weight-bearing gaits (e.g., point gaits) in lower extremity injuries can be used to introduce appropriate levels of mechanoreceptor stimulation while protecting affected joint structures from excessive loading. Progressive mechanoreceptor stimulation can also be introduced by ambulation in water (e.g., a therapeutic pool). Initially, loading of weight-bearing joints can be minimized by walking in deep water, during which external hydrostatic forces are applied to the injured joint. Progression to ambulation in shallow water permits gradual tissue loading and increased mechanoreceptor stimulation.

Surgical Considerations in Proprioception

To an increased extent, preservation of joint receptors and their afferent nerve fibers has become an important consideration in surgical repair and reconstruction of articular structures, notwithstanding selection of the most appropriate surgical procedure to restore the mechanical integrity of static joint restraints (Safran, Caldwell, and Fu 1994). Investigations and clinical observations after hip and knee joint arthroplasty, anterior cruciate ligament (ACL) reconstruction, and glenohumeral joint repair have added to a growing body of knowledge regarding the effect of surgery on mechanoreceptor function. Although surgery lies beyond the domain of the certified athletic trainer and sports therapist, awareness of the anatomical and biomechanical alterations that result from surgery is essential to development of appropriate rehabilitation protocols. As research further clarifies the effect of various surgical procedures on preservation of mechanoreceptors and restoration of proprioceptive mechanisms, it may be equally important for the sports health care clinician to associate particular surgical techniques with anticipated proprioceptive outcomes in order that effective therapeutic protocols can be developed.

Postoperative Mechanoreceptor Repopulation

A review of the literature indicates that most postoperative proprioceptive studies have involved the knee, especially the ACL-reconstructed knee. As summarized by Barrack, Lund, and Skinner (1994), investigators generally agree that most patients with functional instability of the knee after ACL rupture experience proprioceptive deficits that persist to varying degrees after surgical reconstruction. During threshold to detection of passive motion (TTDPM) assessment, Lephart, Kocher et al. (1992) found kinesthetic deficits after ACL reconstruction using patellar tendon autografts and allografts. Bilateral comparisons revealed decreased kinesthetic awareness in surgical knees at the near-terminal range of joint motion in patients who had undergone arthroscopic reconstruction during the previous 11 to 26 months. Presumably, the proprioceptive deficits that remained after surgery were due to preexisting mechanoreceptor disruption.

Despite evidence indicating that proprioceptive deficits persist after surgery, postoperative histological studies have demonstrated repopulation of joint mechanoreceptors after ACL reconstruction. The regeneration process appears to be slow, however. With regard to ACL reconstruction involving a graft replacement, Barrack, Lund, and Skinner (1994) cited histological evidence of mechanoreceptor repopulation and, thus, the potential for return of sensation. However, these processes may require a minimum period of one year. Goertzen et al. (1992) assessed the neurohistological changes in bone-ACL-bone allografts in animal models at 3, 6, and 12 months after surgery. This investigation indicated no evidence of joint receptors at 3 months but did reveal the presence of free nerve endings at 6 months and Golgi tendon organlike endings at 12 months following experimental surgery. Despite documented repopulation of joint receptors in this study, the number of mechanoreceptors in the bone-ACL-bone grafts remained below that of normal anterior cruciate ligaments.

A subsequent histological study of reconstructed anterior cruciate ligaments in animal models revealed somewhat earlier postoperative presence of mechanoreceptors (Denti et al. 1994). These authors found evidence of pacinian corpuscles and free nerve endings at three months after reconstruction with the use of bone-patellar tendon-bone autografts. Mechanoreceptors continued to be present at six and nine months after surgery. Denti et al. also examined two human subjects who had experienced failed ACL reconstruction with semitendinous tendon transfers 9 and 10 years previously. A significant number of Ruffini's corpuscles and pacinian corpuscles, with concentration near the tibial insertion, was found in both patients despite the presence of lax, sclerotic ligaments. This observation appears to contradict the hypotheses of Rowinski (1997), who associated mechanoreceptor deficits with distortion of receptive fields by scar formation.

Discovery of ACL mechanoreceptor repopulation after surgery has led to speculation that restored joint receptors may, in conjunction with musculotendinous mechanoreceptors, contribute to improved proprioception and functional joint stability (Denti et al. 1994). Although the functional significance of mechanoreceptor repopulation is unclear, studies involving comparatively long-term patient follow-up appear more likely to demonstrate restoration of proprioception in postoperative knees (Safran, Caldwell, and Fu 1994). Thus, regeneration of mechanoreceptors and return of proprioceptive sensitivity after surgery is generally considered time dependent. Investigations by Dvir, Koren, and Halperin (1988) suggested that repopulation of mechanoreceptors translates into functional enhancement of proprioception over an extended time period.

Proprioceptive Effects of Surgery

Although histological studies demonstrate repopulation of joint mechanoreceptors after surgery, the effect of surgery on proprioceptive mechanisms is somewhat unclear. This uncertainty is due primarily to a paucity of investigations involving proprioceptive assessment of the same patients before and after surgery (Safran, Caldwell, and Fu 1994). Whether surgery alleviates or exacerbates preexisting proprioceptive deficits appears to be in need of further clarification. In addition, further studies regarding the comparative effects of particular surgical techniques seem to be indicated. Despite a lack of scientific evidence, however, surgery may contribute to preservation or restoration of proprioception through one or a combination of three avenues: (1) selection of surgical techniques that are least disruptive to articular structures and joint afferents, (2) use of graft types that are conducive to repopulation of mechanoreceptors, and (3) selection of surgical procedures that effectively restore tension in lax joint capsules and ligaments. These surgical considerations are reviewed as a basis for development of proprioceptive and sensorimotor training programs for postoperative sports participants.

Preservation of joint afferents

As noted by Safran, Caldwell, and Fu (1994) preservation of joint afferents is a primary objective of surgery. These authors suggested that meticulous surgical techniques are necessary to avoid unnecessary trauma to the joint capsule, ligaments, and other soft tissues that contain mechanoreceptors and afferent nerve fibers. Historically, surgery for sport-related joint injuries has focused on restoration of the structural integrity of capsuloligamentous tissues. Whereas surgical restoration of joint capsules and ligaments is essential to mechanical joint stability, some surgical techniques may involve resection of articular and periarticular tissues without sufficient consideration for retention of mechanoreceptor function. As observed by Safran, Caldwell, and Fu (1994), for example, the infrapatellar fat pad and other periarticular structures have sometimes been removed with impunity in arthroplasty and ACL reconstruction of the knee. Preservation of mechanoreceptors in these structures may be functionally significant. Introduction of arthroscopy several years ago has perhaps made the greatest contribution to preservation of proprioception in sport-related joint injuries. Aside from other advantages, compared to open surgical procedures, arthroscopy results in less disruption of articular and periarticular structures, thereby contributing to retention of proprioception through preservation of mechanoreceptors (Safran, Caldwell, and Fu 1994).

Selection of graft types

In surgical cases involving replacement of ruptured ligaments with grafts (e.g., ACL reconstruction), graft types that have the greatest potential for mechanoreceptor repopulation have received increased attention in the sports medicine literature. Grafts that involve transfer of tissues from one part of a patient's body to another are called *autografts*, whereas grafts obtained from other humans are referred to as *allografts* (Thomas 1993). A third type of graft that has been used for ACL reconstruction consists of synthetic material designed as an artificial ligament, or *prosthesis*. Because of a comparatively high failure rate and the absence of mechanoreceptor repopulation in synthetic ACL prostheses, however, prostheses are not currently recommended (Fu et al. 2000; Safran, Caldwell, and Fu 1994). Although Denti et al. (1994) found mechanoreceptor repopulation after ACL reconstruction using bone-patellar tendon-bone grafts, mechanoreceptors were consistently absent after reconstruction using synthetic ligaments, regardless of the time of postoperative biopsy.

As suggested by Lephart, Kocher et al. (1992), various ACL graft types may have different capacities for mechanoreceptor repopulation and regeneration of afferent neurons. However, with the exception of ACL prostheses, which fail to demonstrate mechanoreceptor repopulation, evidence indicating the comparative potential for restoration of mechanoreceptors in autographs and allografts is limited. Although autografts that employ a portion of the patellar tendon have commonly been used for ACL reconstruction, there appears to be little documentation of their superiority with regard to mechanoreceptor repopulation. In a study of postoperative patients who had undergone arthroscopic ACL reconstruction, Lephart, Kocher et al. (1992) found no significant difference in kinesthetic awareness between a group of subjects having patellar tendon autograft reconstruction and subjects having allograft reconstruction. When tested at 11 to 26 months after surgery, both groups of subjects demonstrated postoperative kinesthetic deficits in the involved knee at the near-terminal range of joint motion. These findings appear to be consistent with the observations of others who have suggested that the mechanoreceptor mechanisms in bone-patellar tendon-bone grafts do not replicate those that exist in a healthy ACL (Nyland et al. 1994). In a study of functional performance after ACL bone-patellar tendon-bone grafts, Lephart et al. (1993) found no significant differences between autograft and allograft groups during a cocontraction test, carioca crossover maneuver, shuttle run, or a single-leg hop test for distance.

Should further research demonstrate the superiority of one type of ACL graft over another with regard to mechanoreceptor repopulation and restoration of proprioception, this may represent a consideration in graft type selection. As acknowledged by Safran, Caldwell, and Fu (1994), however, improved proprioception after ACL reconstruction may be due to sensory input from mechanoreceptors in tissues other than the ACL graft, perhaps enhanced through rehabilitation activities. Denti et al. (1994) also noted the potential contribution of mechanoreceptors in intact articular and periarticular structures to restoration of proprioception after surgery. To the extent that sensory input from mechanoreceptors in intact tissues (e.g., secondary restraints) is compensatory, dependence on ACL autografts and allografts as a source of proprioceptive input may be decreased (Lo and Fowler 2000).

Restoration of capsuloligamentous tension

Surgical procedures designed to restore the mechanical integrity of capsuloligamentous tissues may also contribute to enhanced postoperative proprioception by restoring tension in the affected tissues (Safran, Caldwell, and Fu 1994). As previously noted, mechanical stimulation of articular mechanoreceptors results from deformation of the joint capsules and ligaments that house these sensory organs. Deformation occurs as capsuloligamentous structures are stretched, compressed, or otherwise loaded during joint motion. Several authors have suggested that attenuated capsular or ligamentous structures that demonstrate laxity may not be subjected to sufficient tension to activate afferent neural impulses during normal joint motions (Borsa et al. 1994; Lephart et al. 1994). Hence, surgical techniques that effectively restore capsuloligamentous tension may contribute to restoration of proprioception. Although direct repair of a torn ACL has been suggested by Safran, Caldwell, and Fu (1994) as a test of this hypothesis, these authors acknowledged the mechanical failure rate of direct ACL repair without augmentation. These authors also suggested that suturing of natural ACL ligament stumps to grafts may provide a positive environment for mechanoreceptor repopulation because mechanoreceptors are concentrated at ligament insertions. Complications associated with excessive tissue at the graft-ligament junction were acknowledged, however.

More frequently cited as a potentially effective procedure to restore tension in attenuated articular structures is the use of a capsular shift, commonly used to alleviate instabilities of the glenohumeral joint (Borsa et al. 1994; Lephart et al. 1994). With regard to glenohumeral joint surgery, Borsa et al. (1994) concluded that capsulolabral reconstruction restores both the mechanical and sensory mechanisms that contribute to joint stability. Kinesthesia and joint position sense after reconstructive surgery for glenohumeral instabilities has been studied by Lephart et al. (1994). These authors examined surgical patients after completion of a postoperative rehabilitation program, from 7 to 19 months after surgery. When tested for threshold to detection of passive motion (TTDPM) and reproduction of passive positioning (RPP), no significant mean differences were found between surgically repaired glenohumeral joints and normal contralateral joints. As a result of these findings, the authors suggested that restoration of tension in articular structures, through arthroscopic or open surgery, facilitates deformation of capsuloligamentous tissues and stimulation of mechanoreceptors, thus enhancing the neural mechanisms necessary for proprioception. In recent years, laser energy has been used as an alternative to surgery to shrink and shorten selected portions of the joint capsule. While the histological and biomechanical effects of this procedure have been studied (Hayashi et al. 1999), the effects of thermal capsular shrinkage on joint mechanoreceptors and proprioception present future investigative challenges.

Proprioceptive and Sensorimotor Training

Therapeutic management of deficits in proprioception and neuromuscular control after sport-related injuries is a major component of functional rehabilitation, a concept that has received increased attention during the past several years. In part, functional rehabilitation involves development of muscular strength, power, and endurance in specific movement patterns inherent in a particular sport. Similarly, enhancement of sport-specific motor skills that require neuromuscular coordination, balance, and agility is a primary focus of functional rehabilitation. In contrast, historical approaches to sports injury rehabilitation have been directed to development of muscular strength and power in isolated, one-plane movement patterns. For example, open kinetic chain strengthening of the quadriceps muscles during resisted knee extension and hamstring strengthening during resisted knee flexion exemplify a traditional approach to rehabilitation of knee injuries. Although muscle group isolation for strength development is commonly indicated, especially during the early stages of rehabilitation, functional rehabilitation involving integrated, sport-specific movement patterns is necessary to an athlete's full recovery and safe return to activity (Hillman 1994). In the above example, further strengthening and neuromuscular education of the quadriceps through the use of controlled closed kinetic chain jumping activities (e.g., plyometrics) integrates quadriceps function with the function of synergistic muscle groups to replicate a sport-specific skill. Incorporation of eccentric as well as concentric muscle contractions that normally occur during a particular motor activity demonstrates an additional principle of sport-specific functional rehabilitation.

During the past several years, heightened awareness of the proprioceptive deficits associated with common sports injuries has led to a greater focus on specific proprioceptive and sensorimotor training protocols as important components of functional rehabilitation programs. An increasing amount of evidence indicates that functional rehabilitation may be incomplete and inadequate unless specific attempts to restore the mechanisms associated with proprioception and neuromuscular control are included. Rivera (1994), for example, noted the many physiological, biomechanical, and neurological considerations in functional rehabilitation of an injured athlete that include protocols to optimize proprioceptive mechanisms. The component of functional rehabilitation that focuses on enhancement of proprioceptive input and restoration of appropriate neuromuscular responses has traditionally been referred to as *proprioceptive training*. Considering the integrated neuroanatomy and neurophysiology of the sensory and motor systems described in chapter 8, however, the term *sensorimotor training* is considered more inclusive and, thus, more appropriate to describe this component of functional rehabilitation.

It is important to note that restoration of proprioception and sensorimotor function is consistent with traditional protocols designed to promote muscular strength, power, and endurance. Many therapeutic exercises designed to enhance proprioception and motor control can also be expected to contribute to muscular strength and power. Conversely, traditional methods to develop these components of motor performance contribute to enhanced proprioception and sensorimotor function. Thus, the term *neuromuscular reeducation*, which implies restoration of desired motor responses as well as muscular strength and power, can be appropriately associated with functional rehabilitation of the injured sports participant.

Muscle Strength and Neuromuscular Control

Several studies have provided the sports health care clinician with insight regarding the respective roles of muscular strength and proprioceptive mechanisms in functional joint stability. Lentell, Katzman, and Walters (1990) studied the relationship between chronic ankle instability and strength in the evertors and invertors of the ankle. Although balance asymmetries were found between involved and uninvolved lower extremities in 55% of their subjects with chronic ankle instability, muscular weakness was found to be unrelated to functional instability. These investigators concluded that muscular weakness is not a major factor in chronic ankle instability and suggested that restoration of proprioceptive mechanisms is more important than muscle strengthening. Similar observations have been made regarding the relationship of muscle strength to functional joint stability following injuries of the knee. For example, several investigators have noted that hamstring strengthening alone is not adequate to control anterior tibial translation in ACL-deficient knees (Ihara and Nakayama 1986; Tibone et al. 1986). With regard to joint stability after ACL reconstruction, Wilk et al. (1994) suggested that the ability to stabilize the knee joint during functional activity may be a more critical factor than the amount of force generated by periarticular muscle groups. Other authors have proposed that the most effective protocols for rehabilitation of ACL injuries include both muscle strengthening and dynamic, closed kinetic chain reflex training (Barrack, Lund, and Skinner 1994). With regard to restoration of function after anterior glenohumeral dislocations, observations by Smith and Brunolli (1989) also support incorporation of proprioceptive training into rehabilitation programs, in addition to muscle strengthening. In agreement with Rowinski (1997), these authors contended that neurological dysfunction is a component of glenohumeral dislocation. Consequently, restoration of motor skills based on new, and probably abnormal, sensory input most likely requires extensive proprioceptive training.

Sensorimotor Training: A Conceptual Model

A review of the neuroanatomy and neurophysiology presented in chapter 8 indicates that the peripheral proprioceptive system, the vestibular system, and the visual system provide the integrated sensory information that influences the motor systems of the body. Processing of sensory input to effect appropriate neuromuscular responses is facilitated by a hierarchical organization of the motor system that includes the spinal cord, the brain stem, and the cerebral cortex (figure 9.3). In addition, a parallel organization of motor control allows integration

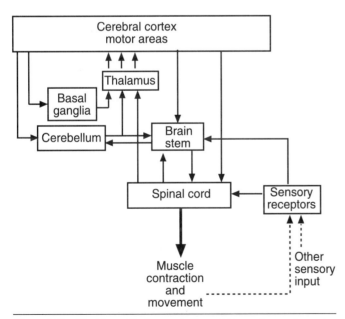

Figure 9.3 The hierarchical organization of the motor systems, including the cerebral cortex (with indirect regulation by the basal ganglia and cerebellum), the brain stem, and the spinal cord.

Reprinted from E.R. Kandel, J.H. Schwartz, and T.M. Jessell, 1991, *Principles of neural science*, 3rd ed. (Norwalk, Connecticut: Appleton & Lange), 429. Reproduced with the permission of The McGraw-Hill Companies.

of sensory information and coordination of motor activities at various levels of the central nervous system (Kandel, Schwartz, and Jessell 1995). The hierarchical organization of motor function, along with the three primary sources of sensory input (i.e., the peripheral proprioceptive, vestibular, and visual systems), provides a simplified yet clinically useful conceptual framework for development of proprioceptive and sensorimotor training programs (Lephart 1994).

The lowest hierarchical level of motor function is the spinal cord where spinal reflexes, the simplest form of motor activity, occur (e.g., the stretch reflex). For example, muscle spindle excitation, initiation of a monosynaptic reflex arc, and reflex muscle contraction form the neural basis for protective periarticular muscle splinting and functional joint stability (see chapter 8). At the second-highest level of motor control, the brain stem functions as the site of several nuclei from which indirect descending motor pathways originate (e.g., the vestibulospinal tract, tectospinal tract). Specific brain stem functions related to control of eye movements, postural control, and balance were discussed in chapter 8. At the highest, most complex level of motor function, voluntary body movements are initiated by the primary motor area of the cerebral cortex, which projects descending motor pathways to the spinal cord (i.e., the corticospinal tracts). Voluntary movements initiated by the motor cortex are indirectly controlled by the basal ganglia and the cerebellum, which influence the planning and coordination of body movements at this level of motor function (see chapter 8). As noted earlier in this chapter, feed-forward mechanisms of dynamic joint control including preactivation, cocontraction, and stiffness of periarticular muscle groups are also mediated at the cortical level (Kandel, Schwartz, and Jessell 1995; Lephart, Riemann, and Fu 2000).

The fundamental clinical challenge in sensorimotor training is to develop and implement therapeutic strategies that optimize the somatosensory, vestibular, and visual input necessary to enhance desired neuromuscular responses at various hierarchical levels of motor control. With specific regard to functional rehabilitation of a sports participant with proprioceptive deficits due to joint trauma, the desired proprioceptive and sensorimotor responses commonly translate into three primary therapeutic objectives: the enhancement of (1) joint position sense and kinesthesia, (2) dynamic joint stabilization, and (3) postural control and balance. Which of these objectives becomes paramount, however, depends in part on the involved extremity. Optimal rehabilitation of lower extremity injuries (i.e., the ankle or knee), for example, typically necessitates attention to all three therapeutic objectives. Injuries to the upper extremities (e.g., the glenohumeral joint), on the other hand, may present therapeutic challenges related to improvement of joint position sense, kinesthesia, and dynamic joint stabilization, but they do not necessarily require restoration of postural control and balance.

Sensorimotor Manipulation and Therapeutic Progression

Throughout the progressive sequence of proprioceptive and sensorimotor training, alteration of somatosensory, vestibular, or visual input is commonly used to challenge a particular source of sensory information or a particular sensorimotor mechanism. Alteration of one or more of the three primary sources of sensory information has been referred to as *sensory manipulation*. A form of sensory manipulation, sometimes referred to as *sensory filtering*, is accomplished by elimination of a particular source of sensory information in order to focus demands on another sensory system, commonly with accompanying changes in the environmental conditions under which a sports participant is asked to perform a particular motor task. For example, standing balance training with progression from single-leg balancing on a hard, stable surface (e.g., the floor) with the eyes open to single-leg balancing on an unstable surface (e.g., a foam mat) with the eyes closed illustrates the use of sensory manipulation, as well as a change in environmental conditions. Generally, elimination of a source of sensory input presents an added challenge to the remaining operative sensory systems. In the previous example, the disadvantaged visual system with elimination of visual clues results in increased reliance on the somatosensory and vestibular systems for maintenance of standing balance, which is made more difficult by progression from a stable surface to an unstable surface.

Although sophisticated commercial devices have been developed for lower extremity sensorimotor training, sports health care clinicians frequently utilize comparatively inexpensive balance boards (e.g., wobble boards, ankle disks), foam mats, Swiss balls, and similar devices. Because these devices permit perturbation in joint position, and thus stimulation of joint and musculotendinous mechanoreceptors, while presenting challenges to the vestibular system, they provide opportunities for sensory manipulation and changes in environmental training conditions. These sensorimotor training devices have proved useful in enhancement of dynamic joint control (Ihara and Nakayama 1986) as well as dynamic balance (Hoffman and Payne 1995; Mattacola and Lloyd 1997). Over the past several years, dynamic joint control training for the shoulder complex has received increased attention through closed kinetic chain exercises with wobble boards, minitrampolines, Swiss balls, and slide boards (Stone et al. 1994).

Although proprioceptive and sensorimotor training have been addressed as a component of functional rehabilitation, which typically characterizes the final stage of sports injury rehabilitation, proprioceptive training may begin shortly after injury as permitted by the degree of injury and the extent of tissue healing. Thus, proprioceptive and sensorimotor training commonly transcend all phases of the rehabilitation process and are characteristically progressive in nature, generally proceeding from performance of simple to more complex motor tasks. For example, as clinical signs and symptoms subside, proprioceptive training after an acute ankle or knee injury may begin with simple open kinetic chain joint repositioning exercises to preserve or enhance cortical perception of joint position and kinesthesia. Subsequent proprioceptive training on a wobble board, ankle disk, or other unstable surface in the seated position represents a progression that further stimulates joint and musculotendinous receptors and begins to incorporate demands for dynamic neuromuscular control, but without challenge to the vestibular system. With permissible weight bearing, sensorimotor training can be progressed from double-leg to single-leg static balancing and from static balancing to dynamic balancing, thereby incorporating vestibular mechanisms operating at the brain stem level as well as dynamic joint control mechanisms that are mediated at the spinal cord and cortical levels. Filtering of visual clues by closing the eyes places further demands on the somatosensory and vestibular systems during controlled dynamic balancing activities.

As sensorimotor training continues into more advanced stages, dynamic balancing activities with incorporation of locomotor skills are commonly used to incorporate input from all sensory systems, thereby promoting neuromuscular responses at all hierarchical levels of motor control. Plyometrics and sport-specific functional activities may be added during this phase. Sport-related activities, such as those described earlier as tests of dynamic balance (e.g., shuttle run, figure eight running, carioca maneuver), provide a variety of sensorimotor challenges. Difficulty can be added to these activities by increasing the speed or varying the direction of movement, increasing the abruptness of cutting maneuvers, or altering the predictability of environmental demands. The predictability of demands on the sensorimotor systems, and thus the challenge to neuromuscular control mechanisms, can be altered by incorporation of sport-specific activities during dynamic balance training, as is frequently done during the late phases of functional rehabilitation. For example, asking a football receiver to catch a ball while performing lateral movements on a slide board challenges the vestibular and visual systems and may invoke the vestibuloocular reflex that operates at the brain stem level (see chapter 8). Meanwhile, the neural feedback and feed-forward systems operating at the spinal cord and cortical levels of motor control are challenged to provide dynamic lower extremity joint control during lateral body movements. Other activities that integrate dynamic balance with sport-specific motor tasks include dribbling a basketball during four-corner or figure eight running, receiving a football while running and cutting, and fielding ground balls in baseball or softball (Lephart 1994). As categorized by Guskiewicz (1999), these types of drills are referred to as *functional balance tasks*.

Proprioceptive Effects of External Support Devices

Adhesive tape, elastic bandages, and a variety of other supportive devices have been used in the management of sports injuries for many years. With the development of products such as neoprene sleeves, functional knee braces, and ankle orthotics, an increased array of protective devices has become available to the sports health care clinician. Historically, the efficacy of most of these products has been judged primarily on the basis of their ability to provide mechanical support for joint capsules and ligaments or alleviation of potentially injurious musculotendinous strain. In recent years, however, the effect of external compression and support devices on somatosensory proprioceptive mechanisms has received increased attention, particularly as related to stimulation of cutaneous mechanoreceptors and facilitation of protective neuromuscular responses. Considering the neurophysiology of cutaneous mechanoreceptors (see chapter 8), enhancement of proprioceptive input through the use of external compression devices is based on plausible rationale. At the current time, however, research regarding the contribution of cutaneous receptors to proprioception and neuromuscular control, and thus the benefits of external compression devices, remains inconclusive.

Whereas some studies have indicated positive effects of adhesive tape, elastic bandages, and orthotic devices on proprioception (Feuerbach et al. 1994; Perlau, Frank, and Fick 1995; Simoneau et al. 1997), other investigations have failed to demonstrate proprioceptive benefits of braces and orthotic devices (Branch, Hunter, and Donath 1989; Kaminski and Perrin 1996; Kinzey, Ingersoll, and Knight 1997). In a study of the effect of a rigid ankle orthosis on proprioception in noninjured subjects, Feuerbach et al. (1994) reported that errors in active joint repositioning were less frequent in subjects who wore an ankle brace compared to subjects who were not braced. A subsequent study indicated that knee joint position sense improved by an average of 25% in 54 uninjured subjects who wore an elastic bandage and that the improvement was lost after bandage removal (Perlau, Frank, and Fick 1995). Of this group, subjects who were determined to have "poor" joint position sense prior to application of an elastic bandage improved by 66%, whereas no improvement was seen in subjects with "good" joint position sense. These investigators suggested that pressure on superficial cutaneous mechanoreceptors (e.g., Merkel's discs) and, to a lesser extent, deeper-lying skin receptors (e.g., end organs of Ruffini) was the most plausible explanation for enhanced proprioception in subjects with poor proprioception (see chapter 8, figure 8.7). A unique study by Simoneau et al. (1997) demonstrated that 5-inch strips of athletic tape applied to the anterior surface of the ankle and, posteriorly, over the Achilles tendon and calcaneus in healthy subjects significantly improved plantar flexion joint position sense in a non-weight-bearing position, but not during weight bearing. Application of these tape strips, however, did not alter perception of passive joint motion (i.e., kinesthesia) in either the weight-bearing or the non-weight-bearing position.

In contrast to studies demonstrating a positive effect of braces and other external compression devices on proprioception, Kaminski and Perrin (1996) concluded that a prophylactic knee brace (McDavid Knee Guard, McDavid Knee Guard, Inc., Chicago, Illinois) had no significant effect on active or passive knee joint repositioning sense in healthy subjects. While double-leg dynamic balance under plantar flexion/dorsiflexion conditions was improved by a knee brace in this study, no improvement was observed during double-leg or single-leg balancing under other unstable or stable test platform conditions. In a study comparing single-leg postural control measurements in healthy subjects with and without ankle braces, Kinzey, Ingersoll, and Knight (1997) reported that their findings did not support or refute the benefits of ankle braces in enhancement of proprioception.

While most studies regarding the proprioceptive effect of braces and other external devices have involved uninjured subjects, some investigators have assessed the benefits of supportive devices on proprioception in subjects with anterior cruciate ligament (ACL) deficiencies. For example, Beynnon et al. (1999) observed that the ability to detect passive joint motion by subjects with ACL deficiencies and accompanying proprioceptive deficits was not significantly changed when either a functional knee brace or a neoprene sleeve was applied, although some improvement was noted. In an earlier study, Branch, Hunter, and Donath (1989) demonstrated that, when compared to unbraced knees, a derotation knee brace significantly reduced quadriceps and hamstring EMG activity in subjects with ACL deficiencies during the stance phase of a sidestep cutting maneuver. These investigators concluded that knee braces do not function proprioceptively to enhance dynamic joint control. Instead, it was suggested that the mechanical efficacy of knee braces may reduce the need for dynamic joint stabilization during a cutting maneuver.

To the extent that braced joints rely on neuromuscular control for stabilization, the effect of braces and other supportive devices on muscle fatigue may be an important consideration. Muscle fatigue has been shown to have a negative effect on knee joint position sense and kinesthesia (Skinner et al. 1986) and glenohumeral position sense (Myers et al. 1999) in healthy subjects. These observations, in combination with research indicating premature muscle fatigue in braced joints, suggest that braces may have a detrimental effect on dynamic joint control. For example, Styf, Lundin, and Gershuni (1994) demonstrated that the time to elicit tibialis anterior muscle fatigue was 35% less when subjects wore a hinged neoprene knee brace compared to unbraced legs. This effect was attributed to external compression and increased intramuscular pressure distal to the brace. Whereas Myers et al. (1999) did not find muscle fatigue to be a factor in neuromuscular control in the shoulder complex, Styf, Lundin, and Gershuni (1994) suggested that premature fatigue of leg muscles brought on by a knee brace may, in part, explain an increase in reported ankle injuries while wearing a brace. In general, a comparison of research results indicates that the interrelationships among proprioception, dynamic joint control, and the use of braces and other support devices remain unclear and in need of further study.

Effects of Sensorimotor Training

As a parallel to heightened awareness of the positive relationship between sensorimotor deficits and sport-related musculoskeletal injuries, an increased amount of clinical research has addressed the effect of sensorimotor training on various parameters of proprioception and neuromuscular control. While several early studies provided a basis for the current understanding of the neuroanatomy and neurophysiology of proprioception (e.g., Freeman and Wyke 1967; Clark et al. 1979; Kennedy, Alexander, and Hayes 1982), research regarding the effects of exercise and sensorimotor training on proprioception began to proliferate in the 1980s. In general, these studies involved the effect of various training protocols on joint position sense and kinesthesia, dynamic joint stabilization, and postural control and balance in both healthy and injured sports participants.

Joint position sense and kinesthesia

While most research regarding the effect of various rehabilitation protocols on proprioception and sensorimotor function has focused on dynamic joint stabilization, postural control, and balance, some investigators have attempted to determine the effect of physical activity and sensorimotor training on joint position sense and kinesthesia. Although various investigators have studied the relationship between physical activity and proprioception in healthy sports participants, a review of the sports medicine literature indicates the need for additional research regarding the effect of proprioceptive training on the specific parameters of joint position sense and kinesthesia in injured athletes. Nevertheless, a study by Docherty, Moore, and Arnold (1998) provided some insight. These investigators reported that active joint repositioning sense in subjects with functional ankle instability was significantly improved during a six-week strength training program compared to subjects with functional instability who received no training. Although simple passive and active joint repositioning exercises have been advocated to enhance conscious awareness of joint position sense after injury (Borsa et al. 1994), evidence exists that traditional active and resistive exercise contributes to joint position sense and kinesthesia. Rogol, Ernst, and Perrin (1998), for example, compared the effects of open and closed kinetic chain resistive exercise on shoulder joint position sense in healthy subjects. These investigators reported that subjects who completed a six-week program of closed kinetic chain exercises (standard push-ups) and subjects who completed a program of open kinetic chain exercises (supine dumbbell presses) of the same duration both demonstrated significant improvement in passive and active joint reposition sense when compared to a control group. Additionally, no significant difference was found between the open and closed kinetic chain exercise groups with regard to enhancement of joint position sense.

On cursory comparison, studies indicating positive effects of therapeutic exercise and physical activity on somatosensory proprioception appear to be inconsistent with studies that demonstrated deficits in joint position sense and kinesthesia in healthy, trained athletes. For example, Barrack et al. (1983) demonstrated deficits in joint position sense in the knees of professional ballet dancers. Similarly, Allegrucci et al. (1995) reported kinesthetic deficits in the dominant shoulder of overhand-throwing athletes. However, the investigators in both of these studies attributed the proprioceptive deficits to chronic capsular laxity and joint hypermobility, which perhaps negated enhancement of proprioception that otherwise may have occurred as the result of active exercise. In a more recent study, Loudon (2000) found diminished active knee joint repositioning ability in 24 healthy women with genu recurvatum, particularly at the near-terminal range of extension (i.e., 10° knee flexion). The extent of proprioceptive deficits found in this study correlated positively with the degree of recurvatum. Lack of tension in the posterior joint capsule was suggested as a possible explanation for decreased joint position sense toward the extended range. In general, comparison of studies regarding the effect of exercise on joint position sense and kinesthesia suggest a potential for enhancement of proprioception, with the possible exception of joints with inherent or acquired hypermobility.

Dynamic joint control

In one of the earliest investigations regarding the effects of sensorimotor training on dynamic joint control, Freeman, Dean, and Hanham (1965) subjected patients with ligamentous injuries and proprioceptive deficits of the foot and ankle to a program of coordination exercises involving repeated attempts at single-leg balancing on unstable balance boards. These investigators reported that patients who completed their exercise program demonstrated a significantly lower incidence of proprioceptive deficits and functional joint instability as compared to two reference groups that were treated with immobilization and conventional physical therapy, respectively. In a subsequent study, Freeman and Wyke (1967) used electromyography to demonstrate the effect of proprioceptive training on reflex muscle activity. Results of their study indicated that balance training on an unstable board had a positive effect on reflex activity of the leg muscles, thus enhancing dynamic joint control following ligamentous injuries of the ankle.

During the 1980s, several investigators noted the value of proprioceptive training on reflex hamstring activity and control of anterior tibial translation in ACL-deficient knees. Ihara and Nakayama (1986), for example, studied the effect of dynamic joint control training on reflex hamstring contraction in four patients with functionally unstable knees. At the end of a three-month training program using various types of unstable exercise platforms, the experimental group demonstrated significantly decreased hamstring reaction time in response to a sudden knee extension force compared to a control group of healthy subjects that received no training. As a result of these findings, the investigators suggested a strong possibility that dynamic joint control training is effective in shortening the lag time between proprioceptive stimulation and neuromuscular response. As a concomitant finding in this study, no correlation was found between hamstring reaction time and isometric muscle strength. This observation appears to be consistent with the observations of Walla et al. (1985), who concluded that hamstring strength and power, as measured isokinetically, is only minimally related to functional stability of the knee. These investigators suggested that muscle coordination is a more important predictor of functional success than the degree of mechanical stability. In general agreement with previous investigators, Tibone et al. (1986) observed that nearly normal isokinetic hamstring strength (a 4% deficit) was inadequate to allow subjects to compensate for ACL deficiency.

Postural control and balance

In addition to research regarding the efficacy of sensorimotor training on joint proprioception (i.e., joint position sense and kinesthesia) and dynamic joint stability, an increasing number of studies in recent years has addressed the effect of various training protocols on postural control and balance. After a 10-week program of single-leg balance training using the Biomechanical Ankle Platform System, or BAPS board (Spectrum Therapy Products, Jasper, Mich.), Hoffman and Payne (1995) found significant postural sway decreases in healthy male and female high school students when compared to a randomly selected control group from the same population. The experimental group in this study demonstrated significant decreases in both anterior-posterior and medial-lateral postural sway in their dominant lower extremity as determined by forceplate measurements. Studies involving subjects with injuries of the ankle and knee have revealed similar positive effects of proprioceptive training on reduction of postural sway. Using a single-case experimental design, Mattacola and Lloyd (1997) studied the effect of a strength and proprioceptive training program on dynamic balance in three male boarding school students with a history of recurrent inversion ankle sprains. These investigators reported significant improvement in the subjects' dynamic balance during a six-week program of manually resisted ankle movements and repetitive single-leg balancing on an unstable single-plane balance board. In another study, Zatterstrom et al. (1994) assessed postural control in 26 ACL-deficient patients with bilateral standing balance deficits. After a three-month training period, normal forceplate values were found in the uninjured leg in both of two groups of subjects who performed either open kinetic chain resisted knee extension exercises or closed kinetic chain activities compared to a reference group of healthy subjects. However, standing balance deficits remained in the injured leg at three months, after which all subjects performed both types of training exercises. Standing postural sway values in the injured leg were normalized when tested at 12 months. Bilateral improvement was found to persist when standing balance was tested at 36 months after initiation of training.

Summary

Proprioceptive and sensorimotor deficits resulting from sport-related musculoskeletal injuries are commonly attributed to disruption of joint capsules and ligaments that house the somatosensory receptors for proprioception. The neuropathology of proprioceptive deficits associated with joint injuries may involve acute disruption of joint mechanoreceptors as well as degeneration of their afferent neurons, resulting in articular deafferentation, a pathological condition. Sensorimotor manifestations of articular deafferentation include impaired joint position sense and kinesthesia, diminished dynamic joint control, and deficits in postural control and balance. Clinical assessment of these proprioceptive and sensorimotor deficits is typically accomplished through the use of proprioceptive testing protocols to assess reproduction of joint positioning or threshold to detection of passive joint motion, electromyographic assessment of periarticular muscle activity, and tests of static and dynamic balance.

Therapeutic intervention in the management of proprioceptive and sensorimotor deficits includes control of effusion and edema in acute injuries, consideration of surgical procedures that are conducive to preservation or restoration of proprioceptive mechanisms, and proprioceptive and sensorimotor training. Intervention in the acute stage of sports injuries through the use of pressure, cold applications, and elevation is directed to the control of effusion, edema, and joint capsule distention that contribute to mechanoreceptor dysfunction. Within the limits imposed by acute tissue damage, early active joint motion is indicated as a means of preserving joint and muscle mechanoreceptor function. To an increased extent, preservation and restoration of proprioceptive mechanisms have become a consideration in the surgical repair and reconstruction of damaged articular structures. Preservation of articular tissues that house joint mechanoreceptors, surgical procedures that effectively restore capsuloligamentous tension, and selection of graft types that are conducive to mechanoreceptor repopulation represent primary considerations related to the role of surgery in proprioception and sensorimotor function.

While sport-specific functional rehabilitation is generally accepted as necessary for full recovery from sports injuries, an increased amount of evidence indicates that functional rehabilitation may be incomplete without incorporation of specific protocols to restore proprioceptive and sensorimotor function. Whereas muscular strength, power, and endurance provide a foundation for motor performance, restoration of neuromuscular function through proprioceptive and sensorimotor training is a prerequisite to optimal sports performance. The hierarchical organization of the motor system including the spinal cord, brain stem, and cerebral cortex provides a conceptual model for development of sen-

Problem-Solving Scenario

After reconstructive surgery for an anterior cruciate ligament-deficient knee with a patella tendon autograft, a 21-year-old college football player, a wide receiver, has achieved a level of rehabilitation that indicates readiness for progression to controlled functional activities. Preliminary proprioceptive testing, however, indicates diminished kinesthetic awareness of knee joint motion while a single-leg balance test demonstrates a deficiency in static balance. Although a clinical assessment reveals acceptable strength levels in the muscle groups responsible for dynamic joint stabilization, the athlete demonstrates poor functional performance on tests involving a carioca maneuver, shuttle run, and a single-leg hop test for distance.

Problem-Solving Questions

- What are the most likely reasons for the proprioceptive and sensorimotor deficits demonstrated by the athlete in this case?

- What was the most likely effect of surgery in preservation and restoration of proprioceptive input?

- What is the most plausible explanation for the athlete's poor performance on tests of functional ability despite acceptable strength levels in the dynamic joint stabilizers?

- Based on the clinical assessment, what specific short-term rehabilitation goals would be most appropriate during the next three weeks of the athlete's recovery period?

- What sensorimotor training activities would be most appropriate for restoration of the athlete's functional abilities in this case? What sequence of activities best demonstrates progression to sport-specific functional activities and return to competition for the athlete in this case?

sorimotor training programs. Commonly, the primary therapeutic objectives of sensorimotor training include enhancement of joint position sense and kinesthesia, dynamic joint stabilization, and postural control and balance. These objectives are typically accomplished through a progressive sequence of sensorimotor activities that incorporate sensory manipulation and changes in the environmental conditions under which the sports participant is asked to perform motor tasks. Pending further research, functional braces, orthotics, and external compression devices may prove to be useful adjuncts to enhancement of dynamic joint control and functional joint stabilization. For the most part, research has supported the effectiveness of contemporary sensorimotor training protocols in restoration of proprioception and neuromuscular control.

References

Allegrucci, M., S.L. Whitney, S.M. Lephart, J.J. Irrgang, and F.H. Fu. 1995. Shoulder kinesthesia in healthy unilateral athletes participating in upper extremity sports. *Journal of Sports Physical Therapy* 21:220-26.

Allen, A.A. 2000. Neuromuscular contributions to normal shoulder joint kinematics. In *Proprioception and neuromuscular control in joint stability*, edited by S.M. Lephart and F.H. Fu. Champaign Ill.: Human Kinetics.

Andriacchi, T.P., and D. Birac. 1993. Functional testing in the anterior cruciate ligament-deficient knee. *Clinical Orthopaedics and Related Research* 288:40-47.

Arnold, B.L., and R.J. Schmitz. 1998. Examination of balance measures produced by the Biodex Stability System. *Journal of Athletic Training* 33:323-327.

Barber, S.D., F.R. Noyes, R.E. Mangine, J.W. McCloskey, and W. Hartman. 1990. Quantitative assessment of functional limitations in normal and anterior cruciate ligament-deficient knees. *Clinical Orthopaedics and Related Research* 255:204-14.

Barrack, R.L., P.J. Lund, and H.B. Skinner. 1994. Knee joint proprioception revisited. *Journal of Sport Rehabilitation* 3:18-42.

Barrack, R.L., H.B. Skinner, and S.L. Buckley. 1989. Proprioception in the anterior cruciate deficient knee. *The American Journal of Sports Medicine* 17:1-6.

Barrack, R.L., H.B. Skinner, M.E. Brunet, and S.D. Cook. 1983. Joint laxity and proprioception in the knee. *The Physician and Sportsmedicine* 11:130-35.

Barrett, D. 1991. Proprioception and function after anterior cruciate reconstruction. *Journal of Bone and Joint Surgery* 73B:833-37.

Berchuck, M., T.P. Andriacchi, B.R. Bach, and B. Reider. 1990. Gait adaptations by patients who have a deficient anterior cruciate ligament. *Journal of Bone and Joint Surgery* 72A:871-77.

Bernier, J.N., D.H. Perrin, and A. Rijke. 1997. Effect of unilateral functional instability of the ankle on postural sway and inversion and eversion strength. *Journal of Athletic Training* 32:226-32.

Beynnon, B.D., S.H. Ryder, L. Konradsen, R.J. Johnson, K. Johnson, and P.A. Renstrom. 1999. The effect of anterior cruciate ligament trauma and bracing on knee proprioception. *The American Journal of Sports Medicine* 27:150-55.

Bierdert, R.M. 2000. Contributions of the three levels of nervous system motor control: Spinal cord, lower brain, cerebral cortex. In *Proprioception and neuromuscular control in joint stability*, edited by S.M. Lephart and F.H. Fu. Champaign, Ill.: Human Kinetics.

Borsa, P.A., S.M. Lephart, M.S. Kocher, and S.P. Lephart. 1994. Functional assessment and rehabilitation of shoulder proprioception for glenohumeral instability. *Journal of Sport Rehabilitation* 3:84-104.

Branch, T.P., R. Hunter, M. Donath. 1989. Dynamic EMG analysis of anterior cruciate deficient legs with and without bracing during cutting. *The American Journal of Sports Medicine* 17:35-41.

Clark, F.J., K.W. Horch, S.M. Bach, and G.F. Larson. 1979. Contributions of cutaneous and joint receptors to static knee-position sense in man. *Journal of Neurophysiology* 42:877-88.

DeMont, R., and S. Lephart. 1998. Repetition drives neuromuscular recovery after ACL injury. *Biomechanics* (April): 31-37.

Denti, M., M. Monteleone, A. Berardi, and A.S. Panni. 1994. Anterior cruciate ligament mechanoreceptors: Histological studies on lesions and reconstruction. *Clinical Orthopaedics and Related Research* 308:29-32.

Docherty, C.L., J.H. Moore, and B.L. Arnold. 1998. Effects of strength training on strength development and joint position sense in functionally unstable ankles. *Journal of Athletic Training* 33:310-14.

Dvir, A., E. Koren, and N. Halperin. 1988. Knee joint position sense following reconstruction of the anterior cruciate ligament. *Journal of Orthopedic Physical Therapy* 10:117-20.

Fahrer, H., H.U. Rentsch, N.J. Gerber, C. Beyeler, C.W. Hess, and B. Grunig. 1988. Knee effusion and reflex inhibition of the quadriceps. *Journal of Bone and Joint Surgery* 70B:635-38.

Feuerbach, J.W., M.D. Grabiner, T.J. Koh, and G.G. Weiker. 1994. Effect of an ankle orthrosis and ankle ligament anesthesia on ankle joint proprioception. *The American Journal of Sports Medicine* 22:223-29.

Freeman, M.A.R., M.R.E. Dean, and I.W.F. Hanham. 1965. The etiology and prevention of functional instability of the foot. *Journal of Bone and Joint Surgery* 47B:678-85.

Freeman, M.A.R., and B. Wyke. 1967. Articular reflexes of the ankle joint: An electromyographic study of normal and abnormal influences of ankle joint mechanoreceptors upon reflex activity in leg muscles. *British Journal of Surgery* 54:990-1001.

Fu, F.H., C.H. Bennett, C.B. Ma, J. Menetry, and C. Latterman. 2000. Current trends in anterior cruciate ligament reconstruction. *American Journal of Sports Medicine* 28:124-30.

Garn, S.N., and R.A. Newton.1988. Kinesthetic awareness in subjects with multiple ankle sprains. *Physical Therapy* 68:1667-71.

Glencross, D., and E. Thornton. 1981. Position sense following joint injury. *American Journal of Sports Medicine* 21:23-27.

Goertzen, M., J. Gruber, A. Dellmann, H. Clahsen, and K.P. Schulitz. 1992. Neurohistological findings after experimental anterior cruciate ligament allograft transplantation. *Archives of Orthopaedic and Trauma Surgery* 111:126-29.

Goldbeck, T.G., and G.J. Davies. 2000. Test-retest reliability of the closed kinetic chain upper extremity stability test: A clinical field test. *Journal of Sport Rehabilitation* 9:35-45.

Grigg, P. 1994. Peripheral neural mechanisms in proprioception. *Journal of Sport Rehabilitation* 3:2-17.

Guskiewicz, K.M. 1999. Regaining balance and postural equilibrium. In *Rehabilitation techniques in sports medicine*, 3rd ed., edited by W.E. Prentice. Boston: WCB McGraw-Hill.

Harter, R.A., L.R. Osternig, K.M. Singer, S.L. James, R.L. Larson, and D.C. Jones. 1988. Long-term evaluation of knee stability and function following surgical reconstruction for anterior cruciate ligament insufficiency. *American Journal of Sports Medicine* 16:434-43.

Hayashi, K., K.L. Massa, G. Thabit III, G.S. Fanton, M.F. Dillingham, K.W. Gilchrist, and M.D. Markel. 1999. Histologic evaluation of the glenohumeral joint capsule after the laser-assisted capsular shift procedure for glenohumeral instability. *American Journal of Sports Medicine* 27:162-67.

Hillman, S. 1994. Principles and techniques of open kinetic chain rehabilitation: The upper extremity. *Journal of Sport Rehabilitation* 3:319-30.

Hoffman, M., and V.G. Payne. 1995. Effects of proprioceptive ankle disk training on healthy subjects. *Journal of Sports Physical Therapy* 21:90-93.

Hoffman, M., J. Schrader, T. Applegate, and D. Koceja. 1998. Unilateral postural control of the functionally dominant and nondominant extremities of healthy subjects. *Journal of Athletic Training* 33:319-22.

Ihara, H., and A. Nakayama. 1986. Dynamic joint control training for knee ligament injuries. *American Journal of Sports Medicine* 14:309-15.

Irrgang, J.J., S.L. Whitney, and E.D. Cox. 1994. Balance and proprioceptive training for rehabilitation of the lower extremity. *Journal of Sport Rehabilitation* 3:68-83.

Johannson, H., J. Pederson, M. Bergenheim, and M. Djupsjobacka. 2000. Peripheral afferents of the knee: Their effects on central mechanisms regulating muscle stiffness, joint stability, and proprioception and coordination. In *Proprioception and neuromuscular control in joint stability*, edited by S.M. Lephart and F.H. Fu. Champaign, Ill.: Human Kinetics.

Kaminski, T.W., and D.H. Perrin. 1996. Effect of prophylactic knee bracing on balance and joint position sense. *Journal of Athletic Training* 31:131-36.

Kandel, E.R., J.H. Schwartz, and T.M. Jessell, eds. 1995. *Essentials of neural science and behavior.* Norwalk, Conn.: Appleton and Lange.

Kennedy, J.C., I.J. Alexander, and K.C. Hayes. 1982. Nerve supply of the human knee and its functional importance. *American Journal of Sports Medicine* 10:329-35.

Kinzey, S.J., C.D. Ingersoll, and K.L. Knight. 1997. The effects of selected ankle appliances on postural control. *Journal of Athletic Training* 32:300-303.

Lentell, G.L., L.L. Katzman, and M.R. Walters. 1990. The relationship between muscle function and ankle stability. *Journal of Orthopaedic and Sports Physical Therapy* 11:605-11.

Lephart, S. 1994. Reestablishing proprioception, kinesthesia, joint position sense, and neuromuscular control in rehabilitation. In *Rehabilitation techniques in sports medicine,* 2nd ed., edited by W.E. Prentice. St. Louis: Mosby-Year Book.

Lephart, S.M., M.S. Kocher, F.H. Fu, P.A. Borsa, and C.D. Harner. 1992. Proprioception following anterior cruciate ligament reconstruction. *Journal of Sport Rehabilitation* 1:188-96.

Lephart, S.M., M.S. Kocher, C.D. Harner, and F.H. Fu. 1993. Quadriceps strength and functional capacity after anterior cruciate ligament reconstruction. *The American Journal of Sports Medicine* 21:738-43.

Lephart, S.M., D.H. Perrin, F.H. Fu, J.H. Gieck, F.C. McCue III, and J.J. Irrgang. 1992. Relationship between selected physical characteristics and functional capacity in the anterior cruciate ligament-insufficient athlete. *Journal of Sports Physical Therapy* 16:174-81.

Lephart, S.M., D.H. Perrin, F.H. Fu, and K. Minger. 1991. Functional performance tests for the anterior cruciate ligament insufficient athlete. *Athletic Training* 26:44-50.

Lephart, S.M., B.L. Riemann, and F.H. Fu. 2000. Introduction to the sensorimotor system. In *Proprioception and neuromuscular control in joint stability,* edited by S.M. Lephart and F.H. Fu. Champaign, Ill.: Human Kinetics.

Lephart, S.M., J.J.P. Warner, P.A. Borsa, and F.H. Fu. 1994. Proprioception of the shoulder joint in healthy, unstable, and surgically repaired shoulders. *Journal of Shoulder and Elbow Surgery* 3:371-80.

Limbird, T.J., R. Shiavi, M. Frazer, and H. Borra. 1988. EMG profiles of knee joint musculature during walking: Changes induced by anterior cruciate ligament deficiency. *Journal of Orthopaedic Research* 6:630-38.

Lo, I.K.Y., and P.J. Fowler. 2000. Surgical considerations related to proprioception and neuromuscular control. In *Proprioception and neuromuscular control in joint stability,* edited by S.M. Lephart and F.H. Fu. Champaign, Ill.: Human Kinetics.

Loudon, J.K. 2000. Measurement of knee-joint-position sense in women with genu recurvatum. *Journal of Sport Rehabilitation* 9:15-25.

Mattacola, C.G., and J.W. Lloyd. 1997. Effects of a 6-week strength and proprioception training program on measures of dynamic balance: A single-case design. *Journal of Athletic Training* 32:127-35.

Myers, J.B., K.M. Guskiewicz, R.A. Schneider, and W.E. Prentice. 1999. Proprioception and neuromuscular control of the shoulder after muscle fatigue. *Journal of Athletic Training* 34:362-67.

Myers, J.B., and S.M. Lephart. 2000. The role of the sensorimotor system in the athletic shoulder. *Journal of Athletic Training* 35:351-53.

Nitz, A.J., J.J. Dobner, and D. Kersey. 1985. Nerve injury and grades II and III ankle sprains. *American Journal of Sports Medicine* 13:177-82.

Nyland, J., T. Brosky, D. Currier, A. Nitz, and D. Caborn. 1994. Review of the afferent neural system of the knee and its contribution to motor learning. *Journal of Sports Physical Therapy* 19:2-11.

Osternig, L. 2000. The role of coactivation and eccentric activity in the ACL-injured knee. In *Proprioception and neuromuscular control in joint stability,* edited by S.M. Lephart and F.H. Fu. Champaign, Ill.: Human Kinetics.

Parkhurst, T.M., and C.N. Burnett. 1994. Injury and proprioception in the lower back. *Journal of Sports Physical Therapy* 19:282-95.

Perlau, R., C. Frank, and G. Fick. 1995. The effect of elastic bandages on human knee proprioception in the uninjured population. *The American Journal of Sports Medicine* 23:251-55.

Perrin, D.H., and S.J. Shultz. 2000. Models for clinical research involving proprioception and neuromuscular control. In *Proprioception and neuromuscular control in joint stability*, edited by S.M. Lephart and F.H. Fu. Champaign, Ill.: Human Kinetics.

Rivera, J.E. 1994. Open versus closed kinetic chain rehabilitation of the lower extremity: A functional and biomechanical analysis. *Journal of Sport Rehabilitation* 3:154-67.

Rogol, I.M., G. Ernst, and D.H. Perrin. 1998. Open and closed kinetic chain exercises improve shoulder joint reposition sense equally in healthy subjects. *Journal of Athletic Training* 33:315-18.

Rowinski, M.J. 1997. Neurobiology for orthopedic and sports physical therapy. In *Orthopedic and sports physical therapy*, 3rd ed., edited by T.R. Malone, T.G. McPoil, and A.J. Nitz. St. Louis: Mosby-Year Book.

Safran, M.R., G.L. Caldwell Jr., and F.H. Fu. 1994. Proprioception considerations in surgery. *Journal of Sport Rehabilitation* 3:105-15.

Sale, D.G. 1992. Neural adaptations to strength training. In *Strength and power in sport*, edited by P.V. Komi. Cambridge, Mass.: Blackwell Science.

Simoneau, G.G., R.M. Denger, C.A. Kramper, and K.H. Kittleson. 1997. Changes in ankle joint proprioception resulting from strips of athletic tape applied over the skin. *Journal of Athletic Training* 32:141-47.

Skinner, H.B., M.P. Wyatt, J.A. Hodgdon, D.W. Conrad, and R.L. Barrack. 1986. Effect of fatigue on joint position sense of the knee. *Journal of Orthopaedic Research* 4:112-18.

Smith, R.L., and J. Brunolli. 1989. Shoulder kinesthesia after glenohumeral joint dislocation. *Physical Therapy* 69:106-12.

Solomonow, M., R. Baratta, B.H. Zhou, H. Shoji, W. Bose, C. Beck, and R. D'Ambrosia. 1987. The synergistic action of the anterior cruciate ligament and thigh muscles in maintaining joint stability. *The American Journal of Sports Medicine* 15:207-13.

Spencer, J.D., K.C. Hayes, and I.J. Alexander. 1984. Knee joint effusion and quadriceps reflex inhibition in man. *Archives of Physical Medicine and Rehabilitation* 65:171-77.

Stone, J.A., N.B. Partin, J.S. Lueken, K.E. Timm, and E.J. Ryan. 1994. Upper extremity proprioception training. *Journal of Athletic Training* 29:15-18.

Styf, J.R., O. Lundin, and D.H. Gershuni. 1994. Effects of a functional knee brace on leg muscle function. *The American Journal of Sports Medicine* 22:830-34.

Tegner, Y., J. Lysholm, M. Lysholm, and J. Gillquist. 1986. A performance test to monitor rehabilitation and evaluate anterior cruciate ligament injuries. *American Journal of Sports Medicine* 14:156-59.

Thomas, C.L., ed. 1993. *Taber's cyclopedic medical dictionary*, 17th ed. Philadelphia: Davis.

Tibone, J.E., T.J. Antich, G.S. Fanton, D.R. Moynes, and J. Perry. 1986. Functional analysis of anterior cruciate ligament instability. *The American Journal of Sports Medicine* 14:276-84.

Tropp, H., and P. Odenrick. 1988. Postural control in single-limb stance. *Journal of Orthopaedic Research* 6:833-39.

Tropp, H., P. Odenrick, and J. Gillquist. 1985. Stabilometry recordings in functional and mechanical instability of the ankle joint. *International Journal of Sports Medicine* 6:180-82.

Voss, D.E., M.K. Ionta, and B.J. Myers. 1985. *Proprioceptive neuromuscular facilitation: Patterns and techniques*, 3rd ed. Philadelphia: Harper and Row.

Walla, D.J., J.P. Albright, E. McAuley, R.K. Martin, V. Eldridge, and G. El-Khoury. 1985. Hamstring control and the unstable anterior cruciate ligament-deficient knee. *The American Journal of Sports Medicine* 13:34-39.

Wilk, K.E., W.T. Romaniello, S.M. Soscia, C.A. Arrigo, and J.R. Andrews. 1994. The relationship between subjective knee scores, isokinetic testing, and functional testing in the ACL-reconstructed knee. *Journal of Sports Physical Therapy* 20:60-73.

Wilkerson, G.B. 1991. Treatment of the inversion ankle sprain through synchronous application of focal compression and cold. *Athletic Training* 26:220-37.

Wilkerson, G.B., and A.J. Nitz. 1994. Dynamic ankle stability: Mechanical and neuromuscular interrelationships. *Journal of Sport Rehabilitation* 3:43-57.

Zatterstrom, R., T. Friden, A. Lindstrand, and U. Mortiz. 1994. The effect of physiotherapy on standing balance in chronic anterior cruciate ligament insufficiency. *The American Journal of Sports Medicine* 22:531-36.

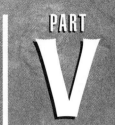

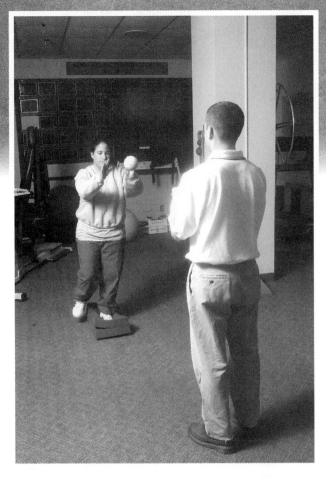

Problem Solving in Sports Injury Management

Previous parts of this book have addressed sport-related soft tissue injuries, fractures, and proprioceptive and sensorimotor deficits with corresponding implications for therapeutic management. Application of the problem-oriented approach to therapeutic management of these conditions is the primary purpose of this part. Chapter 10, Sports Injury Assessment and Problem Identification, is an introduction to the problem-oriented medical system with particular emphasis on use of the problem-oriented medical record, or SOAP notes. The SOAP note format is discussed as a framework for documenting information derived from logical decision making in injury management. Whereas clinical assessment and identification of a patient's health-related problems are emphasized in chapter 10, development of treatment and rehabilitation plans is the primary focus in chapter 11, Sports Injury Treatment and Rehabilitation Planning. This chapter addresses formulation of long-term and short-term rehabilitation goals and presents a conceptual model for rehabilitation of sports injuries. Together, these two chapters provide a comprehensive review of the problem-oriented approach to injury management, from the time of injury to resumption of sports activities.

Sports Injury Assessment and Problem Identification

The Problem-Oriented Medical Record
SOAP Notes
Clinical Assessment
and Problem Identification

Initial Clinical Assessment
The Problem List

Summary

Learning Objectives

After completion of this chapter, the reader should be able to

1. describe the benefits of using the problem-oriented medical record (SOAP notes) for documentation of sports health care information,

2. identify and describe the appropriate type of health care information to be documented in each of the four categories of a SOAP note,

3. describe the primary purposes of an initial clinical assessment as a basis for development of sports injury rehabilitation programs, and

4. describe the purposes and benefits of developing a patient problem list as a component of SOAP note documentation.

The sports injury pathology, tissue-healing mechanisms, and therapeutic challenges discussed throughout previous chapters indicate a clear need for a coordinated, focused approach to injury management involving the collective expertise of the sports health care team. Issues regarding coordination of services and communication among health care providers are not unique to sports health care, however. Although applied in one form or another for many years, the concept referred to as the *problem-oriented medical system* (POMS) emerged in the late 1960s as an effort to provide a uniform approach to health care delivery, patient treatment, and outcomes assessment in the medical arena (Gabriel 1992). With individualized modifications, the POMS has been implemented in hospitals, clinics, and other health care facilities throughout the United States. In a broad sense, the POMS includes three basic components: (1) a problem-oriented medical record that facilitates standardized documentation of medical information and rehabilitation progress, (2) a criterion-referenced auditing system that permits evaluation of treatment effectiveness, and (3) an educational program designed to correct deficiencies and improve health care services. While an auditing system to monitor the quality of health care delivery and an educational program to enhance health care services are integral components of the problem-oriented medical system, the problem-solving approach to sports injury management can best be clarified by a discussion of the problem-oriented medical record.

The Problem-Oriented Medical Record

Despite its widespread adoption in the general medical community, use of the problem-oriented medical record (POMR), commonly referred to as *SOAP notes*, evolved at a slower pace in traditional sports health care settings (e.g., high schools, colleges, professional sports). Incorporation of the POMR in a sports health care facility requires conscientious commitment to an organized system of injury evaluation, treatment planning, and outcomes assessment. Although personnel shortages, time constraints, and other difficulties in fully implementing the POMR system in the athletic setting are acknowledged, contemporary thought supports the view that if sports health care clinicians are providing services in traditional athletic training rooms and treatment centers, they are operating in a health care facility that should be subject to appropriate standards of operation analogous to those applied to health care facilities in the public domain (National Athletic Trainers' Association Board of Certification 2000). Aside from enhancing compliance with professional standards, as well as state and federal legislation and third-party payer requirements, the POMR format provides the clinician with a systematic guide to sports injury rehabilitation that facilitates achievement of positive functional outcomes (e.g., successful return to sports activities). The organizational format of the POMR represents a system for documentation of data that parallels a logical sequence of clinical assessment, identification of health problems related to a patient's injury status, and development of corresponding treatment plans. Additionally, the POMR format facilitates subsequent documentation of rehabilitation progress, continuation or resolution of particular health problems, and modification of treatment plans. Thus, the POMR transcends the sports participant's entire recovery period, from initial clinical assessment to discharge. Ideally, it provides a standardized, uninterrupted reference for all members of the sports health care team, thereby enhancing communication and coordination of health care services.

SOAP Notes

Based on the acronym SOAP, a major feature of the POMR is organization of documented information in four primary categories: (1) subjective information (S), (2) objective information (O), (3) assessment (A), and (4) treatment plans (P) (Kettenbach 1995). Thus, the POMR has traditionally been referred to by health care providers as *SOAP notes*. Figure 10.1 is an

University of _____
Department of Intercollegiate Athletics

Injury evaluation/Treatment record

Name _____ Date of birth _____

Date of injury _____ Sport _____

Diagnosis (Medical):

Subjective (S)

History (medical treatment, surgery, etc.):

Chief complaint (e.g., pain):

Objective (O)

Functional status (ambulation, mobility, etc.):

Physical status (ROM, muscle strength, etc.):

Assessment (A)

Patient problems:

Long-term goals:

Short-term goals:

Plan (P)

Clinician signature _____ Date _____

Figure 10.1 Sample of sports injury evaluation and treatment record (SOAP note format).

From *Musculoskeletal Trauma: Implications for Sports Injury Management* by Gary Delforge, 2002, Champaign, Ill.: Human Kinetics.

example of a sports injury evaluation and treatment record that incorporates the SOAP note format. As computer technology continues to enhance the efficiency and consistency of health care documentation, particular methods of recording data will no doubt change accordingly. Nevertheless, the thought processes and problem-solving sequence that characterize use of the SOAP format will most likely withstand the test of time. An overview of the SOAP note format is warranted as an illustration of the problem-oriented approach to sports injury management.

The first two sections of the SOAP note format provide for documentation of subjective (S) and objective (O) information gathered during the clinician's assessment of the patient. In the initial clinical assessment, this data complements information gleaned from the patient's medical history, laboratory reports, surgical reports, and similar sources. When combined, the accumulated information forms the *database*. Data entered in the subjective section of the SOAP note is provided by the patient and commonly includes, but is not limited to, the patient's symptoms. For example, subjective information is exemplified should a patient with a knee injury state, "The pain wakes me up at night." A SOAP note to this effect clearly indicates something the patient tells the examining clinician, as opposed to information gathered through objective clinical assessment of various physical parameters (e.g., strength levels, joint mobility). An expression of pain, for example, may warrant subsequent inclusion on the patient's *problem list*. The problem list, which may appear in the assessment (A) section of the SOAP note, is a concise listing of the patient's primary health-related problems that become a focus of therapeutic intervention. Other appropriate data in the subjective section might include information related to the patient's goals, feelings and attitude, social environment, and response to previous treatment (e.g., pain relief) (Kettenbach 1995).

In contrast to subjective information (S), objective information (O) in the SOAP note is illustrated by the results of clinical examinations and observations such as goniometric measurements of joint motion, isokinetic strength testing, and limb girth measurements. In the previous example of a patient with a knee injury, quantitative goniometric verification of limited joint motion may suggest a second entry on the patient's problem list, pending further clinician analysis and determination of the cause of restricted movement. As these examples illustrate, objective data are measurable and testing procedures to collect the data are repeatable (Kettenbach 1995), thus providing a baseline for subsequent progress evaluation. In some facilities, relevant information taken from the patient's medical record is included in the objective (O) section of a SOAP note.

The third component of the SOAP note format, the assessment (A) section, provides an opportunity for the clinician to document his or her professional analysis of the patient's health condition based on information in the database, including the subjective and objective data in the first two sections (S and O). In the assessment section, the sports health care clinician's synthesis and analysis commonly reflect identification of the patient's health problems that become the focus of therapeutic intervention. As summarized by Kettenbach (1995), the assessment section of the SOAP note format includes the problem list, long-term goals, short-term goals, and a summary of the clinician's professional judgment regarding the patient's health problems, goals, and treatment plans.

The fourth component of the SOAP note format, documentation of treatment plans (P) that address each of the patient's problems, represents a logical extension of the examining clinician's thought processes during completion of the first three SOAP note sections (S, O, and A). As discussed further in chapter 11, treatment plans typically address short-term goals (i.e., interim goals) rather than long-term goals (e.g., return to activity). As such, they indicate the specific type, frequency, and progression of treatment. Plans for referral to other services or consultation with other health care providers may also be included in this section.

It is significant to note that the SOAP note format does not represent a treatment method but rather an organized system of documenting sequential steps in the decision-making process. As applied to clinical decision making in sports health care, the SOAP note format involves development of a database (accumulation of information), clinical assessment and identification of health problems (problem analysis), consideration of various treatment strategies (alternative actions), and finally, determination of therapeutic objectives and selection of therapeutic agents (course of action). Thus, adoption of the SOAP documentation format compels the sports health care clinician to employ fundamentally sound decision-making skills in injury management. As illustrated throughout the following discussion of clinical assessment and problem identification, sound decision making is an inescapable challenge in effective sports injury management.

Clinical Assessment and Problem Identification

As the term implies, the problem-oriented approach to health care is based on identification and resolution of a patient's health "problems," which traditionally are stated in specific clinical terms (e.g., restricted joint motion, strength loss). With respect to sports medicine, however, Gabriel (1992, p. 42) offered a more global definition, stating that "a problem is any significant deviation from the norm that has influenced, is influencing, or may influence the athlete's health or capacity to perform at the level of ability demanded by the sport." As this broad definition suggests, a sports participant's health problems may involve multifaceted physical, psychological, or sociological dimensions that necessitate clear, specific problem identification and a coordinated team approach to resolution.

Before embarking on a treatment regimen, it behooves the sports health care clinician to assess an injured sports participant's medical, physical, and psychological status for four primary purposes: (1) identification of specific health problems, and thus a focus of therapeutic intervention, (2) formulation of realistic, attainable goals and objectives, (3) establishment of baseline parameters for subsequent evaluation of rehabilitation progress (e.g., initial strength levels, range of joint motion), and (4) selection of appropriate and effective treatment protocols. A review of the SOAP note format indicates provision for documentation of information related to each of these functions.

Initial Clinical Assessment

Experience has indicated a need for clarification of the concept *initial clinical assessment* as interpreted by various sports health care providers. In a general sense, an initial clinical assessment is that which occurs during the clinician's first encounter with the patient. As such, the initial assessment is designed to elicit information upon which subsequent decisions are based (e.g., a course of treatment). In the sports health care setting, however, the initial patient encounter varies with the circumstances. Correspondingly, the decisions to be made also differ. For example, a certified athletic trainer's initial encounter with an injured athlete commonly occurs on the playing field or in the athletic training room before a physician's examination and diagnosis. In this scenario, an injury evaluation (i.e., an initial clinical assessment) is indicated for the primary purpose of decision making related to emergency care, acute injury management, and medical disposition. In contrast, the sports health care clinician's initial patient encounter in a sports medicine clinic typically follows a physician's diagnosis and referral for treatment. Consequently, the decisions to be made in these circumstances differ from those required during emergency management and disposition in the athletic setting. Although similar evaluation techniques are commonly used in both scenarios (e.g., subjective and objective data collection), the fundamental purpose of an initial clinical assessment after a physician's diagnosis and referral to the sports health care clinician is to establish a basis for decision making regarding therapeutic intervention and rehabilitation.

Clinical assessment as a basis for development of therapeutic strategies and treatment protocols is the relevant discussion topic in this chapter. In this regard, it is important to note that clinical assessment is a continuing process throughout the patient's recovery period. While clinicians strive for identification and assessment of all relevant health factors during the initial patient encounter, complicating factors (e.g., pain, swelling) may, in some cases, preclude valid assessment of some parameters, muscle strength for example. In this example, baseline strength measurements may be postponed, out of necessity, to subsequent treatment sessions, after which the complicating signs and symptoms have subsided. In other cases, signs and symptoms that appear after the initial patient encounter may indicate a need for follow-up assessment. For example, joint stiffness that commonly exists after removal of an immobilization device may require assessment and therapeutic attention. In the event that follow-up evaluations identify clinically significant problems, in addition to those identified during the initial assessment, the new problem should be added to the patient's problem list as a focus for therapeutic intervention.

Before further discussion, it is important to emphasize that a broad interpretation of the term *clinical assessment* has been adopted to include consideration of relevant information obtained from various sources. For example, data collected during the initial patient encounter should be complemented by information obtained from diagnostic reports, laboratory tests, surgical reports, and similar sources, as well as information obtained through consultation with attending physicians. Despite legitimate confidentiality issues, the sports health care clinician who is responsible for prudent therapeutic intervention should strive to establish "need to know" medical information that may have an impact on therapeutic protocols. In this context, the actual clinical assessment is one of several sources, albeit a critical source of information.

As an additional consideration, it is important to recognize that a clinical examination may elicit only signs and symptoms of underlying pathology. In a previously cited example, a patient's expression of pain is a typical symptom of underlying pathology that commonly warrants inclusion on the patient's problem list. In this example, symptomatic treatment (i.e., for pain) may be appropriate pending further analysis. In other cases, however, the sports health care clinician's analytical skills are frequently challenged to identify the cause of a particular sign or symptom before proceeding with treatment. Although a simple goniometric measurement, for example, may quantify a loss of physiological joint motion (a clinical sign), it does not necessarily reveal the underlying cause of restricted motion. On the premise that acute inflammatory responses (e.g., pain, joint effusion) have subsided and, consequently, have been ruled out as contributing factors in this example, the clinician may attribute loss of joint motion to contractures or adhesions in noncontractile articular tissues (e.g., joint capsules), contractile periarticular tissues (i.e., muscles), or both (see chapter 5). A treatment approach that addresses only the most obvious clinical sign in this case (i.e., restricted physiological joint motion) with traditional passive range of motion exercises may produce less than optimal results if, in fact, the accessory joint motions (e.g., roll, spin, slide) that permit normal physiological movements are restricted. In this case, selection of an appropriate treatment method (e.g., joint mobilization techniques) is dependent on determination of the restricting tissues (i.e., capsuloligamentous structures) in addition to identification of the clinical sign (i.e., limited physiological movement).

Although a discussion of specific examination techniques is beyond the scope of this chapter, a summary of factors that commonly necessitate assessment is presented in table 10.1. This summary is not meant to imply that all parameters need to be addressed in individual cases, nor is the categorization intended to be exhaustive. Rather, the assessment categories are intended to identify typical parameters that the sports health care clinician should be prepared to address should assessment be indicated by the patient's medical history or current signs and symptoms. As presented in table 10.1, general evaluation categories are summarized with identification of specific corresponding factors that may be in need of assessment.

Table 10.1   Sports Injury Assessment Categories

Assessment category	Specific parameters
Inflammatory responses	Effusion/edema Erythema Hyperthermia Pain/muscle spasm
Surgical results	Surgical procedure Fixation/immobilization devices Anatomical/biomechanical alterations
Joint mobility	ROM (degrees) Physiological movements Accessory joint motions Pain (end range pain, painful arc, etc.) Capsuloligamentous integrity
Flexibility	Muscle shortening Bilateral imbalances/asymmetry
Muscle strength/atrophy	Muscle/muscle group strength levels Bilateral imbalances Agonist/antagonist strength ratios Limb girth
Neurological status	Sensation (pain, temperature, touch, paresthesia) Motor function (tendon reflexes, paresis, etc.)
Pain	Onset/duration Location (local, referred, radiating) Type (sharp, dull, aching, etc.) Nature (constant, intermittent) Intensity Behavior (exacerbating factors, etc.)
Posture/gait	Structural/functional postural deviations Walking/running gait
Physical fitness	Body weight/composition Cardiovascular fitness Muscular strength/endurance
Psychological/emotional status	Self-concept Emotions (fear, anxiety, etc.) Coping skills Motivation

The Problem List

In the problem-oriented system, as applied to sports injury management, a patient's problem list is derived from a synthesis and analysis of information included in the database. A problem list is simply a listing of health problems related to the patient's current injury status. The problem list includes major parameters that are not within normal limits (e.g., the typical range of motion in a normal, healthy joint). Hence, each problem becomes a focus of therapeutic attention until resolved during treatment. As such, the problem list is a critical component of the problem-oriented medical record (POMR) that provides organization, direction, and continuity to therapeutic intervention by members of the sports health care team, each of whom focus their respective areas of expertise on resolution of particular problems. For example, a problem list for a patient who is recovering from knee surgery may include (1) joint pain, (2) disturbed sleep patterns, (3) limited joint motion, and (4) muscle weakness (e.g., quadriceps muscles, hamstrings). Each of these problems suggest a need for formulation of specific short-term goals and a treatment plan to resolve the problem.

In some health care settings, each entry on a patient's problem list is numbered, typically on a priority basis. In the above case, for example, a team physician may prescribe an analgesic medication to address the joint pain (i.e., problem number one). If pain is the reason the patient is awakened at night, pain medication may also resolve the second problem (i.e., disturbed sleep pattern). Should alleviation of pain and restoration of normal sleep patterns result from the physician's treatment, resolution of these two problems is noted and dated in the SOAP note. The third and fourth problems on the list, limited joint motion and muscle weakness, however, remain in need of resolution, most likely through intervention by a certified athletic trainer or physical therapist. As resolution of these problems occurs, additional notes to this effect are entered and dated in the SOAP note.

As previously indicated, the SOAP format allows for documentation of progress toward resolution of each problem identified on the patient's problem list. Ideally, progress notes address each problem separately. Depending on the circumstances, however, progress notes after a particular treatment session do not necessarily need to address all problems on the list. Professional judgment and practicality typically guide the experienced clinician's decision with regard to timely entry of progress notes. Even though SOAP note documentation may eventually indicate resolution of all problems on a patient's initial problem list, it does not necessarily follow that discharge and return to sports activities is indicated. As noted earlier, problems identified subsequent to the initial clinical assessment should be added to the problem list and addressed accordingly. In the event of knee surgery, for example, proprioception testing may reveal postoperative proprioceptive and sensorimotor deficits that require therapeutic intervention and resolution before return to sports activities (see chapter 9). As this scenario suggests, identification and resolution of all problems that may preclude safe and successful sports participation is a critical consideration. Use of a problem list not only enhances this process but also facilitates decisions regarding resumption of sports activities based on resolution of each particular problem.

Summary

The problem-oriented medical system (POMS) represents an organized approach to health care delivery designed to enhance coordination of services and communication among health care providers. Over the past several years, concepts inherent in this system have been increasingly applied to sports injury management. As an integral component of the problem-oriented approach, the problem-oriented medical record (POMR or, more commonly, SOAP notes) provides an organized format for documentation of information related to clinical assessment of a patient's injury, identification of the patient's health problems that become the focus of therapeutic intervention, and formulation of treatment plans. The format, based on the acronym SOAP, guides documentation of relevant information in four primary categories: subjective information (S), objective information (O), assessment (A), and treatment plans (P). Implementation of the SOAP note format provides a standardized reference for all members of the sports health care team, thus promoting communication and coordination of services.

The clinician's clinical assessment and identification of a patient's relevant health problems are fundamental to the problem-oriented approach to sports injury management. Accurately identified heath problems and determination of causative factors provide a focus for therapeutic intervention throughout the sports participant's recovery period. These processes are facilitated by development of a problem list that documents the primary health-related problems to be resolved.

References

Gabriel, A.J. 1992. The problem-oriented approach to sports injury evaluations. *Journal of Athletic Training* 27:40-42.

Kettenbach, G. 1995. *Writing SOAP notes*, 2nd ed. Philadelphia: Davis.

National Athletic Trainers' Association Board of Certification. 2000. *Standards of professional practice.* Omaha, Neb.: National Athletic Trainers' Association Board of Certification.

Sports Injury Treatment and Rehabilitation Planning

Rehabilitation Goals and Objectives
    Long-Term Rehabilitation Goals
    Short-Term Rehabilitation Goals
    Therapeutic and Behavioral Objectives
    Behavioral Approach
**Principles and Concepts
in Rehabilitation Planning**
    Elements of Sports Injury Rehabilitation
    Sports Injury Rehabilitation: A Conceptual
    Model

Early Rehabilitation Phase (Phase I)
Intermediate Rehabilitation Phase (Phase II)
Late Rehabilitation Phase (Phase III)
    Resumption of Activity
    and Treatment Discharge
Summary

Learning Objectives

After completion of this chapter, the reader should be able to

1. describe the purposes and benefits of formulating long-term and short-term goals in sports injury rehabilitation,

2. differentiate between a therapeutic objective and a behavioral objective as applied to rehabilitation of sports injuries,

3. write short-term treatment goals that incorporate the four basic elements of a behavioral objective, and

4. describe the three major phases of a sports injury rehabilitation program and relate the primary therapeutic objectives in each phase.

Clinical assessment, including accumulation of subjective and objective data, and identification of a patient's health problems are the fundamental initial steps in the problem-oriented approach to sports injury management. Whereas these steps were discussed in chapter 10, this chapter addresses subsequent steps in the problem-oriented approach, specifically formulation of rehabilitation goals and development of treatment plans. A review of the SOAP note format discussed in chapter 10 indicates that therapeutic strategies begin with development of long-term and short-term goals, which the clinician begins to formulate and document in the assessment (A) section of the SOAP note (Kettenbach 1995).

Rehabilitation Goals and Objectives

The scope of rehabilitation planning in sports health care characteristically ranges from global conceptualization of the overall rehabilitation plan, including the general time frame, to determination of therapeutic strategies to resolve specific health problems during each phase of the recovery period. Consequently, effective planning not only requires identification of long-term rehabilitation goals but also necessitates development of short-term (i.e., interim) goals to provide direction to attainment of desired functional outcomes throughout the recovery period.

Long-Term Rehabilitation Goals

After a sports injury, most highly motivated competitive and recreational athletes have an inherent long-term goal of returning to sports participation. Fortunately, given the quality of current sports health care practices, resumption of sports activities is an attainable goal in most cases. Although a long-term goal, including return to sports participation, may be attainable, it must also be realistic with regard to the length of time necessary for full recovery. For example, it may be unrealistic for a college football player who sustains an anterior cruciate ligament (ACL) injury during the latter part of the fall season, consequently requiring surgery, to recover in time for spring practice. With exceptions, however, resumption of competition during the following fall season is typically a realistic expectation. In comparison, return to sports activities within a few weeks after a grade II ankle sprain, for example, is commonly a realistic expectation.

As these examples illustrate, long-term rehabilitation goals are relative, with time frames typically dependent on the nature and severity of specific injuries. As team physicians, certified athletic trainers, and other sports health care clinicians encounter injuries of a similar type and severity, they become particularly adept in counseling injured athletes with regard to attainable goals and realistic time frames. Although the long-term goal of a motivated athlete (i.e., return to sports activities) is commonly taken for granted, adherence to the SOAP note format described in chapter 10 requires documentation in the assessment (A) section (Kettenbach 1995).

Short-Term Rehabilitation Goals

Because long-term goals are often too general to provide meaningful day-to-day direction and patient motivation during recovery from a sports injury, specific short-term (i.e., interim) goals are a primary characteristic of effective rehabilitation programs, especially if a prolonged recovery is anticipated. Like long-term rehabilitation goals, the time frames specified in short-term goals are relative, ranging from days to weeks, or longer. Regardless of the time frame, however, short-term goals represent interim goals to be achieved at particular intervals during the rehabilitation program. Clearly identified short-term goals serve several purposes. First, specific interim goals related to each of the health problems identified in a patient's problem list provide a focus for coordinated treatment by members of the sports health care team. Second, clear short-term goals establish a basis for selection of appropriate therapeutic agents (i.e., pharmacological and physical agents). Third, appropriately stated short-term goals identify criteria for the patient's progression throughout various phases of the rehabilitation program. Finally, realistic and attainable but challenging short-term goals provide a motivational basis for the patient.

Therapeutic and Behavioral Objectives

With regard to sports injury management, short-term rehabilitation goals may represent therapeutic objectives or behavioral objectives. For clarification purposes, a distinction is made between the terms *therapeutic objectives and behavioral objectives.* As discussed in previous chapters, particular treatment modalities, heat applications for example, produce predictable physiological responses (e.g., increased blood flow) that are conducive to connective tissue repair. In this example, the objective (i.e., increased blood flow) is therapeutic in nature. In another example, use of physical agents that evoke "gating" mechanisms of pain control represents a treatment strategy to achieve a therapeutic objective (i.e., pain reduction). While therapeutic objectives guide selection of particular treatment modalities throughout the recovery period, achievement of the desired therapeutic effects (e.g., pain relief, edema reduction) facilitates the patient's attainment of specified behavioral objectives. In this context, therapeutic objectives identify a treatment effect to be achieved by the attending clinician, whereas behavioral objectives represent challenges to be met by the patient. In the case of an athlete with a lower extremity injury for example, progression from an antalgic walking gait to successful performance of sport-related motor tasks (e.g., running, cutting, jumping) necessitates the patient's active involvement in achievement of a behavioral objective. The behavioral change in this example is obviously functional in nature. Thus, establishment of behavioral objectives in sports injury management is consistent with current concepts of sport-specific functional rehabilitation.

The five primary categories of therapeutic intervention in connective tissue repair introduced in chapter 1 (i.e., control of hemorrhage and edema, alleviation of pain and muscle spasm, and so on) are most appropriately viewed as therapeutic objectives. In comparison, however, the functional nature of proprioceptive and sensorimotor training, previously identified as a sixth major category of intervention in sports injury management, suggests a patient's achievement of behavioral objectives (i.e., functional outcomes). As a recovering patient becomes progressively active throughout the rehabilitation process, progress is most appropriately assessed in terms of functional (i.e., behavioral) achievements.

Behavioral Approach

As described by DePalma and DePalma (1989), the behavioral approach to sports injury management is characterized by establishment of short-term subgoals (i.e., behavioral objectives) that culminate in achievement of long-term goals (e.g., return to sports activity). Effective short-term behavioral objectives, or subgoals, have several defining characteristics. First, as noted earlier, the objective is stated in terms of what the patient is to accomplish, rather than what the clinician does to assist in the process. For example, a short-term goal stated in behavioral terms is illustrated by a SOAP note entry such as "Patient will demonstrate active terminal knee extension to 0° flexion in the sitting position within two weeks." In this example, the four basic elements of a properly stated behavioral objective are included. First, the *audience,* or the person to perform the task, is identified (the patient). Second, the expected *behavior* is specified (demonstration of active terminal knee extension). Third, the *condition* under which the task is to be performed is identified (the sitting position). Last, the *degree* to which the task is to be performed is specified (knee extension to 0° flexion within two weeks).

As the above example illustrates, effective short-term rehabilitation goals are specific and measurable. In this regard, it is significant to note that the short-term goal stated earlier (active terminal knee extension) corresponds to a specific entry on the patient's problem list (i.e., limited joint motion). In addition, a well-conceived short-term goal is not only measurable, but the assessment techniques to determine progress toward achievement are repeatable. As exemplified by the previous example, knee extension can be measured quantitatively and repeatedly by the use of a goniometer. Because achievement of short-term (i.e., interim) goals commonly becomes a criterion for progression through various phases of the rehabilitation program, measurability and repeatability become important characteristics. In many instances, subjective determination of a patient's readiness for progression based on the knowledge and experience of a physician or sports health care clinician is appropriate and justifiable. Nevertheless, subjective decision making based on quantitative clinical assessment is desirable.

In addition to specificity and measurability, appropriate short-term goals are characteristically realistic and attainable. In this regard, DePalma and DePalma (1989) described an "optimal" short-term subgoal as a challenge that does not doom the patient to failure; nor is it easy enough to guarantee success. As these authors noted, achievement of optimal short-term goals provides the greatest amount of reinforcement and motivation for the recovering patient, thereby enhancing the likelihood of accomplishing long-term goals. A key factor in establishing realistic and attainable short-term goals is the clinician's knowledge of the tissue-healing process, the time factors involved, and the effect of treatment methods on body tissues at any particular stage of recovery. In a general sense, formulation of realistic short-term goals throughout the recovery period parallels but does not surpass the sequential events of tissue-healing. In this regard, flexibility in modifying time frames as the circumstances indicate is another feature of effective goal setting (DePalma and DePalma 1989).

Principles and Concepts in Rehabilitation Planning

The three fundamental steps in the problem-oriented approach to sports injury rehabilitation involve clinical assessment and problem identification, formulation of long-term and short-term rehabilitation goals, and development of treatment plans. Previous discussion of the SOAP note format indicated that treatment plans are a logical outgrowth of short-term goals that address specific health problems during particular stages of the rehabilitation program. Whereas the assessment (A) section of the SOAP note provides for documentation of short-term goals, corresponding treatment plans are documented in the treatment plan (P) section as the final step in the planning process. While treatment plans that specify particular therapeutic modalities, dosages, and frequency of treatment provide direction and continuity in short-term patient care, treatment plans should also be viewed in a broader context, particularly as related to the overall rehabilitation program and expected functional outcomes. Hence, the remainder of this chapter is devoted to a discussion of basic principles and concepts in comprehensive rehabilitation program planning in sports injury management. This includes presentation of a conceptual model that provides a framework for development and incorporation of short-term goals and criteria for the patient's progression throughout the recovery period.

Elements of Sports Injury Rehabilitation

In general, a well-planned sports injury rehabilitation program demonstrates three primary characteristics. The first characteristic is overlapping, but identifiable, sequential *phases* that reflect the patient's progression. As discussed shortly, an early, intermediate, and late phase of injury rehabilitation can be identified. In a general sense, these three phases parallel the three primary stages of soft connective tissue repair discussed in chapter 3 (i.e., inflammation, scar formation, and scar maturation) and the analogous stages of fracture healing reviewed in chapter 6 (i.e., hematoma formation and inflammation, cellular proliferation and callus formation, and remodeling). Thus, the extent of tissue repair and the structural and biomechanical integrity of healing tissues are primary determinants of the therapeutic strategies and protocols that characterize each phase of the rehabilitation program.

While the overall sports injury rehabilitation model described later in this chapter is characterized by three primary sequential phases, each phase includes two basic components: (1) short-term (i.e., interim) goals and (2) corresponding criteria for the patient's progression to the subsequent rehabilitation phase. Development of short-term rehabilitation goals is a fundamental step in the problem-solving approach to sports injury management. Ideally, well-stated short-term goals inherently reflect measurable criteria that, if achieved, guide decision making regarding the patient's progression throughout the recovery period. In many cases, particularly during the early and intermediate stages of rehabilitation, quantitative determination of goal achievement is comparatively uncomplicated (e.g., joint range of motion, muscle strength levels). However, as a patient progresses through the rehabilitation program, criteria for progression inherently become more functional in nature, ultimately culminating in successful performance of sport-specific motor tasks. Consequently, quantitative progress assessment becomes more challenging, often necessitating an interpretation of the term *functional* as related to sports activities. For example, in the 1960s and 1970s, isokinetic testing of muscle group strength, power, and endurance (e.g., the quadriceps muscles, hamstrings) was projected as a measure of functional ability. Consequently, considerable credence was given to isokinetic strength levels as an indicator of "complete" rehabilitation and readiness for sports participation. Although isokinetic strength testing was highly touted, experienced sports health care clinicians recognized that isokinetic tests offer only limited assessment of the parameters that indicate readiness for resumption of sports activities.

While individual muscle and muscle group strength levels commonly serve as a useful criterion for progression from the intermediate phase to the late phase of rehabilitation, successful performance of sport-related motor tasks that require neuromuscular joint control and dynamic balance (e.g., figure eight running, carioca crossover maneuver) represents a more functional criterion for return to full sports participation (Lephart et al. 1991). These examples of progression criteria illustrate a basic principle of rehabilitation planning in sports injury management. That is, the criteria for progression from one phase of rehabilitation to the next should reflect the demands to be placed on the recovering patient during the subsequent phase. Consequently, the sports health care clinician is presented with two primary challenges. First, it behooves the clinician to be knowledgeable about the physical demands of a particular sport and, specifically, the effect of these demands on recovering body structures. Second, the sports health care clinician is challenged to quantify and validate the assessment techniques used to determine the patient's preparedness to meet anticipated demands. As noted earlier, this challenge increases as rehabilitation activities become more functional in nature. The objective criteria for progression described by Lephart et al. (1991) for the anterior cruciate ligament (ACL)-deficient athlete represents an excellent example of relating progression criteria to anticipated sport-specific demands. The functional performance tests described by these authors (cocontraction test, carioca crossover maneuver, shuttle run) are designed to elicit pathological joint motions typically associated with ACL deficiency (e.g., anterior tibial translation, pivot shift), thereby requiring dynamic joint control to meet the demands of sports participation.

Sports Injury Rehabilitation: A Conceptual Model

The conceptual model for sports injury rehabilitation presented in this section incorporates characteristic rehabilitation phases, short-term (i.e., interim) goals, and progression criteria that provide a framework for program planning. Because rehabilitation programs are most appropriately designed on an individual basis, it would be presumptuous to suggest a definitive plan that accommodates all cases. Nevertheless, sports injury rehabilitation programs have several defining characteristics that, collectively, provide a useful conceptual model that can be adapted to individual cases, particularly if a prolonged recovery period is anticipated. The proposed model is based on the premise that team physicians, certified athletic trainers, and other sports health care providers who function in an athletic setting are involved in the patient's entire recovery process, from the time of injury through resumption of sports activities. Consequently, a comprehensive model that transcends all phases of the recovery period is presented.

As indicated earlier, three primary rehabilitation phases provide the general framework for more definitive program planning in sports injury rehabilitation. These phases include an early phase (Phase I), an intermediate phase (Phase II), and a late phase (Phase III). Table 11.1 provides an overview of the proposed rehabilitation model, including a general description of each sequential phase as related to the progressive stages of soft connective tissue repair. Although changing interim goals and treatment protocols provide distinguishing characteristics for each of these phases, it is important to emphasize that effective sports injury rehabilitation proceeds on a continuum of uninterrupted medical and clinical services. Thus, considerable overlap exists between each phase. Progressive short-term goals and changing treatment protocols facilitate a smooth transition from one phase to the next. As an introduction to each phase of the rehabilitation model, a descriptive summary is offered as a prelude to identification of short-term goals and criteria for progression. Although the goals that define each phase function as interim goals, they are summarized in nonspecific terms without regard to duration of the rehabilitation phase. Thus, in the following discussion, the goals identified for each phase are presented as guides to formulation of short-term goals with appropriate relevancy, specificity, and clarity. Likewise, the corresponding progression criteria are summarized in a nonspecific context and, as such, are offered as a framework for development of quantitative criteria wherever possible.

Early Rehabilitation Phase (Phase I)

The early phase of sports injury rehabilitation is described as the period following an acute injury, or surgery, during which movement in the affected body part is involuntarily limited by acute inflammatory responses (i.e., swelling, pain, muscle spasm) or purposely restricted by medically indicated protective devices (e.g., casts, splints). During the early rehabilitation phase, exercise of the affected body part involving joint motion is restricted or completely contraindicated, although exercise of unaffected body parts may be indicated. In general, the early phase of rehabilitation corresponds with the inflammatory stage of tissue healing and the early stages of scar formation (see chapter 3). The implications for therapeutic management of inflammation and scar formation were reviewed in chapter 4 and chapter 5, respectively.

Short-term goals during the early phase of sports injury rehabilitation include therapeutic intervention to

- control the primary inflammatory responses to tissue trauma (hemorrhage, effusion/ edema),
- alleviate the secondary inflammatory responses to tissue trauma (pain, muscle spasm),
- facilitate the rate and quality of tissue repair,

Table 11.1   A Conceptual Model for Sports Injury Rehabilitaiton

Early phase (Phase I)

Primary characteristics	Tissue healing stage
Involuntary movement restriction (due to pain, swelling, etc.) and/or prescribed movement restriction (e.g., protective devices); maintenance of physical fitness parameters.	Inflammation/early fibroplasia (scar formation)

Progression criteria (to intermediate phase): Resolution of inflammatory responses (pain, swelling, etc.) and acceptable level of tissue healing to permit initiation of therapeutic exercise/sensorimotor training.

Intermediate phase (Phase II)

Primary characteristics	Tissue healing stage
Controlled progressive therapeutic exercise to optimize tissue structure and function (affected tissues), physical fitness parameters (muscle strength/endurance, cardiovascular fitness, etc.), and sensorimotor function.	Late fibroplasia (scar formation)/early scar maturation.

Progression criteria (to late phase): Acceptable restoration of tissue structure and function (affected tissues) to permit introduction of sport-specific sensorimotor training and functional activities.

Late phase (Phase III)

Primary characteristics	Tissue healing stage
Sport-specific sensorimotor training/functional activities.	Intermediate/late scar maturation

Progression criteria (to full activity): Optimal restoration of tissue structure and function (affected tissues), physical fitness parameters (muscle strength/endurance, cardiovascular fitness, etc.), and sensorimotor function.

- prevent development of soft tissue contractures and adhesions,
- minimize muscular strength loss and muscle atrophy,
- preserve somatosensory proprioceptive input and sensorimotor function, and
- maintain optimal levels of physical fitness (e.g., body weight, cardiovascular fitness).

Criteria for progression from the early phase to the intermediate phase of sports injury rehabilitation (Phase II) are based to a large extent on the sports health care clinician's knowledge of sequential tissue repair mechanisms, including the typical time frames associated with particular injuries. Aside from removal of protective devices (if used), criteria for progression to the intermediate phase of rehabilitation typically include the reduction of clinical signs and symptoms (e.g., pain, effusion/edema) and a level of tissue repair (i.e., restoration of structural and functional integrity) that permit initiation of therapeutic exercise.

Intermediate Rehabilitation Phase (Phase II)

The intermediate phase of sports injury rehabilitation is identified by initiation of controlled, progressive therapeutic exercise, although therapeutic protocols may continue to address lingering inflammatory responses (e.g., pain) and enhancement of tissue repair. For the most part, the intermediate phase of rehabilitation represents a restorative phase during which the consequential effects of tissue trauma and the detrimental effects of restricted movement are addressed. As related to soft connective tissue repair, the intermediate phase of rehabilitation typically transcends the late events of scar formation, the second major stage of tissue repair, and the early events of scar maturation, the third major stage of connective tissue healing (see chapter 3). Implications for therapeutic intervention in these stages of connective tissue repair were discussed in chapter 5.

Short-term goals that characterize the intermediate phase of rehabilitation include therapeutic strategies to

- enhance the definitive structural and functional properties of scar tissue (e.g., plasticity, tensile strength),
- restore optimal joint mobility (i.e., accessory joint motions, physiological movements),
- restore optimal musculotendinous extensibility and general flexibility,
- restore optimal muscle strength and appropriate strength balances (i.e., bilateral strength balance, agonist-antagonist strength ratio),
- restore optimal muscular endurance,
- restore proprioceptive and sensorimotor function (i.e., joint position sense and kinesthesia, dynamic joint control, and balance),
- restore normal gait patterns, and
- maintain optimal levels of physical fitness (e.g., body weight and composition, cardiovascular fitness).

Criteria for progression from the intermediate phase to the late phase of sports injury rehabilitation (Phase III) are based on the estimated structural and functional integrity of the affected tissues, as well as quantitative clinical assessment of relevant physical parameters (i.e., parameters that were the focus of intervention during the intermediate phase). Basic criteria for progression to the late phase of rehabilitation commonly include

- absence of complicating clinical signs and symptoms (e.g., pain, swelling),
- restoration of the structural and functional properties of the affected tissues (e.g., plasticity, tensile strength) to permit introduction of sport-related functional activities, and
- restoration of relevant physical parameters (e.g., joint motion, flexibility, muscular strength) to permit initiation of sport-related functional activities.

Late Rehabilitation Phase (Phase III)

Optimal restoration of sensorimotor function and sport-specific motor skills is the primary defining characteristic of the late phase of sports injury rehabilitation. Thus, this phase is commonly referred to as *functional rehabilitation*. Generally, the functional phase of rehabilitation is initiated as permitted by soft tissue scar maturation (i.e., tissue plasticity and tensile strength). Sport-specific activities that characterize the functional phase of rehabilitation can be expected to contribute to optimal connective tissue properties during the maturation phase of tissue repair. As defined in this model, the functional phase of sports injury rehabilitation begins with introduction of monitored sensorimotor training activities in the clinical setting (e.g., balancing activities, slide board exercises) and, thus, may overlap considerably with the intermediate phase. Progression through the functional phase of rehabilitation includes the use of controlled sport-related motor activities (e.g., figure eight running, cutting maneuvers, overhead ball tosses) with subsequent selective integration of the recovering athlete into regular conditioning drills and practice activities. Termination of the functional rehabilitation phase is marked by resumption of unrestricted sports participation. The primary goals of the functional phase of sports injury rehabilitation include

- optimal restoration of connective tissue structural and functional properties (e.g., tensile strength, plasticity);
- optimal restoration of neuromuscular coordination, dynamic joint control, and dynamic balance;
- establishment of normal sport-specific motor patterns (e.g., running, jumping, throwing);
- optimal restoration of sport-related physical fitness parameters (e.g., muscular strength and endurance, cardiovascular fitness); and
- satisfactory restoration of the athlete's confidence and freedom from apprehension.

Resumption of Activity and Treatment Discharge

The final phase of sports injury rehabilitation involves progressive integration of the recovering athlete into regular conditioning drills and practice activities with unrestricted sports participation as the expected outcome. Regardless of the particular sport, this transition is a critical period during the functional phase of rehabilitation. As return to full activity becomes imminent, it behooves the sports health care clinician to consider several factors that may influence the athlete's exposure to reinjury. Assurance of a safe practice environment (e.g., practice field surfaces), effectiveness of protective equipment, and the athlete's confidence level are relevant considerations. Aside from these factors, judicious selection of practice activities that involve minimal injury risk yet are conducive to optimal recovery is one of the most critical factors. Given the multitude of loading mechanisms imposed on body structures during sports activities, the sports health care clinician is challenged to determine if particular drills and motor tasks are indicated or contraindicated. A coach's cooperation in allowing and monitoring selective practice activities can be a critical factor in an athlete's successful return to sports participation.

As an athlete resumes unrestricted sports participation, discharge from treatment becomes a consideration. In many cases, however, an athlete's progressive return to activity is accompanied by continuation of specific exercises designed to minimize the risk of reinjury. On occasion, exacerbation of an injury after resumption of activity indicates further treatment. Given the progressive nature of a recovering athlete's transition to full participation, determination of a specific discharge date becomes somewhat difficult in the athletic setting. Nevertheless, professional standards for patient care in a health care facility specify dated documentation of patient discharge. With regard to health care services rendered by certified athletic trainers, for example, the *Standards of Professional Practice* (National Athletic Trainers' Association Board of Certification 2000) specifies dated documentation of discontinued services at such a time that the patient has received optimal benefits from the treatment program. While successful resumption of sports participation functions inherently as an indicator of positive treatment outcomes, documentation of functional outcomes in sports health care is essential if third-party payment for services is a relevant consideration.

Protocol for termination of patient care in a health care facility typically requires documentation in a written discharge summary. The SOAP note format described in chapter 10 accommodates inclusion of a discharge summary in the patient's record. Professional and legal considerations, as well as third-party payer requirements, indicate specific data to be included. Typically, the contents of a discharge summary include data related to the patient's attainment of rehabilitation goals (i.e., functional outcomes) and current health status, as well as information regarding the reason for discharge, the type and number of treatments given, recommendations for follow-up care, and referrals to other health care providers (Kettenbach 1995).

Summary

After a clinical assessment and identification of an injured sports participant's relevant health problems, formulation of rehabilitation goals and development of treatment plans are the next two steps in the problem-oriented approach to sports injury management. Rehabilitation goals include long-term goals as well as short-term (i.e., interim) goals to be achieved at particular intervals throughout the recovery period. Typically, the long-term goal, or expected functional outcome, of a highly motivated athlete is resumption of sports activity. Short-term goals that provide direction to attainment of expected outcomes provide a basis for formulation of therapeutic strategies and treatment plans, thereby providing a focus for coordinated health care services. Successful attainment of realistic but challenging short-term goals provides a motivational basis for the recovering patient.

Short-term rehabilitation goals may reflect a therapeutic objective or a behavioral objective. Whereas a therapeutic objective, such as alleviation of pain or edema reduction, represents a treatment effect to be achieved through the clinician's use of therapeutic agents, a behavioral objective specifies a challenge to be met by the patient. As applied to sports injury rehabilitation, a meaningful behavioral objective is stated in terms of desired functional behavior such as demonstration of normal gait patterns, proper throwing mechanics, or other sport-related motor tasks. The behavioral approach to rehabilitation involves formulation of short-term goals that identify the audience, the expected functional task, the conditions under which the task is to be performed, and the degree to which the task is to be accomplished. Meaningful short-term goals identify criteria for rehabilitation progression that are quantitative and measurable.

Sports injury rehabilitation programs have several characteristic elements that provide a conceptual framework for program planning. The basic elements include three identifiable sequential phases, which are characterized by short-term (i.e., interim) goals and criteria for progression to the next phase. The primary phases include an early phase, an intermediate phase, and a late phase, which generally parallel the sequence of normal connective tissue repair. As resumption of full sports participation becomes imminent, the sports health care clinician is challenged to monitor the recovering athlete's integration into regular practice activities that not only involve minimal risk of reinjury but also contribute to the recovery process. As unrestricted participation occurs, appropriate protocols for documentation of treatment discharge become a consideration.

References

DePalma, M.T., and B. DePalma. 1989. The use of instruction and the behavioral approach to facilitate injury rehabilitation. *Athletic Training* 24:217-19.

Kettenbach, G. 1995. *Writing SOAP notes*, 2nd ed. Philadelphia: Davis.

Lephart, S.M., D.H. Perrin, F.H. Fu, and K. Minger. 1991. Functional performance tests for the anterior cruciate ligament insufficient athlete. *Athletic Training* 26:44-50.

National Athletic Trainers' Association Board of Certification. 2000. *Standards of professional practice.* Omaha, Neb.: National Athletic Trainers' Association Board of Certification.

Appendix

Select Terms

This appendix is intended to serve as a reference for further clarification of subject matter discussed in this book. It is not all-inclusive and does not necessarily include all key concepts or terms highlighted in each chapter.

accessory joint motions—Involuntary movements between joint surfaces that allow unrestricted physiological movements (i.e., spin, roll, slide).

acoustic streaming—Mechanical effect of nonthermal, pulsed ultrasound involving movement of fluids away from the source of energy.

action potential—Electric impulse transmitted across the cell membrane of a nerve fiber during transmission of a nerve impulse.

adaptation—The rate of decline in an afferent nerve impulse (i.e., number of impulses per second) following stimulation of a sensory receptor.

adhesion—Fibrous bands between adjacent tissue surfaces that are normally separated.

agranulocyte—A white blood cell that does not contain granules (monocytes and lymphocytes).

allograft—Surgical transplantation of tissues obtained from another individual.

analgesic—A drug that relieves pain.

angiogenesis—Formation of new blood vessels.

antibody—Glycoproteins (protein and carbohydrate compounds) produced by lymphocytes in the immune response to specific antigens.

antipyretic—A drug that reduces fever.

autogenic inhibition—A reflex inhibitory neural response that causes relaxation of a muscle following stimulation of its mechanoreceptor (i.e., Golgi tendon organ).

autograft—Surgical transplantation of tissues from one part of a patient's body to another.

body righting reflex—A reflex neuromuscular response to restore the body to its normal upright position after sudden perturbation (e.g., a fall).

cavitation—Mechanical effect of nonthermal, pulsed ultrasound involving vibration of small gas pockets, or bubbles, in tissue fluids.

chemoreceptor—A sensory nerve ending that is activated by a chemical stimulus.

chemotaxis—Unidirectional movement of white blood cells toward an area of inflammation in response to a chemical mediator.

chondroblast—A cell that forms cartilage.

chondroclast—A giant multinucleated cell associated with absorption of cartilage.

coagulation—Transformation of blood from a liquid into a semisolid gel (i.e., blood clotting).

coagulation factor—One of several elements in the blood that interact to complete the blood-clotting process.

coagulum—A blood clot.

cocontraction—Simultaneous contraction of two or more muscles, or muscle groups (e.g., agonists and antagonists).

collagen fibers—Inelastic connective tissue fibers that provide tensile strength to the tissues.

conjugate gaze—Simultaneous movement of both eyes in the same direction.

connective tissue—Tissue that connects and supports other body tissues and parts.

contractility—Having the ability to contract, or shorten (e.g., muscle tissue).

contracture—Abnormal formation of fibrous connective tissue characterized by shortening, loss of elasticity, and limitation of mobility.

coping skills training—Teaching specific techniques and behaviors to enable a patient to cope with a pain experience.

creep—The capability of body tissues to elongate as the result of prolonged stretching.

deafferentation—An interruption in afferent (sensory) nerve impulses.

delayed union—Retardation of bone healing in which a bone eventually heals following a fracture, but not within the typical time frame.

elastic fibers—Connective tissue fibers that are capable of returning to their original state after being stretched or otherwise deformed.

elasticity—The ability of tissue to regain its original length after being stretched.

emigration (diapedesis)—Passage of blood cells, especially white blood cells, through the walls of small blood vessels.

endochondral ossification—Bone formation during which cartilage is replaced by osseous tissue.

endomysium—A thin connective tissue sheath that surrounds a muscle fiber and binds muscle fibers together.

endorphins—Natural opiate-like chemicals produced in the brain that act, along with enkephalins, to reduce pain.

enkephalins—Natural opiate-like chemicals produced in the brain that act, along with endorphins, to reduce pain.

epimysium—The outermost connective tissue sheath that surrounds a skeletal muscle.

erythema—Redness of the skin or mucous membranes due to capillary dilatation and increased blood flow.

exteroceptor—A sensory receptor that is activated by stimuli originating from outside the body.

exudate—Accumulation of fluid, proteins, and cells that pass through the walls of small blood vessels into adjoining tissues. See *transudate*.

fibroblast—A cell from which connective tissue is developed.

fibroplasia—The development of fibrous tissue, as in connective tissue healing.

fibrosis—Abnormal formation of fibrous tissue.

formed elements—Components of the blood that include platelets, white blood cells, and red blood cells.

glycoprotein—Any group of compounds in which protein is combined with a carbohydrate.

glycosaminoglycans (GAGs)—Carbohydrate chains attached to a protein core to form proteoglycans. See *proteoglycans*.

granulation tissue—The initial granular, highly vascularized tissue type that forms in connective tissue repair.

granulocyte—A white blood cell that contains granules (i.e., neutrophils, eosinophils, and basophils).

granuloma (foreign body)—A granular mass of chronic inflammatory tissue around a foreign body (e.g., sutures).

ground substance—The fluid, semifluid, or solid material that occupies the intercellular spaces in connective tissue.

hemopoiesis—Formation and development of blood cells.

hemostasis—Arrest of bleeding.

Hilton's law—A nerve trunk sends branches not only to periarticular muscles but also to the underlying joint structures (e.g., ligaments, joint capsule) and the overlying skin.

histology—Study of the microscopic structure of body tissues.

hydrogen bonds—Chemical linkage of hydrogen to other chemicals.

hyperalgesia—Excessive sensitivity to pain.

hyperthermia—Unusually high temperature.

hypertonus—Increased muscle tension (e.g., muscle spasm).

hypertrophic scar—Excessive fibrous tissue formation resulting in increased size and bulk of scar tissue.

hypoxia—Oxygen deficiency.

inflammation—The protective response of body tissues to irritation or injury that represents the initial stage of tissue healing.

interneuron—An intervening nerve cell that mediates transmission of impulses between neurons.

intramembranous ossification—Bone formation during which mesenchyme (embryonic membrane) is replaced by osseous tissue.

imagery—A psychological approach to pain management that involves a patient's calling up of distractive events or mental pictures.

ischemia—Temporary local deficiency of blood supply.

joint position sense—A component of proprioception that involves an individual's ability to perceive the static position of a joint.

keloid—Raised, dense scar tissue due to abnormal collagen deposition and excessive tissue formation. See *hypertrophic scar*.

kinesthesia—A component of proprioception that involves an individual's ability to perceive movement of a joint.

leukocyte—A white blood cell (granulocyte and agranulocyte).

leukocytosis—An increase in the number of leukocytes (white blood cells) in the blood.

lysis—Degradation or decomposition of a substance (e.g., collagen). Compare to *synthesis*.

macrophage—A monocyte that emigrated through the vascular wall into extravascular tissues and matured into a large phagocytic cell.

malunion—Bone healing with union of fracture fragments in a malaligned position.

margination—Alignment of white blood cells along the inner walls of a blood vessel during the early stages of inflammation.

mast cell—A resident connective tissue cell that synthesizes and releases histamine and other mediators of inflammation.

mechanoreceptor—A sensory nerve ending that is activated by a mechanical stimulus (i.e., mechanical deformation).

mesenchyme—Network of embryonic cells that give rise to connective tissues, blood and blood vessels, and lymph tissues.

mineralization—Deposition of minerals in body tissues.

morphology—The study of physical size, form, and structure without regard to function.

myofibroblast—A specialized connective tissue cell that mediates wound contraction.

neurotransmitter—A substance that mediates transmission of nerve impulses from one neuron to the next across a synaptic junction. May be excitatory or inhibitory.

nociceptor—A sensory nerve ending that is activated by a pain stimulus.

nonsteroidal anti-inflammatory drugs (NSAIDs)—A group of drugs that have analgesic, anti-inflammatory, and antipyretic properties.

nonunion—Failure of bone fragments to unite following a fracture.

opioid—A natural substance in the body that acts to decrease pain sensation (e.g., endorphins, enkephalins).

ossification—Formation of bone or conversion of other body tissue into bone. See *osteogenesis*.

osteoblast—Cell concerned with the formation of bone.

osteoclast—Giant multinuclear cell concerned with absorption of unwanted bone tissue.

osteogenesis—Bone formation or development in connective tissue or cartilage. See *ossification*.

osteoporosis—A disease process that results in reduction of bone mass.

osteoprogenitor cell—An ancestor, or precursor, cell that gives rise to bone cells.

osteosynthesis—Surgical fixation of the ends of a fractured bone with mechanical devices.

perimysium—A connective tissue sheath that envelops a bundle of muscle fibers.

phagocytosis—Ingestion and destruction of pathogenic microorganisms and cellular debris.

plasma—Liquid part of the blood or the lymph.

plasma cell—A lymphocyte-like cell found in connective tissue, bone marrow, and lymphoid tissue.

plasticity—The ability of a material to be molded (e.g., plastic deformation of connective tissue).

platelet—A small blood cell concerned with formation of a platelet plug during hemostasis.

platelet adhesion—Adherence of platelets to the inner lining of blood vessels.

platelet aggregation—Clustering or clumping together of platelets.

primary bone healing—The type of fracture healing that occurs directly between bone fragments without callus formation as the result of rigid internal fixation and compression.

proprioception—A sensory modality concerned with perception of joint position and joint movement.

proprioceptor—A sensory nerve ending that is activated by a mechanical stimulus (i.e., a mechanoreceptor). See *proprioception*.

proteoglycans—Molecular compounds consisting of proteins and carbohydrate chains that are constituents of the extracellular ground substance of connective tissue.

receptive field—An area within a particular body structure that, if mechanically distorted, leads to excitation of a particular sensory receptor.

receptors—Afferent (sensory) nerve endings that respond to various kinds of stimuli.

reciprocal inhibition—A reflex neural response that causes contraction of a muscle following stimulation of its mechanoreceptor (i.e., muscle spindle) with simultaneous relaxation of its antagonist.

reflex arc—A neural pathway formed by an afferent (sensory) neuron, a spinal cord synapse, and an efferent (motor) neuron that produces an involuntary reflex response to a stimulus.

regeneration—Tissue healing characterized by restoration of the normal structural and functional properties of body tissues. Compare to *repair*.

relaxation training—A psychological approach to pain management that includes activities to reduce the patient's anxiety.

remodeling—The third major stage of fracture healing during which a bone resumes its normal structure and function.

repair—Tissue healing characterized by formation of fibrotic scar tissue. Compare to *regeneration*.

scar formation—The second major stage of connective tissue repair that is characterized by development of fibrous scar tissue.

scar maturation—The third major stage of connective tissue repair during which scar tissue develops its ultimate structural and functional properties.

secondary bone healing—The type of fracture healing characterized by development of an interfragmentary fibrocartilaginous callus.

secondary hypoxic injury—Ischemic cellular necrosis in tissues adjacent to the tissues disrupted by trauma as the result of impaired circulation.

sensorimotor—Pertaining to both sensory and motor nerve functions.

skeletal muscle relaxant—A drug that reduces the contractility of skeletal muscle fibers.

stress-relaxation—Tissue relaxation that occurs as resistance to constant tensile loading decreases.

stress riser—A bone defect that creates a weakened focal point for stress and thus a propensity for tissue failure.

summation—Cumulative neural response to stimulation of multiple sensory nerve endings or to increased rate of stimulation.

synapse—The junction between two neurons in a neural pathway across which nerve impulses are transmitted.

synthesis—Formation of a complex substance from simpler elements (e.g., collagen synthesis). Compare to *lysis*.

tensile loading—Application of constant tensile strain, or tension, to effect elongation of tissue fibers.

tensile strength—The ability of tissues to resist elongation without tearing.

tensile stress—Tissue resistance to constant tensile loading.

thermoreceptor—A sensory nerve ending that is activated by a thermal stimulus.

transudate—Accumulation of fluids that pass through the walls of small blood vessels into adjoining tissues.

tropocollagen—The basic molecular unit of collagen fibrils.

Wolff's law—Adaptive changes in the structure and biomechanical properties of bone occur in accordance with functional demands placed on the bone.

wound contraction—The tissue-healing mechanism that pulls the margins of a tissue defect toward the center.

woven bone—The initial soft, immature bone that forms during fracture healing.

Index

Note: The italicized *f* and *t* following page numbers refer to figures and tables, respectively.

A

abducens nerve (VI) 181
accessory joint motions 107-108
acetaminophen 79-80
acetylsalicylic acid 79. *See also* aspirin
Achilles tendon stretching 104
acoustic streaming 91
action potential 68, 166
active-assisted stretching 106
acupuncture-like TENS 78
acute inflammation
   about 31
     cellular responses 34-36
     therapeutic objectives 54
     vascular changes 32-34
adaptation 46, 75
adaptive defense system 34, 37
adhesion 34
adhesion molecules 34
adhesion prevention 92-94, 94-97
afferent (sensory) neurons 63, 64f, 170
afferent (sensory) pathways 179-180, 182-183
agonist-contract-relax 106
agranular leukocytes 16
agranulocytes 16
Alexander, I.J. 159
Allegrucci, M 210
Allen, A.A. 193
allografts 202
all-or-none principle 166
alpha motor neurons 162
ambulation in water 200
Amenta, P.S. 30-31
ampulla 180
analgesics 59, 78-80
Andriacchi, T. 93, 99
angiogenesis 41
ankle disks 207
ankle sprains, relationships of 189f
anterior corticospinal tract 177
anterior cruciate ligament injury 188-190
anterior spinothalamic tract 65
anterolateral system 169
   about 62-63
     afferent (sensory) neurons 63
     ascending spinal cord pathways 65
     cerebral cortex 66-68
     spinal cord connections 64-65
     thalamus 66
antibodies 38
anti-coagulation properties 59-60
antigens 37-38
anti-inflammatory drugs 59
antipyretic drugs 59
anxiety, as reaction to pain 81
AO/ASIF system 134-135, 137, 139, 141
arthrokinematic movements 107-108
articular deafferentation 188-189
artificial ligaments 202
ascending spinal cord pathways 170
aspirin 59-60, 79-80
assessment, in SOAP notes 222
Association for Osteosynthesis (AO) 134

Association for the Study of Internal Fixation
    (ASIF) 134
ataxia 175
attention diversion 82
autogenic inhibition 105-106, 164
autografts 202
avascular necrosis 129

B

Baker, R.J. 55
balance boards 207
balance deficits. *See* postural control and
    balance
Barber, S.D. 196
Barrack, R.L. 191, 195, 201, 210
Barrett, D. 192
basal ganglia 172-173, 174f
Bassett, C.A. 147
Becker, R.O. 147
behavioral approach, rehabilitation 231-232
Behrens, T.W. 89
Bell, G.W. 55
Bernier, J.N. 197, 198
beta-endorphin 74
Beynnon, B.D. 209
Biodex Stability System 198
Biomechanical Ankle Platform System 211
blood
blood vessel resorption 43
    cells 15-16, 35f
    coagulation 23-25
    composition 15-16
body righting reflexes 182
bone
    long bone histology 119-121
    long bone morphology 118-119
    primary bone 127
    primary bone healing 122, 134
    secondary bone 128
    secondary bone healing 122, 134
    site-specific bone hypertrophy 149
    woven bone 126
bone abnormal healing
    about 128
    delayed union 129-130
    malunion 130
    nonunion 128-129
bone fatigue 149-151
bone function restoration
    about 146-147
    mechanical loading 147-148
    therapeutic implications 148
    Wolff's law 147
bone plates 138-139
bone regeneration and repair
    about 121-122
    cellular proliferation and callus formation
      123-127
    hematoma formation and inflammation 122
    remodeling 127-128
bone screws 137-138, 138-139
bony labyrinth 179-180
Borsa, P.A. 203

braces 134-135, 141-142, 208-209
Branch, T.P. 209
Brashear, H.R., Jr. 128, 129, 136
breathing exercises 82
brief intense TENS 78
Bristol, H. 106
Brodmann, Korbinian 67
Brodmann's areas 67, 171-172
Brodowicz, G.R. 102
Brunolli, J. 205
Bryant, W.M. 30, 49
Buchanan, W.W. 59-60
Burgess, R.C. 169
Burnett, C.N. 191
buttress plates 138

C

calcium ions 24
Caldwell, G.L., Jr. 199, 202, 203
canaliculi 119-120
cancellous bone screws 137
cancellous (spongy) bone 119
capsuloligamentous tension, restoration of 203-
    204
capsuloligamentous trauma 192
carbohydrates, in tissue healing 17-18
Carlstedt, C.A. 101
cascade concept, coagulation 24
cast-braces 134, 141-142
casts 141
cavitation 90-91
cells
    acute inflammation responses 34-36
    B cells 37-38
    blood cells 15-16, 35f
    classification 10
    connective tissue cells 12, 16-17
    epithelioid cells 47
    hair cells 180
    labile cells 10
    in long bones 119
    mast cells 12, 16
    mesenchymal cells 12
    osteogenic cells 121
    osteoprogenitor cells 121
    permanent cells 10
    plasma cells 12
    satellite cells 10
    stable cells 10
    T cells 37-38, 72
    transmission cells 72
cellular immunity 38
center of gravity maintenance 198
centrifugal pain control 73
cerebellum 172-173, 174-175
cerebral cortex 66-68, 67f, 171-172, 174f
cerebral nuclei 173
cerebrocerebellum 174
chemical mediators 15
chemical synapse 65f, 68
chemoreceptors 61
chemotaxis 35
chondroblasts 124
chondroclasts 124

chronic inflammation 31, 37-38
Ciccone, C.D. 59-60
circumferential compression 57
Clark, F.J. 169
clinical assessment 223-224
clinical decision making 5
clinical signs 5-6
clinical union 125
closed reduction 136
clot retraction 24
coactivation 162, 193
coagulation 23-24
coagulum 24
cocontraction 194-195
codeine 79
coenzymes 17
cognitive therapy 82
cold applications. *See* cryotherapy
collagen
    fiber alignment 45-46
    increased collagen deposition 43
    type I collagen formation 41-42
    type III collagen formation 41-42
collagen cross-linkage 44-45, 93-94
collagen degradation 44
collagen fibers 12-13
collagen synthesis 39-40
collagen turnover 44
collateral compression 57
combined accessory joint mobilization 108f
compact (dense) bone 119
concentric lamellae 119
cones 182
conjugate gaze movement 181
connective tissue
    cells 12, 16-17
    contracture mechanisms 93f
    fibers 12-13
    healing stages 6, 7f
    major components 12f
    relationship of cells, fibers, and ground
        substance 13f
    repair overlapping stages 30f
    structure and function 11-14
    therapeutic intervention in repair 8f
    types 14
connective tissue immobilization
    about 92-93
    adhesions 94
    contractures 93-94
connective tissue repair enhancement
    about 88-89
    electrotherapy 92
    mechanical ultrasound 90-91
    pharmacologic agents 89
    thermotherapy 89-90
connective tissue tensile strength 99-100
connective tissue viscoelasticity 100
continuous passive motion 94-95
contractility 146
contract-relax 105
contract relax, agonist contract 106, 107
contracture prevention 92-94, 94-97
contractures 48-49
controlled breathing exercises 82
coping skills training 81-82
cortex 119
cortical bone 119-120
cortical bone screws 137
corticobulbar tract 177
corticospinal tracts 176-177
corticosteroids 60, 89
creep 100-101

crista ampullaris 180
cryostretching 102
cryotherapy 55-56, 76, 89
Cummings, G.S. 94, 98, 100, 103
Cummings, J.P. 143
cutaneous receptors 164, 165f
Cyriax, J. 109
D
Daly, T.J. 30
Darvon 79
database, SOAP notes 222
Davies, G.J. 196
deafferentation 188-189
Dean, M.R.E. 191, 197, 210
deep-heating modalities 89-90
definitions 239-243
deGroot, J. 74
delayed union 129-130
denaturation 103
Denegar, C. 75
dense connective tissue 14
dense irregular connective tissue 14
dense regular connective tissue 14
Denti, M. 188, 201, 202, 203
deossification 121
DePace, D.M. 71, 77
DePalma, B. 231, 232
DePalma, M.T. 231, 232
depolarization 166
descending (motor) pathways 175-176
descending pain inhibitory pathways 74f
descending pain inhibitory system 71, 73-75
DeVane, D.A. 103
diapedesis 35
diaphysis 119
direct (pyramidal) pathways 175, 176-177
displacement 136
distraction 82
disuse atrophy, muscles 145-146
Dobner, J.J. 189
Docherty, C.L. 210
doctrine of specific nerve endings 71
Donley, P.B. 75
dorsal column-medial lemniscal system
    about 62, 169
    afferent (sensory) neurons 170
    ascending spinal cord pathways 170
    thalamus 170-171
dorsal horn layers 64-65
dorsal spinocerebellar tract 170
Draper, D.O. 103
drug receptors 79
Dvir, A. 201
dynamic balance 198
dynamic compression plates 138
dynamic equilibrium 179
dynamic joint control, sensorimotor training
    effects 210-211
dynamic joint stabilization
    about 191
    cocontraction of periarticular muscles 194-
        195
    functional joint stability 192
    reflex muscle splinting 193-194
    research and clinical observations 195-196
dynamic splinting 96
dynamic stretch reflex 162
Dyson, M. 91, 103
E
early tissue mobilization 200
ecchymosis 25
edema 7, 32, 33-34, 199-200. *See also* hemor-
    rhage and edema management

efferent (motor) projections 180-182, 184
effusion 7, 199-200
elastic fibers 12-13
elasticity 100
elastic stretch 100
electrical muscle stimulation 97
electrical synapse 68
electroanalgesic stimulation methods 77f
electrotherapy 77-78, 92, 143
elevation, of injured extremities 58
embryonic connective tissue 14
emigration 35
emotional status assessment 225t
endochondral ossification 122
endogenous opioids 74-75
endomysium 12
end organs of Ruffini 168
endorphins 74
endosteum 119
endothelial cell budding 91
enkephalins 74
enzymes 15
epimysium 25
epiphyseal plate 119
epiphyses 119
epithelioid cells 47
equilibrium 179
Ernst, G. 210
erythema 7
excitatory neurotransmitters 68
excitatory PNF techniques 104-105
extensibility 100
external callus 124
external compression 57
external mobilization, fractures 140-143
external skeleton fixation 140
external support devices, proprioceptive effects
    of 208-209
exteroceptors 61
extrafusal fibers 161-162
extrinsic fracture healing complications 128
extrinsic pathway 24
exudate 35
exudation 32
eye movement control 181

F
Fahrer, H. 196
Farrar, E.L. 128
fast pain 63
fatigue 150-151
fatigue fractures 150
fear, as reaction to pain 81
Ferreira, E. 106
Feuerbach, J.W. 208
Feuerstein, M. 70
fibers, in long bones 119
fibrillar collagens 39
fibrinogen 24
fibrinolysis 24
fibroblasts 12, 16-17, 38
fibrogenesis 39-40
fibroplasia
    about 38
    collagen synthesis 39-40
    in connective tissue healing 6
    fibroblast proliferation 38
    fibrogenesis 39-40
    fibrous scar formation 42-43
    granulation tissue formation 40-41
    wound contraction 41-42
fibrosis 11
fibrotic contractures 145
fibrous adhesions 49

fibrous layer 119
firing level 166
first order neurons 62, 169
first pain 63
Fischer, E. 76
fixed macrophages 37
flexibility assessment 225t
foam mats 207
foreign body granulomas 47
formed elements 15
fracture, defined 118
fracture fixation
    about 136-137
    external skeleton fixation 140
    internal skeleton fixation 137-140
fracture healing. See also bone regeneration and
        repair
    early phase 123f, 124
    intermediate phase 124-126
    late phase 126-127
fracture reduction 136
fracture treatment
    about 134-135
    electrotherapy 143
    external mobilization and protected
        mobilization 140-143
    function preservation and restoration 143-
        148
    removal of internal fixation devices 151
    special protective devices 142-143
Freeman, M.A.R. 191, 197, 210
free nerve endings 61, 161
functional balance 198-199
functional balance tasks 207-208
functional electrical muscle stimulation 97
functional fracture bracing 134-135
functional joint stability 192
functional rehabilitation 9, 204-205, 236-237
functional tissue loading 109-110
function loss 34

G
Gabriel, A.J. 223
gait assessment 225t
gamma-aminobutyric acid 74
gamma motor (efferent) neurons 69, 162
Ganong, W.F. 74-75
Garn, S.N. 191
gate control theory 71, 72-74
Gibbons, K.T. 106
Gieck, J.H. 103
Gill, K.M. 81
Glencross, D. 191
glenohumeral dislocation 205
glossary 239-243
glycoproteins 13
glycosaminoglycans 13-14
Goertzen, M. 201
Goldbeck, T.G. 196
Golgi, Camillo 161
Golgi ligament endings 161
Golgi tendon organlike endings 161
Golgi tendon organs 105, 163-164
Goodwin, J.S. 89
graft types 202-203
granular leukocytes 16
granulation tissue formation 40, 41-42
granulocytes 16
granulomas 47
granulomatosis 47
granulomatous inflammation 47
gray matter 173
Grigg, P. 160, 168
ground substance 13-14, 119
Guskiewicz, K.M. 197, 198, 208

H
Hageman factor 24
hair cells 180
Hall, J.L. 75
Hanegan, J.L. 70, 72
haversian canal 119
haversian systems 119
Hayes, K.C. 196, 199-200
healing, defined 9
hemarthrosis 25
hematoma 25
hematoma formation 122
hemopoiesis 34
hemorrhage 6
hemorrhage and edema management
    about 54-55
    pharmacologic agents 59-60
    physical agents 55-58
hemorrhagic manifestations 25
hemostasis
    defined 22
    primary hemostasis 22-23
    promotion of 7
    secondary hemostasis 23-25
hemostatic plug formation 22-23
high-voltage, pulsed galvanic stimulation 92
Hilton, John 159
Hilton's law 159
hinged cast-braces 142
Hippocrates 54
histamine 16, 32
histology 118
Hoffman, M. 198, 211
hold-relax 105
hold relax, agonist contract 106, 107
Holm, G. 106
Howship's lacunae 121
humoral immunity 38
Hunter, R. 209
Hutton, R.S. 106, 107
hydrogen bonds 103
hyperalgesia 69
hyperstimulation analgesia 78
hyperthermia 7
hypertonus 69
hypertrophic scars 49-50
hypertrophy 145-146, 149
hypoxia 55

I
ice massage 55, 56
ice pack treatments 55
Ihara, H. 210-211
imagery 82
immobilization
    about 58
    connective tissue immobilization 92-94
    effects of 99
    of fractures 140-143
    modified immobilization 95-97
    relative immobilization 140
    serial static immobilization 96
    tissue immobilization 98-99
immune responses 37-38
index of suspicion 6
indirect (extrapyramidal) pathways 175, 177-
        178
inflammation
    about 31
    acute inflammation 31-36
    assessment 225t
    chronic inflammation 37-38
    in connective tissue healing 6
    granulomatous inflammation 47
    and hematoma formation 122

indications for cryotherapy 56f
and muscle spasm 7, 34
signs of 33-34
subacute inflammation 37
systemic inflammation 31
Ingersoll, C.D. 209
inhibitory association neurons 163, 164
inhibitory neurotransmitters 68
inhibitory PNF techniques 104-105
initial clinical assessment 223-224
innate defense system 34
inner ear 179-180
intensity theory 71
interfragmentary bone screws 137-138
intermuscular hematoma 25
internal callus 124
internal fixation devices, removal of 151
internal health locus of control 81
internal skeleton fixation 137-140
International Association for the Study of Pain 70
interneurons 163, 164
interoreceptors 61
interstitial lamellae 120
intrafusal fibers 161-162
intramedullary nails 139
intramembranous ossification 122
intramuscular hematoma 25
intrinsic fracture healing complications 128
intrinsic pathway 24
Ionta, M.K. 105
ischemia 55

J
Johannson, H. 194
joint afferents, preservation of 202
joint instability, relationships of 189f
joint mobility
    assessment 225t
    restoration of 144-145
joint mobilization 107-109
joint position sense
    about 158
    impairment of 190-191
    sensorimotor training effects 209-210
joint receptors 159-161
joint stabilization. See dynamic joint stabilization

K
Kaltenborn, F. 109
Kaminski, T.W. 208
Kandel, E.R. 194
Katzman, L.L. 197, 198, 205
Kelly, D.D. 64, 72
keloids 49-50
Kennedy, J.C. 159
Kilcoyne, R.F. 128
kinesthesia
    about 158
    impairment of 190-191
    sensorimotor training effects 209-210
Kinzey, S.J. 209
Kirschner wires 139-140
Kocher, M.S. 201, 202-203
Koren, E. 201
Kottke, F.J. 104
Krahl, H. 147-148

L
labile cells 10
labyrinth 179-180
lacunae 119
LaRiviere, J. 169
lateral corticospinal tract 176
lateral gaze centers 181
lateral spinothalamic tract 65
lateral vestibulospinal tract 177

Lentell, G. 102, 103-104
Lentell, G.L. 197, 198, 205
Lephart, S.M. 168, 191, 194, 196, 201, 202-203, 204, 233
leukocytes 15
leukocytosis 34
leukotrienes 16
ligaments
    artificial 202
    collagen fiber alignment 45f
limit detectors 160
lipids, in tissue healing 17
Lloyd, J.W. 198, 211
localization 67
Loitz-Ramage, B.J. 124, 126-127, 129, 149
long bones
    blood supply 120-121
    histology 119-121
    major parts of 118f
    microstructure 120f
    morphology 118-119
    osteogenic cells 121
long-term rehabilitation goals 230
loose connective tissue 14
Loudon, J.K. 210
low-load, prolonged stretching 101, 102-104
Lund, P.J. 195, 201
Lundin, O. 209
lymphadenitis 31
lymphangitis 31
lymphocytes 37-38

M
macrophages 12, 16, 37, 91
macula 180
Maitland, G.D. 108-109
Maitland's grades of oscillatory movement 108t
malalignment 136
malleolar bone screws 137
malunion 130
manipulation 108-109
margination 34
Martin, J.H. 71, 73, 74
Martinez-Hernandez, A. 30-31
mast cells 12, 16
Mattacola, C.G. 198, 211
mature connective tissue 14
mechanical ultrasound 90-91
mechanoreceptor deficits 192
mechanoreceptor degeneration 188-190
mechanoreceptor neurophysiology 164-169
mechanoreceptor repopulation 201
mechanoreceptors 61, 63, 159-164
medial lemniscus 170
medial vestibulospinal tract 177
mediators 15
medullary cavity 119
medullary pyramia 176
Meissner's corpuscles 168
Melzack, R. 71, 72, 73
membranous labryinth 179-180
mesenchymal cells 12, 14
metaphysis 119
Michlovitz, S.L. 76, 77
microcurrent electrical nerve stimulation 77
microstreaming 91
microwave diathermy 76
mineralization 123, 127
minerals, in tissue healing 17
minitrampolines 207
modality of sensation 66, 171
modeling 127
modified immobilization 95-97
modifiers 10-11
mononuclear phagocytes 35, 37
monosynaptic reflex arc 162

Montoye, H.J. 146-147
Moore, J.H. 210
morphology 118
motor circuit 173, 174f
motor control system 172
motor denervation 189
motor end plates 162
motor homunculus 172
motor-level stimulation 77
motor systems, hierarchical organization 205f, 206
movement, restriction of 58
Muller, Johannes 71
muscle atrophy 145-146, 225t
muscle fatigue 150-151
muscle fiber regeneration, retardation of 47-48
muscle hypertrophy 145-146
muscle relaxants 80
muscle spasm 7, 34, 60, 68-70
muscle spasm alleviation. See pain and muscle spasm alleviation
muscle spindle 69-70
muscle spindles 161-163
muscle stiffness 194
muscle strength 205, 225t
muscular strength, restoration of 145-146
musculoskeletal injury, problem identification 5-6
musculotendinous receptors 161-164
Myers, J.B. 191, 209
myofiber regeneration 48
myofibroblasts 17, 41-42
myofilaments 145
myostatic contractures 145

N
Nakayama, A. 210-211
narcotic analgesics 78
nerve endings 61, 62f, 71, 161
nerve impulse 68
neurological status, assessment 225t
neuromuscular control 205
neurons
    afferent (sensory) neurons 63, 64f, 170
    alpha motor neurons 162
    first order neurons 62, 169
    gamma motor (efferent) neurons 69, 162
    inhibitory association neurons 163, 164
    relay neurons 171
    stimulatory association neurons 164
    thalamocortical projection neurons 171
    upper motor neurons 175-176
    wide dynamic range neurons 65
neurotransmitters 68
neutralization plates 138
neutrophils 35
Newton, R.A. 71, 77, 191
Nicholson, G. 109
Nitz, A.J. 189, 196, 197, 200
nociceptors 61, 68-69
nociceptor stimulation 62
noninvasive electroacupuncture 78
nonopioid analgesics 78, 79-80
nonsteroidal anti-inflammatory drugs (NSAIDS) 59, 79-80, 89
nonunion 128-129
Nordin, M. 101
North, R.B. 77
noxious-level electrical stimulation 77, 78
noxious rotations 168
NSAIDS (nonsteroidal anti-inflammatory drugs) 59, 79-80, 89
nutrient arteries 120
nutrient foramen 120

O
objective information, in SOAP notes 222
oculomotor nerve (III) 181

Odenrick, P. 197
O'Donoghue, P.C. 94
open reduction 136
opioid analgesics 78-79
opioid receptors 79
opioids 74
optic nerve 183
orthotic devices 208-209
oscillatory movement, Maitland's grades of 108t
ossification 127
osteoblasts 121, 124
osteoclasts 121
osteocytes 119, 121
osteogenic cells 121
osteogenisis, electrical stimulation of 143
osteons 119
osteoporosis of disuse 139
osteoprogenitor cells 121
osteosynthesis 137
Osternig, L. 194
Osternig, L.R. 106, 169

P
Pacini, Filippo 160
pacinian corpuscles 160
pain
    ascending and descending neural pathways 62f
    assessment 225t
    fast pain 63
    as inflammation characteristic 7, 34
    localization of stimulus 67
    perception of 80
    responses to 81
    slow pain 63
    vicious cycle with muscle spasm 60, 68-70
pain and muscle spasm alleviation
    about 60
    neuroanatomy and neurophysiology 60-68
    pain-spasm-pain cycle 68-70
    psychological strategies 79f, 80-82
    theoretical bases of pain 70-75
    therapeutic strategies 75-82
pain-spasm-pain cycle 60, 68-70
pain theory
    about 70-71
    descending pain inhibitory system 71, 73-75
    early theories 71
    gate control theory 71, 73-74
    pattern theory 71
Parkhurst, T.M. 191
Parkinson's disease 173
passive joint motion 95
patient care, termination of 237
pattern theory 71
Pauley, D.L. 104
pavementing 34
Payne, V.G. 211
Peck, C.L. 81
periaquiductal gray matter 73-75
periarticular muscles, cocontraction of 194-195
perimysium 12
periosteal arteries 120
periosteum 119
peripheral mechanoreceptors 159-164
peripheral proprioceptive system
    about 159
    basal ganglia 172-173
    cerebellum 172-173, 174-175
    cerebral cortex 171-172
    descending (motor) pathways 175-178
    dorsal column-medial lemniscal system 169-171
    neurophysiology of mechanoreceptors 164-169
    peripheral mechanoreceptors 159-164
permanent cells 10
permanent elongation 104
Perrin, D.H. 197, 198, 208

phagocytosis 32-33, 36-37
pharmacologic agents
    analgesic drugs 78-80
    connective tissue repair enhancement 89
    hemorrhage and edema management 59-60
    pain-spasm-pain cycle 78
    skeletal muscle relaxants 80
phonophoresis 60
photoreceptors 182-183
physical fitness assessment 225t
physical therapeutic agents
    about 55
    continuous passive motion 94-95
    cryotherapy 55-56, 76, 89-90
    electrotherapy 77-78, 92, 143
    elevation 58
    external compression 57
    functional electrical muscle stimulation 97
    mechanical ultrasound 90-91
    modified immobilization 95-97
    protected mobilization 95-97
    restricted movement 58
    thermotherapy 76-77, 89-90
piezoelectricity 147
pins 139-140
plasma 15
plasma cells 12
plaster of paris casts 141
plasticity 97-98, 100
plastic stretch, and tensile loading 100-101
platelet adhesion 23
platelet aggregation 23
platelet release reaction 22
platelets 15-16
plyometrics 207
point stimulators 78
polymodal nociceptors 61, 63, 71
polymorphonuclear leukocytes 35
polysynaptic reflex arc 163
pool therapy 200
porosity 119
Portney, L. 109
postoperative mechanoreceptor repopulation 201
postsynaptic membrane 68
postural control and balance
    about 197
    dynamic balance 198
    functional balance 198-199
    semi-dynamic balance 198
    and sensorimotor training 211
    static balance 197-198
posture assessment 225t
premotor area 172
Prentice, W.E. 106
presynaptic membrane 68
primary bone 127
primary bone healing 122, 134
primary motor area 172
primary somatosensory area 171
problem list 225-226
problem-oriented approach 4-6
problem-oriented medical record 220-226
procollagen molecule 39
prolonged loading 104
propoxyphene hydrochloride 79
proprioception 158, 191. See also peripheral
    proprioceptive system
proprioception testing 190-191
proprioceptive deficits
    about 188-190
    acute injury management 199-200
    in cycle with capsuloligamentous trauma
        and recurrent joint injury 192f
    diminished dynamic joint stabilization 191-196
    impairment of joint position sense and
        kinesthesia 190-191

postural control and balance deficits 197-199
    surgery 200-204
proprioceptive neuromuscular facilitation (PNF)
    about 104-105
    autogenic inhibition response 164
    research and clinical observations 106-107
    therapeutic principles and techniques 105-106
    as therapeutic stretching 101
proprioceptive training 9, 204-205, 208-209
proprioceptors 61, 69, 159
prosthesis 202
prostoglandins 59
protected mobilization 95-97, 140-143
proteins, in tissue healing 17
proteoglycans 13
prothrombin 24
prothrombinase 24
provisional callus 125
pseudoarthrosis 129
psychological intervention, for pain 80-82
psychological status assessment 225t
psychological support 81
pus 36
pyramidal decussation 176
pyramidal tract 176

Q
quadriceps avoidance gait 196

R
radiographic union 127
Rainsford, K.D. 59-60
Randall, T. 109
Raney, R.B., Sr. 128, 129, 136
raphe nuclei 73, 74
rapidly adapting receptors 166-167
reactive neuromuscular control 193
receptive fields 164-166
receptor adaptation 166-167
receptors. See also peripheral mechanoreceptors
    cutaneous receptors 164, 165f
    drug receptors 79
    interoreceptors 61
    joint receptors 159-160, 161
    mechanoreceptors 61, 63, 159
    musculotendinous receptors 161-164
    opioid receptors 79
    photoreceptors 182-183
    sensory receptors 61, 62
    skin receptors 164
    thermoreceptors 61, 63
    vestibular receptors 179-180
    visual receptors 182-183
reciprocal inhibition 105-106, 163
recurrent joint injury 192f
Reed, B. 49
reflex arc 162
reflex muscle splinting 193-194
regeneration 9-10
rehabilitation
    behavioral approach 231-232
    functional rehabilitation 9, 204-205, 236-237
    long-term goals 230
    planning principles and concepts 232-237
    short-term goals 230-231
    therapeutic and behavioral objectives 231
relative immobilization 140
relaxation PNF techniques 104-105
relaxation training 82
relay neurons 171
relay nuclei 66, 170-171
remodeling 127-128
Rennie, G.A. 77
repair 9-10
reproduction of active positioning 190-191
reproduction of passive positioning 190-191

research
    dynamic joint stabilization 195-196
    joint mobilization 109
    low-load, prolonged stretching 104
    proprioception 191
    proprioceptive neuromuscular facilitation
        106-107
resting membrane potential 166
reticular fibers 12-13
reticuloendothelial system 37
reticulospinal tract 177-178
retina 182
Rexed, Bror 64
Rexed's laminae 64
rhythmic stabilization 195
Riemann, B.L. 194
Rivera, J.E. 204
rods 182
Rogol, I.M. 210
roll 107-108
Romberg's test 197
Rowinski, M.J. 165, 167, 201, 205
rubrospinal tract 177-178
Rucinski, T.J. 57, 58
Ruffini, Angelo 160
Ruffini's corpuscles 160

S
Safran, M.R. 199, 202, 203
Saliba, E.N. 103
Salter, R.B. 94, 135, 151
Sapega, A.A. 100, 102
satellite cells 10
scar formation 7, 42-43
scar maturation 6, 8, 43-46
scar tissue structure and function enhancement
    about 97-98
    biomechanics of tensile loading and plastic
        stretch 100-101
    tensile loading 98, 99-100
    therapeutic strategies and techniques 101-110
    therapeutic tensile loading 98
    tissue immobilization 98-99
Schrader, J.W. 106
Schwartz, J.H. 194
secondary bone 128
secondary bone healing 122, 134
secondary hypoxic injury 34, 55
secondary inflammatory responses 7
second order neurons 62, 169
selective focal compression 57
semi-dynamic balance 198
sensation 66, 158, 171
sensorimotor deficits 188, 189f
sensorimotor function 158
sensorimotor system 171
sensorimotor training
    about 204-205
    balance 211
    conceptual model 205-206
    dynamic joint control 210-211
    external support devices 208-209
    joint position sense 209-210
    kinesthesia 209-210
    muscle strength 205
    neuromuscular control 205
    postural control 211
    therapeutic progression 206-208
sensory filtering 206
sensory homunculus 68, 171
sensory-level stimulation 77-78
sensory manipulation 206-207
sensory nuclei 66
sensory receptors 61, 62
sensory stimuli, identification of 66
serial static immobilization 96

serotonin 16, 22, 68, 74
short-term rehabilitation goals 230-231
shortwave diathermy 76
Simoneau, G.G. 208
site-specific bone hypertrophy 149
sixth sense 158
skeletal muscle, cross section 48f
skeletal muscle relaxants 80
skeletal muscle tissue, structure and composition 146f
skeletal traction 136
skin, neuroanatomy of 165f
Skinner, H.B. 191
skin receptors 164
slide 107-108
slide boards 207
slowly adapting receptors 166-167
slow pain 63
slow reversal-hold-relax 105
Smith, R.L. 205
Snyder-Mackler, L. 77, 78
SOAP notes 5, 220-223, 226, 230, 232, 237
soft tissue function restoration 144-146
Solomon, S. 76
somatosensory association area 171-172
somatosensory cortex, somatopic organization of 68f
somatotopy 68, 171
specificity theory 71
specific nociceptors 71
Spencer, J.D. 196, 199-200
spin 107-108
spinal cord connections 64-65
spinal cord pathways, ascending 65
spinocerebellar tracts 174
spinocerebellum 170, 174
spinomesencephalic tract 65
spinoreticular tract 65
spinothalamic tract 65, 66f
splinting 96-97, 141
sports injury evaluation and treatment record 221f, 222
sports injury management
    assessment categories 225t
    basic concepts 6-11
    clinical assessment 223-224
    problem identification 223, 225-226
    problem-oriented approach 4-6
    problem-oriented medical record 220-226
    proprioceptive deficits 199-200
    rehabilitation goals and objectives 230-232
    rehabilitation planning 232-237
sports injury rehabilitation
    conceptual model 234, 235f
    early rehabilitation phase 234-235
    elements of 232-233
    intermediate rehabilitation phase 235-236
    late rehabilitation phase 236-237
sports participation, resumption of 142, 148-151, 192, 237
sports trauma 6-8
stable cavitation 91
stable cells 10
Standards of Professional Practice 237
Starkey, C. 58
static balance 197-198
static equilibrium 179
static progressive splinting 96
static stretch reflex 162
Steinman pins 139-140
stimulation analgesia 77
stimulatory association neurons 164
stimuli, receptor adaptation to 75
strength, defined 146
stress, defined 150

stress fractures 149-151
stress reaction 150
stress-relaxation response 100-101
stress-relaxation therapy 101
stress riser 137
stretch, defined 100
stretch reflex 162
Strickland, J.W. 139
structural glycoproteins 13
Styf, J.R. 209
subacute inflammation 37
subjective information, in SOAP notes 222
subsensory electrical stimulation 77
substance P 65, 68
substantia gelatinosa 72-73
summation 71
superficial-heating modalities 89-90
superior colliculus 183, 184
supplementary motor area 172
Surburg, P.R. 106
surgical considerations, proprioception 200-204
surgical results, assessment 225t
Swiss balls 207
symptomatic treatment 224
symptoms 5-6
synapse 68, 169
synaptic bulbs 68
synaptic cleft 68
synaptic junction 68, 169
systemic inflammation 31

T
tactile discs 168
Tanigawa, M.C. 106
T cells 37-38, 72
tectospinal tract 177-178
tectum 184
Tegner, Y. 196
tendons 40f, 43, 45f
tensile loading 98, 99-100, 100-101
tensile strain 97
tensile strength 97-98
tensile stress 101
TENS (transcutaneous electrical nerve stimulation) 77
thalamic nuclei 67f
thalamocortical projection neurons 171
thalamus 66, 170-171, 174f
therapeutic agents 10-11. See also physical therapeutic agents
therapeutic intervention categories 8-9
therapeutic objectives, rehabilitation 231
therapeutic stretching
    about 101-102
    low-load, prolonged stretching 101, 102-104
    proprioceptive neuromuscular facilitation (PNF) 101, 104-107
    stress-relaxation therapy 101
therapeutic tensile loading 98
thermoreceptors 61, 63
thermotherapy 76-77, 89-90
third order neurons 62, 169
Thornton, E. 191
threshold level 166
threshold to detection of passive motion 190-191
thromboplastin 23-24
thromboxane 22-23
Tibone, J.E. 211
Tillman, L.J. 94, 98, 100, 103
Tipton, C.M. 99
tissue
    classification 11
    early mobilization 200
    healing as time dependent 54
    immobilization 98-99
    normal structure and function 11-14

physiological responses to trauma 6-7
    repair complications 46-50
    temperature 90t, 102-104
tissue healing
    blood cells 15-16
    chemical mediators 15
    connective tissue cells 16-17
    essential elements 15
    mechanisms 9-10
    modifiers 10-11
    nutrients 17-18
tonus 69
trabeculae 119
trabecular bone 119
tract of Lissauer 64
transcutaneous electrical nerve stimulation (TENS) 77
transient cavitation 91
transmission cells 72
transudate 32
treatment discharge 237
treatment plan, in SOAP notes 222
trochlear nerve (IV) 181
tropocollagen 39
Tropp, H. 197

U
ultrasound 76, 90-91
unstable cavitation 91
upper motor neurons 175-176

V
Vailas, A.C. 99
vasoconstriction 22-23
ventral posterior nucleus 66, 171
ventral spinocerebellar tract 170
vergence 181
vergence center 181
vestibular labryinth 180
vestibular nuclei 180-182
vestibular receptors 179-180
vestibular system 178-182
vestibulocerebellum 174-175, 182
vestibuloocular reflex 181, 182f
vestibulospinal tract 177, 182
viscoelasticity 100
visual receptors 182-183
visual system 182-184
vitamins, in tissue healing 17
Volkmann's canals 120, 128
VonNieda, K. 76
Voss, D.E. 105

W
Wall, P.D. 71, 72, 73
Walla, D.J. 211
wandering macrophages 37
Waxman, S.G. 74
Weber, C. 106-107
Welsh, R. 102
Wessling, K.C. 103
white blood cells, actions in acute inflammation 35f
Whiting, W.C. 148, 149, 150
wide dynamic range neurons 65
Wilk, K.E. 193, 196, 205
Wilkerson, G.B. 55, 57, 58, 189, 196, 197, 199, 200
wires 139-140
wobble boards 207
Wolff, Julius 147
Wolff, R. 106-107
Wolff's law 46, 128, 147
Woo, S.L-Y. 95
wound contraction 7, 41-42
woven bone 126
Wyke, B 210

Z
Zatterstrom, R. 197, 211
Zernicke, R.F. 124, 126-127, 129, 148, 149, 150

About the Author

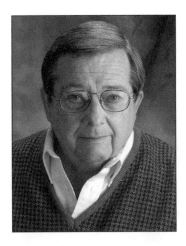

Gary Delforge, EdD, ATC, draws from more than 40 years of experience as a certified athletic trainer and educator. Most recently, he served as director of the sports health care department at the Arizona School of Health Sciences, a division of Kirksville College of Osteopathic Medicine, where he developed an NATA-accredited master's degree program in athletic training. For 32 years he was associated with the University of Arizona, where he served for 7 years as head athletic trainer before devoting his time to curriculum development and teaching in athletic training.

As an active member of the NATA for many years, Dr. Delforge chaired the NATA Professional Education Committee and served as a member of the NATA board of directors. He is also a recipient of the Sayers "Bud" Miller Distinguished Athletic Training Educator award and a member of the NATA Hall of Fame.

He has written many journal articles and book chapters and presented frequently at national and regional meetings. Dr. Delforge earned his EdD in rehabilitation administration at the University of Arizona and a master's degree in health, physical education, and recreation at Kent State University.

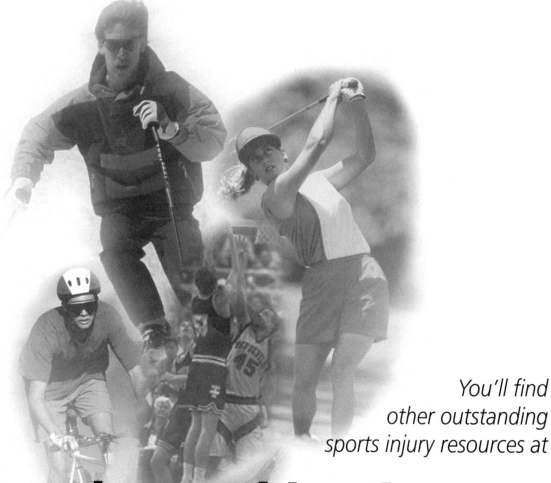

*You'll find
other outstanding
sports injury resources at*

www.humankinetics.com

In the U.S. call

1-800-747-4457

Australia .... (08) 8277-1555
Canada .... (800) 465-7301
Europe .... +44 (0) 113-278-1708
New Zealand .... (09) 309-1890

HUMAN KINETICS
The Information Leader in Physical Activity
P.O. Box 5076 • Champaign, IL 61825-5076 USA